DNA Repair- An Update

Edited by Maddalena Mognato

Published in London, United Kingdom

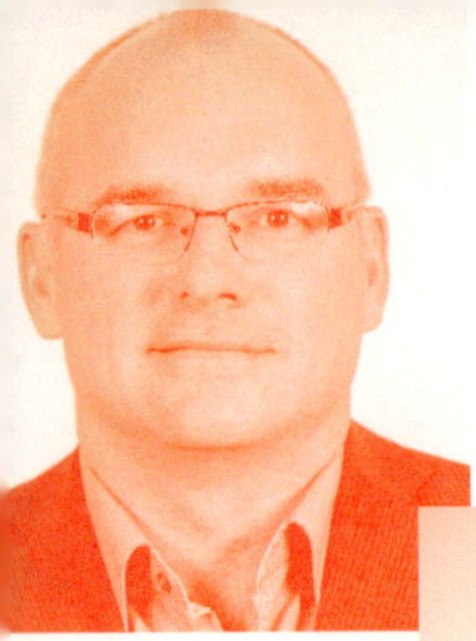
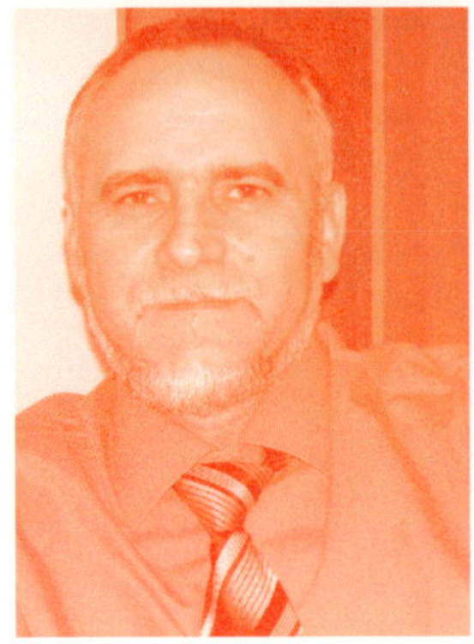
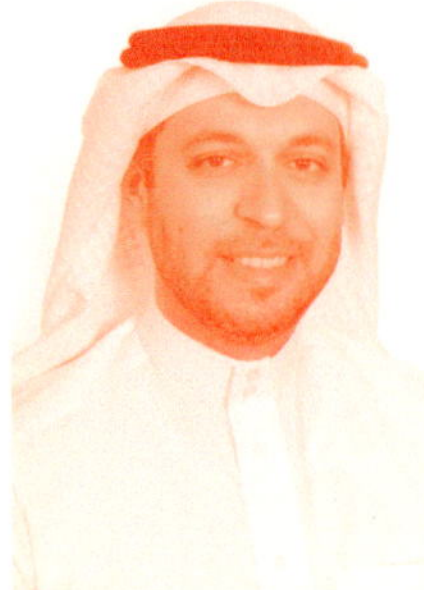
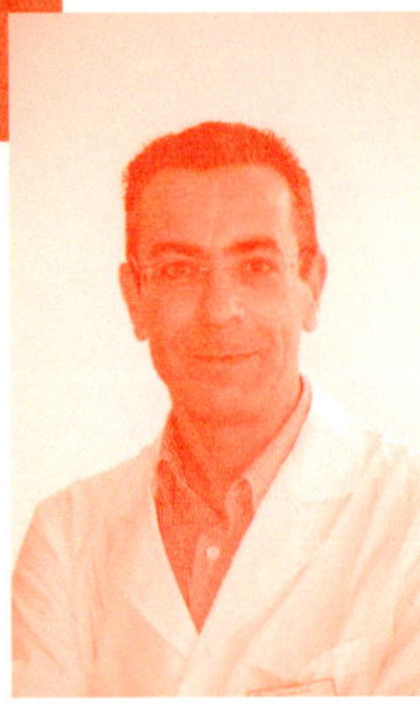
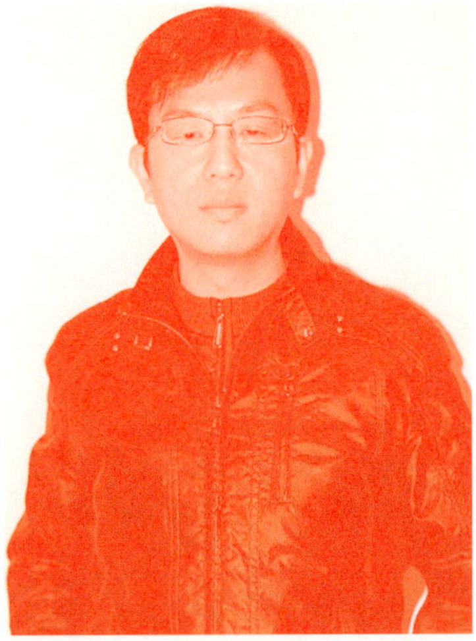
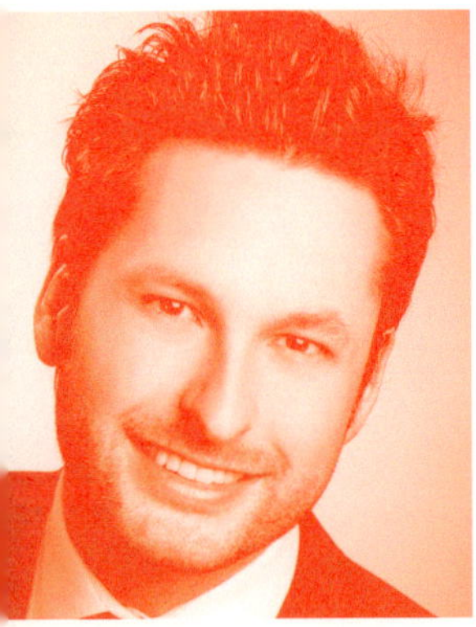
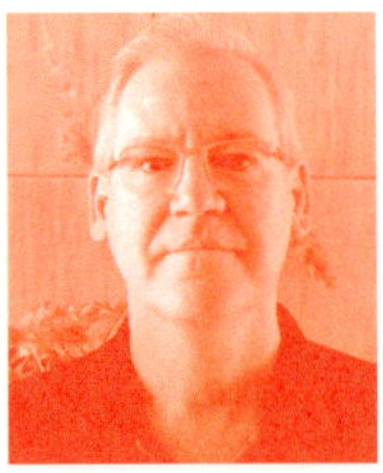

IntechOpen

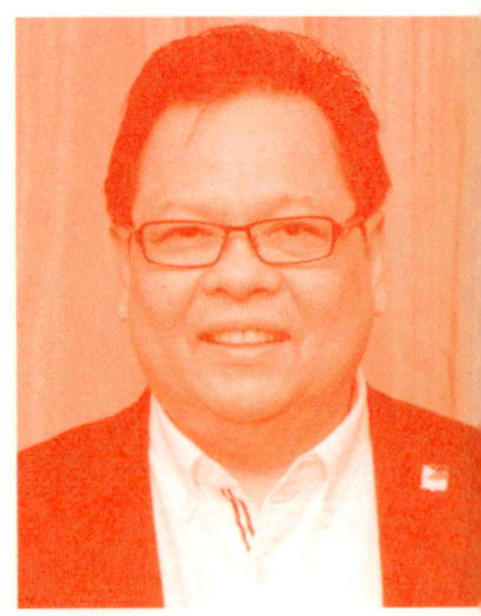
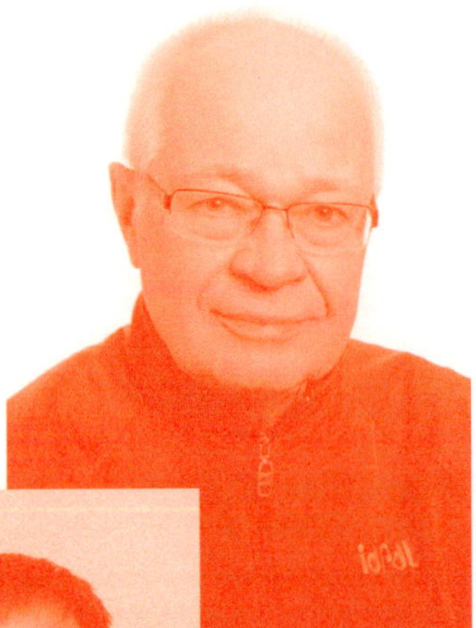
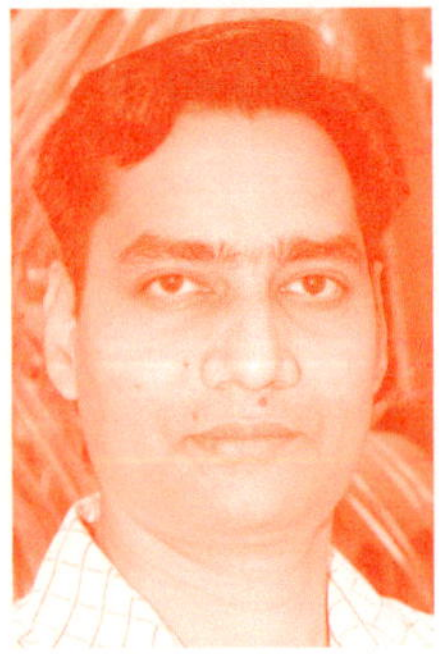
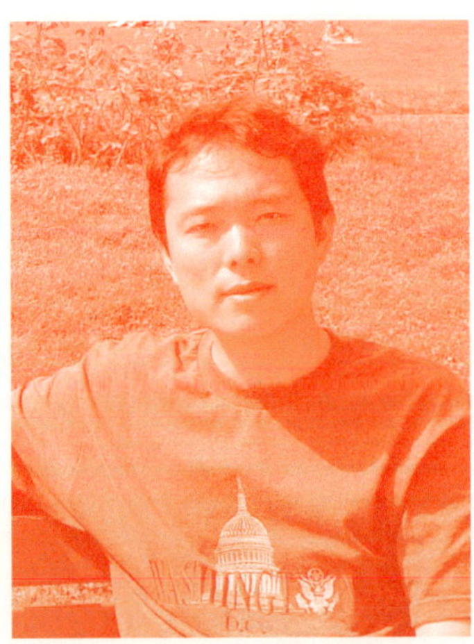
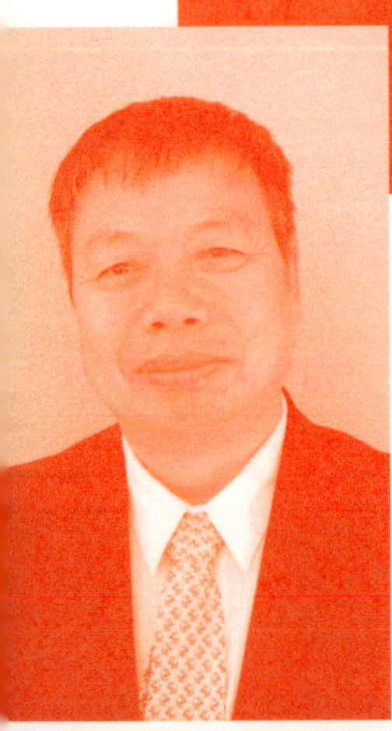
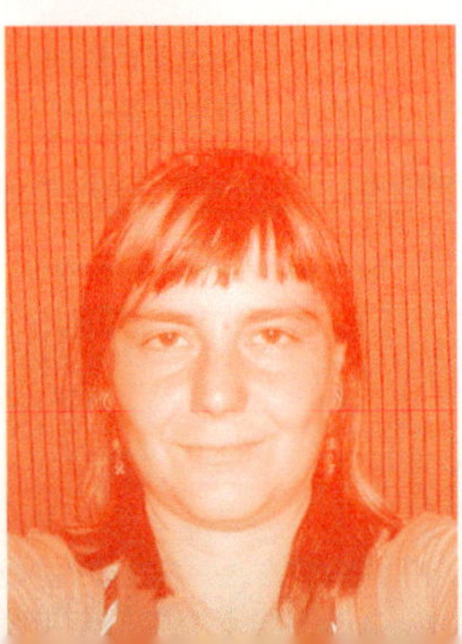

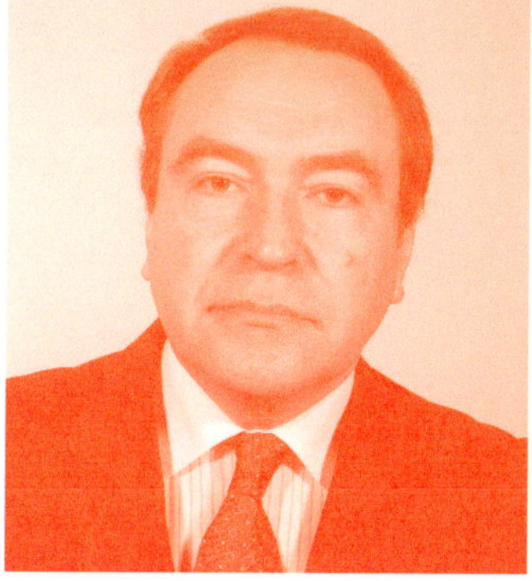
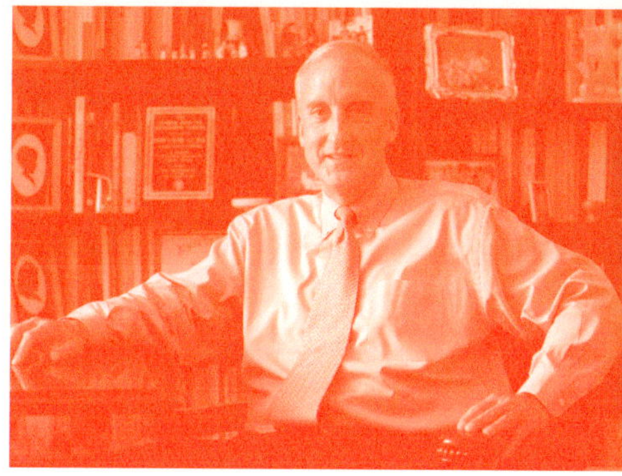
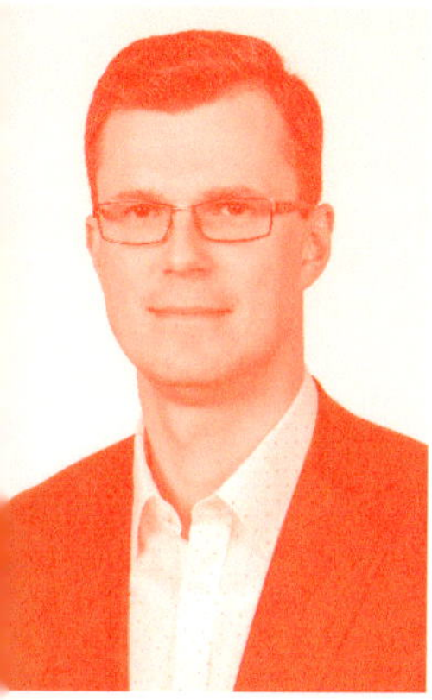
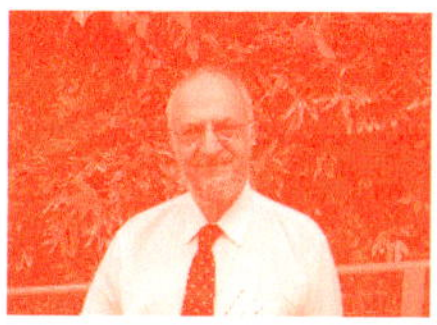
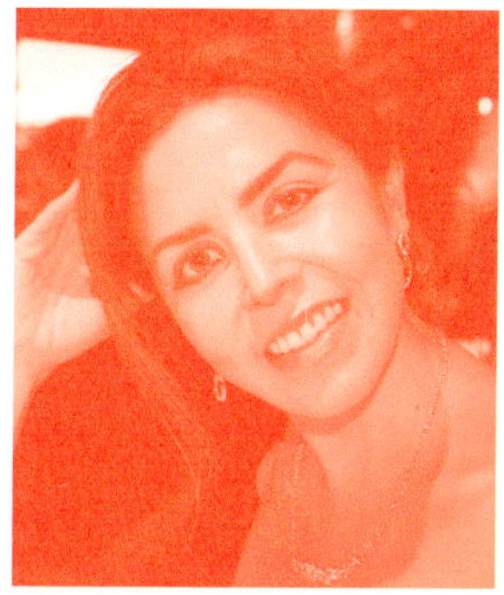

Supporting open minds since 2005

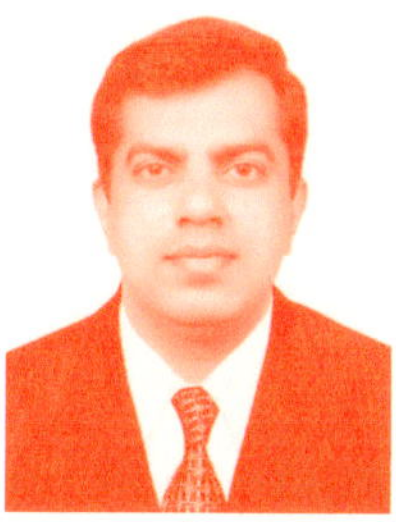
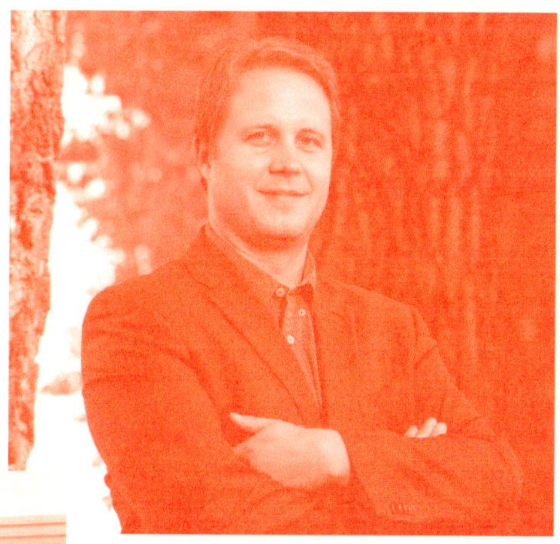
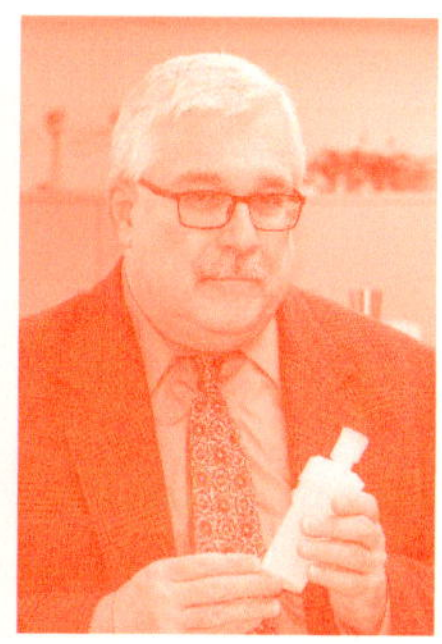
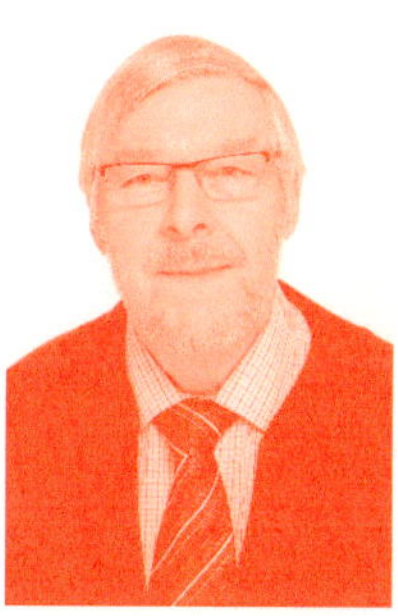
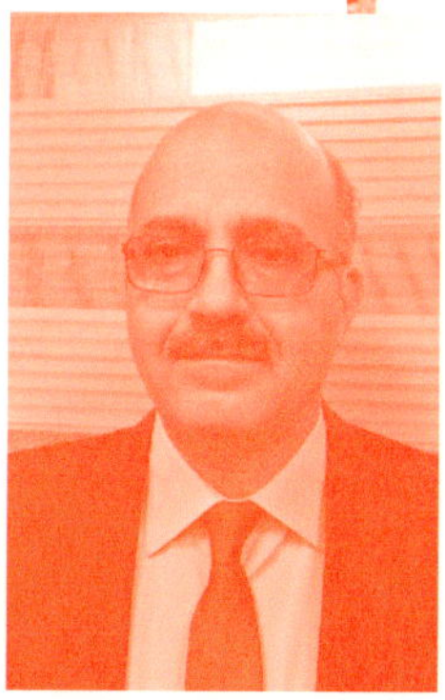
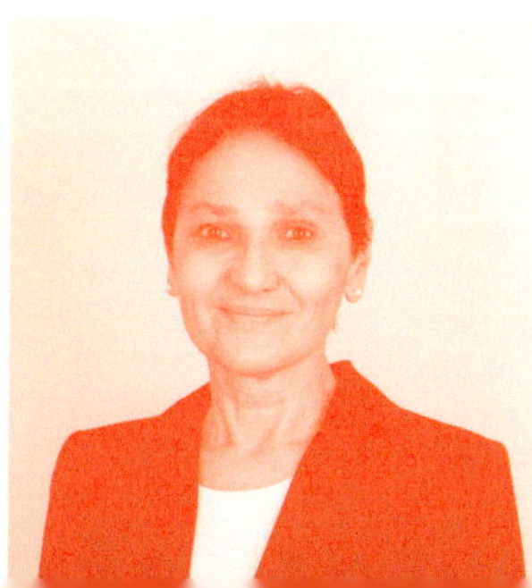
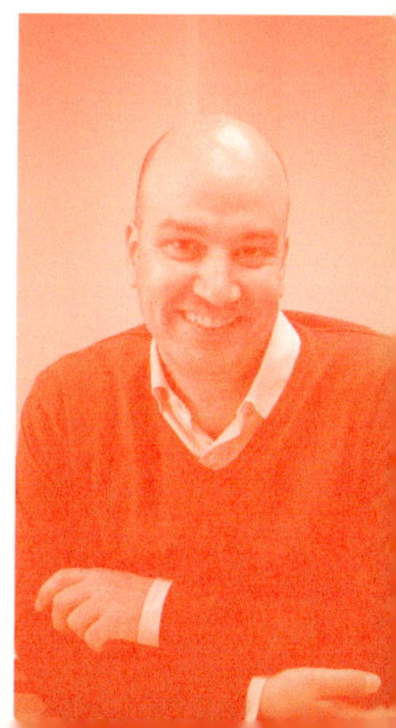

DNA Repair- An Update
http://dx.doi.org/10.5772/intechopen.79123
Edited by Maddalena Mognato

Contributors
Martin Berger, Alia Abukiwan, Xi-Dai Long, Maddalena Mognato, Shiladitya Sengupta, Chunying Yang, Muralidhar L. Hegde, Sankar Mitra, Bradley Eckelmann, Michael Fasullo, Thulasi Pillai, Cherupally Krishnan Krishnan Nair, Uma Devi, Olga Lavrik, Nina Moor, Harris Bernstein, Carol Bernstein, Rosa Bermudez, Francisco-Alejandro Lagunas-Rangel, Ulises Omar Garcia-Lepe

First published in London, United Kingdom, 2019 by IntechOpen
IntechOpen is the global imprint of INTECHOPEN LIMITED, registered in England and Wales, registration number: 11086078, The Shard, 25th floor, 32 London Bridge Street
London, SE19SG - United Kingdom
Printed in Croatia

British Library Cataloguing-in-Publication Data
A catalogue record for this book is available from the British Library

Additional hard and PDF copies can be obtained from orders@intechopen.com

DNA Repair- An Update
Edited by Maddalena Mognato
p. cm.
Print ISBN 978-1-83880-782-5
Online ISBN 978-1-83880-783-2
eBook (PDF) ISBN 978-1-83880-784-9

For EU product safety concerns:
IN TECH d.o.o., Prolaz Marije Krucifikse Kozulić 3, 51000 Rijeka, Croatia, info@intechopen.com or visit our website at intechopen.com.

Meet the editor

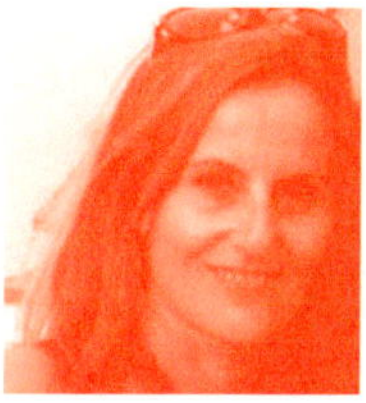

Dr. Maddalena Mognato is a researcher in cell biology at the Department of Biology, University of Padova (Italy). She obtained a master's degree in Biological Sciences from the University of Padova in 1996 and received her PhD in Environmental Medicine in 2001. Her research activity is focused on cytotoxic and genotoxic effects induced by physical and chemical agents in human and mammalian cells, both primary and established. Her research is mainly focused on the DNA-damage response signaling pathway, in particular on the repair of radio-induced DNA double-strand breaks and on gene expression modulation mediated by microRNAs. Her research activity is documented in international peer-reviewed articles and numerous abstracts in international and national congresses. Since 2007, she has held courses for the students of molecular biology at the University of Padova.

Contents

Preface

During the last few years, many advances in the knowledge of DNA repair mechanisms were made in eukaryotic cells, thanks to innovative technologies in cellular and molecular biology. However, due to the complexity of cellular physiology, the whole mechanism is still under investigation, highlighting different factors that affect DNA repair efficiency in human cells. The role of proteins involved in DNA repair has been widely studied, but the modality and power of extrinsic and intrinsic factors in influencing protein functionality and correct protein-protein interactions represent a research area under constant investigation. Among intrinsic factors affecting DNA repair processes, there is epigenetics, which strongly impacts on gene expression regulation of DNA repair genes and the complex network of DNA-damage response-related genes. The structure and function of the epigenome under physiological and pathological conditions in the presence of DNA damage are an open and rapidly growing research field. Moreover, in mammalian aged cells, accumulated DNA damage is a source of genomic instability if proper repair is not carried out.

The book is divided into four sections with chapters describing different topics connected to DNA repair in human cells. The first section contains the introductory chapter dealing with the subjects of the book. The second section is dedicated to the role of protein-protein interactions during DNA repair in nuclear and mitochondrial compartments. The third section is dedicated to the relationship between the epigenome and DNA repair in normal and cancer cells. The fourth section is about the interconnection between aging and DNA repair. This last section also contains a chapter on the relationship between the angiogenesis of cancer cells and DNA damage repair and a chapter on the DNA repair-enhancing property of glucan.

I acknowledge the authors that contributed to this book and hope that the topics here discussed may suggest readers to explore new avenues and aspects of the interconnection between different DNA lesions and responses essential for the maintenance of nuclear and mitochondrial genome stability.

Maddalena Mognato, PhD
Department of Biology,
University of Padova,
Italy

Section 1

Introduction

Chapter 1

Introductory Chapter: DNA Repair in Human Cells - A Daily Challenge

Maddalena Mognato

1. Introduction

The faithful repair of DNA is a challenge that human cells have to fight every day to maintain genomic stability. The type and frequency of DNA lesions are related to both endogenous and exogenous sources of DNA damage. In addition to normal metabolism, which is responsible for a great number of DNA lesions (approximately 70,000 per cell) [1, 2], environmental agents (i.e., ionizing radiation, UV light, and chemicals) contribute to enhance such number. The capacity of cells to faithfully repair their proper DNA is the primary goal to safeguard the genome integrity. To this purpose, eukaryotic cells have evolved accurate repair systems to overcome the different lesions induced by both external and internal sources of DNA damage. A lot of information is now available for most repair systems, and in the last decades, a lot of efforts have been made in the comprehension of the role of DNA repair proteins, in relation to the type of damage and the effectiveness of repair carried out by different complexes. Besides the molecular role of proteins in such pathways, several other important factors can affect the efficiency of DNA repair, including epigenetics, chromatin structure, mitochondrial function, and aging.

Epigenetics regulate gene function through posttranslational modifications of histones, DNA methylation noncoding RNAs, and when DNA is damaged, epigenetic alterations can occur at sites of lesions. Epigenetic alterations that occur during DNA repair are mostly transient, being the original epigenetic marker restored. However, sometimes, epigenetic alterations can persist after DNA repair as a sort of "scars" [3]. What is the role of such epigenetic markers left after repair? Epigenetic modifications occur either in normal cells or in cancer cells, representing a further element for cancerogenesis in this last case. Numerous studies reported gene expression changes in human cancers and found signature for specific type of tumors. Each cancer has its own genetic and epigenetic profile, which increases the difficulty to comprehend the process of tumorigenicity. In this regard, the response to each tumor to different DNA-damaging agents is related to the characteristics of its genetic and epigenetic landscape.

The structure of chromatin around DNA damage changes significantly to promote DNA repair proteins accessibility. During DNA repair, the structure of chromatin is modified as a consequence of new histone incorporation, replacement, and modification. The coordination of DNA repair protein interactions is a critical process which needs to be fully elucidated, also in relation to the specific DNA-damaging agent.

Mitochondria, with their own DNA, are organelles that are on the rise for several reasons, including the repair of their proper DNA, the mtDNA. Mitochondrial DNA is different from the nuclear one, being circular, without histones, and present in multiple copies. The repair of mtDNA relies on the activity of proteins encoded by

IntechOpen

nuclear DNA, and the efficiency of repair is crucial for the maintenance of mtDNA integrity. What happens when the mitochondrial genome is affected by improper DNA repair and mutations arise? To address this question, studies should take into account that the multiplicity of mtDNA genomes inside the same cell originates a coexistence of mutant and wild-type genomes [4].

Notably, the accumulation of DNA damages during the cell lifespan threatens the fidelity of repair. According to the candidate hallmarks of aging in mammalian cells, recently reviewed by Lopez-Otin et al. [4], it appears evident how the process of DNA repair is tightly linked to genomic instability, cellular senescence, epigenetic alterations, and mitochondrial dysfunction. In humans, alterations in nuclear DNA repair are present in several syndromes characterized by premature aging, and epigenetic modifications in histones and histone-modifying enzymes affect chromatin structure in an age-related manner. Several studies attempted to elucidate the linkage between mitochondria dysfunction and aging. Indeed, when the mitochondrial function is impaired, the result is an increase of oxidative stress that triggers a cascade of toxic effects on cellular environment.

Finally, the connection between DNA repair process and angiogenesis is another open research field. Angiogenesis is a physiological process that allows the regeneration of blood vessels following injuries. However, angiogenesis is extremely harmful in pathological conditions, such as in tumoral tissues, characterized by the uncontrolled growth of new blood vessels. Mutations or alterations in genes involved in the cellular response to DNA damage can affect the angiogenic response.

Many questions are still open and further investigations are needed to shed light on the whole mechanism of DNA repair, either nuclear or mitochondrial. To this purpose, the present book offers a collection of chapters dedicated to the interplay between DNA repair and epigenetics under physiological and pathological conditions, aging, mitochondrial function, angiogenesis, and the contribution of base excision repair process to oxidative damage, giving a contribution to cancer biology and clinical management. **Figure 1** shows some of the principal aspects discussed in this book.

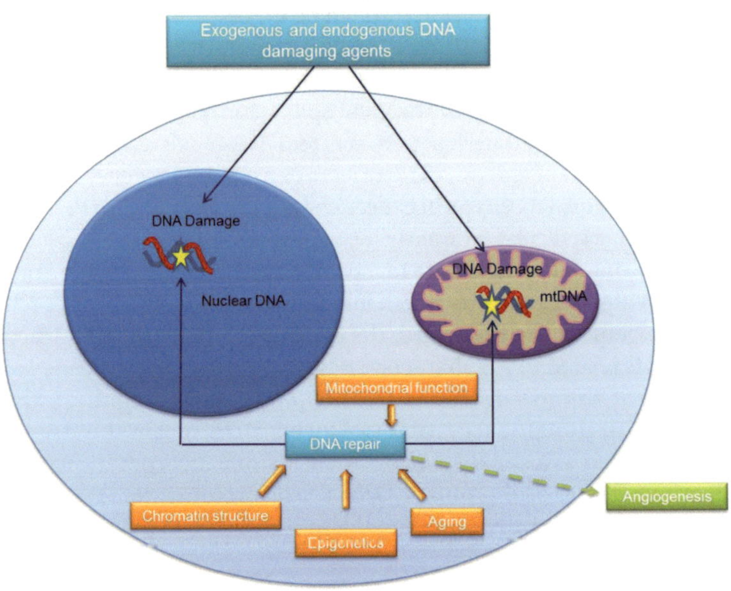

Figure 1.
Example of intrinsic factors affecting the repair of DNA damage induced by exogenous and endogenous sources in nucleus and mitochondria of eukaryotic cells.

Author details

Maddalena Mognato
Department of Biology, School of Sciences, University of Padova, Italy

*Address all correspondence to: maddalena.mognato@unipd.it

References

[1] Lindahl T, Barnes DE. Repair of endogenous DNA damage. Cold Spring Harbor Symposia on Quantitative Biology. 2000;**65**:127-133

[2] Tubbs A, Nussenzweig A. Endogenous DNA damage as a source of genomic instability in cancer. Cell. 2017;**168**(4):644-656. DOI: 10.1016/j.cell.2017.01.002

[3] Dabin J, Fortuny A, Polo SE. Epigenome maintenance in response to DNA damage. Molecular Cell. 2016;**62**(5):712-727. DOI: 10.1016/j.molcel.2016.04.006

[4] López-Otín C, Blasco MA, Partridge L, Serrano M, Kroemer G. The hallmarks of aging. Cell. 2013;**153**(6):1194-1217. DOI: 10.1016/j.cell.2013.05.039

Section 2

DNA Repair Protein Interactions

Chapter 2

Coordination of DNA Base Excision Repair by Protein-Protein Interactions

Nina Moor and Olga Lavrik

Abstract

The system of base excision repair (BER) evolved to correct the most abundant DNA damages in mammalian cells is the most essential for maintaining the genome integrity. The multistep BER process involves several enzymes and protein factors functioning in a coordinated fashion that ensures the repair efficiency. The coordination is facilitated by the formation of protein complexes stabilized via either direct or indirect DNA-mediated interactions. This review focuses on direct interactions of proteins participating in BER with each other and with noncanonical factors found recently to modulate the efficiency of BER. All the known partners of main BER participants, the sites responsible for their interaction, and the characteristics of protein-protein affinity are summarized. Well-documented evidences of how DNA intermediates and posttranslational modifications of proteins modulate protein-protein interactions are presented. The available data allow to suggest that the multiprotein complexes are assembled with the involvement of a scaffold protein XRCC1 and poly(ADP-ribose) polymerase 1, a key regulator of the BER process, irrespective of the DNA damage; the composition and the structure of the complexes are dynamically changed depending on the DNA damage, its chromatin environment, and the step of BER process.

Keywords: base excision repair, protein-protein interactions, noncanonical factors, posttranslational modifications of proteins, coordination of DNA repair

1. Introduction

Many forms of DNA damage are generated due to permanent action of endogenous and exogenous factors. In order to maintain genome integrity, cells have evolved several specific pathways to repair DNA lesions. Base excision repair (BER), which ensures correction of the most abundant damages—modified nitrogenous bases and apurinic/apyrimidinic (AP) sites—is critically important for survival of human cells [1–3]. Enzyme and protein factors of BER also participate in the repair of DNA single-strand breaks (SSBs) considered as a separate pathway of the BER system [4, 5]. The other repair systems (**Figure 1**) deal with bulky nucleobase lesions (NER), DNA double-strand breaks (HR; NHEJ), and mismatched bases (MMR). Impaired DNA repair is associated with embryonic lethality, rapid aging, and a variety of severe human hereditary diseases as well as development of cancer [7, 8]. The balance of DNA damage and DNA repair is highly relevant to both

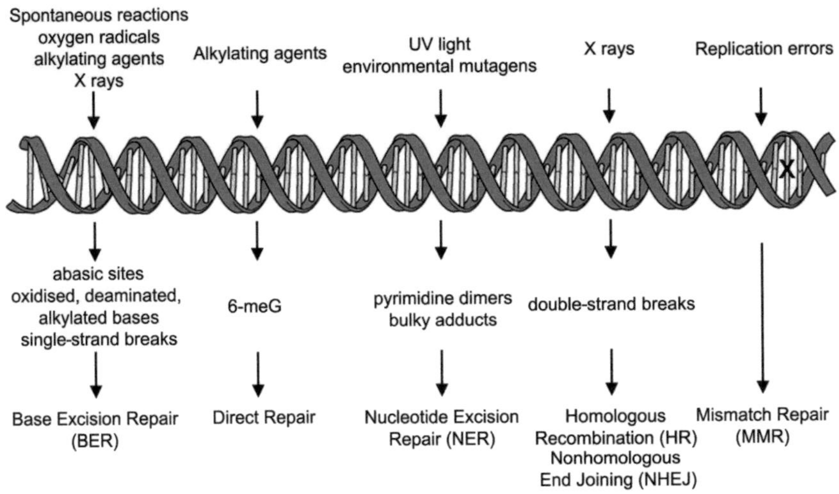

Figure 1.
DNA damages generated by endogenous and exogenous factors and specific systems of their repair. Letter X in DNA duplex marks mismatched base pair. Reproduced with modification from [6] with permission of Pleiades Publishing, Ltd.

cancerogenesis and effective anti-cancer therapy due to the ability of cancer cells to repair therapeutically induced DNA damage and impact therapeutic efficacy [9]. Hence, intensive investigation of DNA damage repair is essential to advance our understanding of molecular mechanisms maintaining genome integrity and to develop cancer therapy.

2. Main steps of BER and proteins involved

The widely accepted model for mammalian BER involves several sub-pathways presented schematically in **Figure 2**. The damaged bases are removed by DNA glycosylases specific to the certain type of damage; mono- and bifunctional DNA glycosylases form an intact or cleaved (via β- or β/δ-elimination mechanism) AP site, respectively [10]. The intact AP site is further processed by the main enzymatic activity of multifunctional AP endonuclease 1 (APE1) producing the one-nucleotide gap with 3′-hydroxyl and 5′-deoxyribose phosphate residue (5′-dRp) at the gap margins. Terminal blocking groups in the DNA intermediates produced by bifunctional DNA glycosylases are removed by the phosphatase activity of polynucleotide kinase/phosphatase (PNKP) or 3′-phosphodiesterase and 3′-phosphatase activities of APE1. At the next step, a bifunctional DNA polymerase β (Polβ) catalyzes the removal of the 5′-dRp residue by its dRp-lyase activity and one-nucleotide gap filling by the nucleotidyl transferase activity. The repair of DNA chain integrity via joining of the single-strand break is completed by DNA ligase IIIα (LigIIIα) acting in the complex with X-ray repair cross-complementing protein 1 (XRCC1). This main BER sub-pathway is known as a short-patch repair (SP BER). When the 5′-dRp residue is modified, it cannot be removed by the Polβ-lyase activity, and a long-patch sub-pathway of BER (LP BER) is realized. Polβ initiates the DNA strand displacement synthesis continued by replicative DNA polymerases δ and ε (Polδ and Polε) acting in the complexes with protein factors PCNA and RFC. The flap structure produced at this step is removed by the flap endonuclease 1 (FEN1). According to another model, FEN1 is capable of sequential removing nucleotides at the 5′-end of the break, and the produced gap is filled by the activities of Polβ or

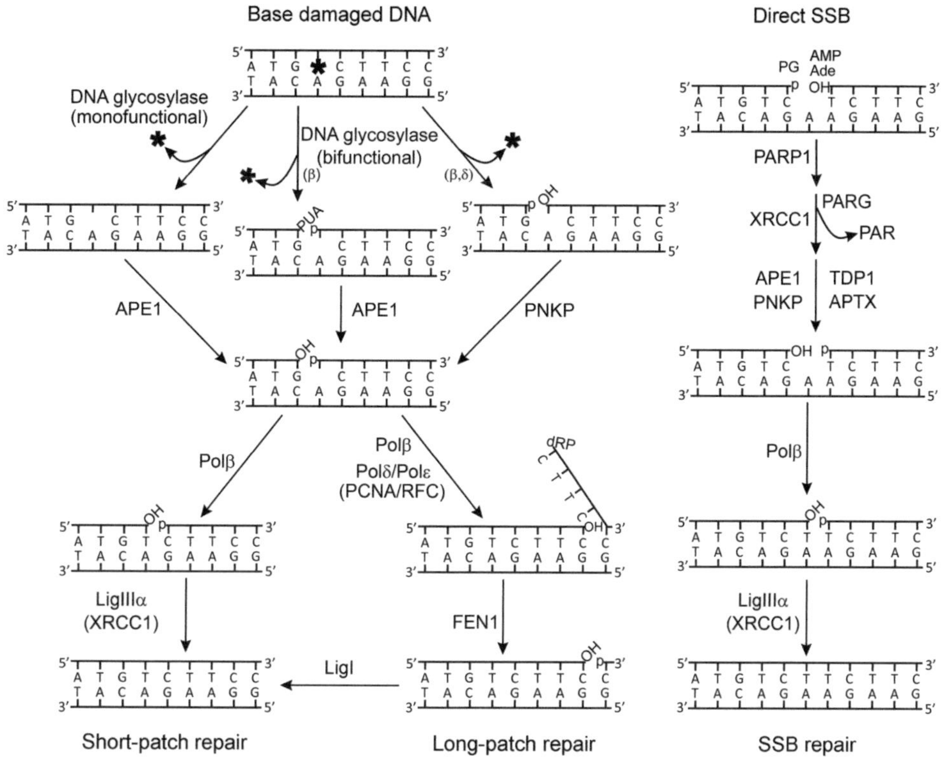

Figure 2.
BER sub-pathways for repair of damaged bases and DNA SSBs. Catalytic steps and proteins involved are schematically presented. The terminal groups in DNA intermediates and SSBs are designated as follows: PUA, 3′-phospho-α,β-unsaturated aldehyde; p, 3′-/5′-phosphate; OH, 3′-/5′-hydroxyl; dRP, 5′-deoxyribose phosphate; PG, 3′-phosphoglycolate; Ade, 5′-aldehyde group; and AMP, 5′-AMP. Reproduced with modification from [6] with permission of Pleiades Publishing, Ltd.

Polλ [11, 12]. Final ligation of the break is catalyzed by DNA ligase I (LigI). A new long-patch sub-pathway of BER that involves formation of a 9-nucleotide gap 5′ to the lesion has been recently discovered; it is mediated by DNA helicase RECQ1 and ERCC1-XPF endonuclease in cooperation with PARP1 and replication protein A (RPA) [13].

Repair of DNA SSBs arising directly via disintegration of the oxidized sugar and as a result of erroneous activity of DNA topoisomerase 1 involves the following steps: (1) detection of the break, (2) removal of blocking groups, (3) filling the gap, and (4) ligation of the break (**Figure 2**). The DNA breaks are detected primarily by poly(ADP-ribose) polymerase 1 (PARP1); the unblocking of 3′- and 5′-ends in breaks is catalyzed by specific activities of APE1, PNKP, aprataxin (APTX), and tyrosyl-DNA phosphodiesterase 1 (TDP1); gap filling and ligation are catalyzed by the same set of enzymes that participate in the respective steps of the short-patch repair of the damaged DNA bases (Polβ and LigIIIα). PARP1 is activated via the interaction with the damaged DNA; it catalyzes the synthesis of poly(ADP-ribose) (PAR) and covalent attachment of the PAR polymer to PARP1 itself and other proteins involved in the DNA repair [4, 5]. The XRCC1 protein is considered to be a main target of PARP1 catalyzed poly(ADP-ribosyl)ation. PARP1 has been suggested to play the main role in recruitment of the XRCC1 protein to the damages of chromosomal DNA [4, 5]. XRCC1 displays no enzymatic activity and is proposed to function as a scaffold protein of the BER process. PARP2 is another enzyme from the PARP family that is activated via binding with DNA SSB and catalyzes PAR synthesis [14, 15]. The importance of both PARP1 and PARP2 for DNA repair is indicated by knockout studies revealed that knocking out the *parp1* gene activity increased the sensitivity of cells to DNA-damaging agents, while *parp1* and *parp2* double knockouts caused early embryonic lethality [16]. The role of PARP2 in BER processes and its possible synergism with PARP1 action are under intensive investigation [17, 18]. Poly(ADP-ribosyl)ation of proteins is a transient modification that turns over rapidly due to the enzymatic activity of poly(ADP-ribose) glycohydrolase (PARG) [19]. Another important function of PARP1 in DNA repair is remodeling of chromatin structure via poly(ADP-ribosyl)ation of histones and binding of the remodeling proteins with the synthesized PAR polymer [20].

Coordinated action of the enzymes catalyzing the sequential individual reactions of the multistep BER process is required for efficient repair of damaged DNA. One of the coordination mechanisms proposed previously is the "passing the baton," that implies the transfer of the DNA intermediate from the enzyme remaining bound to the product to the next enzyme [1, 21]. This model is supported by numerous data on mutual modulation of activities of the BER enzymes [2, 21]. The stimulating effect of APE1 on the catalytic activity of DNA glycosylase OGG1 explored in detail recently does not require direct interaction between the proteins and is adequately described by the "passing the baton" model [22]. Another mechanism of coordination implies the formation of multiprotein complexes (so-called repairosomes) composed of enzymes and scaffold proteins [2]. XRCC1 is a striking example of the scaffold protein involved in BER. The existence of "repairosomes" is evidenced by multiple interactions between enzymes and protein factors of BER detected even independent of the DNA damage. Most likely both mechanisms are relevant to coordination of the BER process.

3. Proteins involved in BER interact directly with each other

Many protein participants of BER have been shown to interact physically with each other. Data on their direct interactions and structural domains involved are summarized in **Table 1**. Interactions of the XRCC1 protein with multiple partners have been explored in the greatest detail. The structure of XRCC1 is composed of three domains linked with disordered fragments (linkers XL1 and XL2), one of which (XL1) contains a nuclear localization signal (**Figure 3**) [23]. The availability of two BRCT domains (BRCTa and BRCTb) mediating protein-protein interactions (for review, see [24]), in addition to the N-terminal domain (NTD) involved in DNA binding, favors the main function of XRCC1 as scaffold in structural organization of "repairosomes". Interestingly, the binding sites of four enzymes catalyzing sequential steps of BER—APE1, PNKP (N-terminal domain), Polβ, and LigIIIα—are localized in different structural modules of XRCC1 (**Figure 3**). A second PNKP interaction site localized recently in XRCC1 (linker XL1) binds PNKP (catalytic domain) with lower affinity; this interaction has been proposed to stimulate PNKP activity, in contrast to the high-affinity interaction responsible for PNKP recruitment to DNA damage [25]. At the same time, the binding sites of various DNA glycosylases in XRCC1 overlap with those for APE1, Polβ, and PARP1 (**Figure 3**). It is likely that the enzymes initiating the repair of damaged bases form dynamic contacts with XRCC1 and other constituents of "repairosome." Direct interactions of DNA glycosylases NEIL1, NEIL2, and MYH with other enzymes of SP and LP BER (APE1, PNKP, Polβ, LigIIIα, Polδ, FEN1, and LigI) have been shown (**Table 1**). The multiprotein complexes of XRCC1 detected in many studies to be formed by recombinant proteins and cell extracts contain Polβ, PNKP, and LigIIIα as stable partners, and their presence enhances the interaction of XRCC1 with

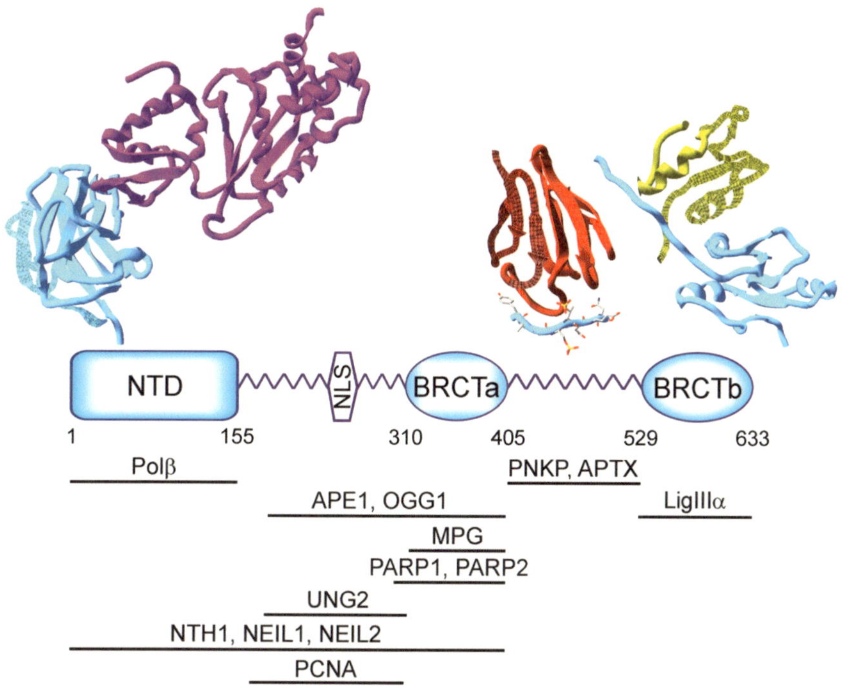

Figure 3.
The multidomain structure of XRCC1 and specific regions responsible for its scaffold function in BER. Protein partners and their binding sites in XRCC1 are shown schematically in the upper part of the figure. At the top, 3D structure models determined for the N-terminal domain, a fragment of XL2 linker, and the BRCTb domain crystallized as complexes with the respective domains of Polβ, PNKP, and LigIIIα (PDB codes: 3K75, 2W3O, and 3QVG) are presented. Reproduced with modification from [6] with permission of Pleiades Publishing, Ltd.

DNA glycosylases [30, 31, 33, 52]. PNKP and LigIIIα are the constituents of another multiprotein complex containing XRCC1 and TDP1 [53].

The PARP1 protein consists of multiple structural modules constituting an N-terminal DNA-binding domain and a C-terminal catalytic domain in addition to the central BRCT domain [55, 57]. The coordinating function of PARP1 in BER can be realized via direct interaction with some enzymes (PNKP, Polβ, LigIIIα, and TDP1) or indirect interaction mediated by the XRCC1 protein. The binding sites for main BER enzymes (Polβ and LigIIIα) and the scaffold XRCC1 protein are localized in the DNA binding and BRCT domains, while that for TDP1 is completed by the catalytic domain of PARP1 (**Table 1**). As a consequence, TDP1 is capable of the formation of a stable ternary complex with PARP1 and XRCC1 [53]. The overlapped binding sites for the majority of PARP1 partners create prerequisites for dynamic contacts in the preformed multiprotein assemblies, which can be stabilized in the complex with automodified PARP1 (PAR-PARP1). Many BER participants such as XRCC1, Polβ, PNKP, APTX, TDP1, LigIIIα, and LigI contain PAR-binding motifs, and some of them (XRCC1, LigIIIα, and TDP1) have been shown to interact with PAR-PARP1 more efficiently than with the unmodified PARP1 [46, 47, 58, 59]. The poly(ADP-ribose) acceptors have been identified in all the structural domains of PARP1; this expands significantly the platform for the formation of the "repairosomes" [60]. In contrast to PARP1, PARP2 does not have the BRCT domain and specialized zinc-fingers for DNA binding [15, 61]. The nonconserved WGR domain of PARP2 is responsible for the interaction with proteins (**Table 1**) as well as for DNA break detection [15]. The function of PARP2 (similar to that of PARP1) in coordination of the DNA repair process can be further mediated through its interaction with XRCC1 [17].

Protein (domain)[a]	Protein partner (domain)[a,b]
XRCC1 (NTD)	Polβ (CD) [23, 26–28]
XRCC1 (NTD + XL1)	NTH1 (CTD); NEIL1 (CTD); NEIL2 (NTD) [29–31]
XRCC1 (XL1)	PCNA [32]; UNG2 (CD) [33]; PNKP (CD) [25]
XRCC1 (XL1 + BRCTa)	APE1, OGG1 [34]
XRCC1 (BRCTa)	MPG, NTH1 (CTD), NEIL1 (CTD), NEIL2 (NTD) [29–31]; PARP1 (DBD, BRCT), PARP2 (WGR) [35, 36]
XRCC1 (XL2)	PNKP (NTD), APTX (FHA) [23, 37–39]
XRCC1 (BRCTb)	LigIIIα (BRCT) [40–42]
XRCC1	TDP1 [43]
PARP1 (DBD + BRCT)	Polβ (CD), PARP1, PARP2 (WGR) [36, 44, 45]; LigIIIα (55–122) [46]
PARP1 (CD)	TDP1 (NTD) [47]
APE1 (CTD)	MYH (293–351) [48]
NEIL1 (CTD)	PNKP, Polβ, FEN1, LigI [49]
Polβ (NTD)	NEIL1 (CTD), NEIL2 (NTD) [30, 31]; LigI (NTD) [50]
Polβ (CD)	PARP2 (WGR) [36]
Polβ	APE1 [51]; PNKP [52]
LigIIIα (BRCT)	NEIL1 (CTD), NEIL2 (NTD) [30, 31]; PARP2 (WGR) [36]; PNKP [52]; TDP1 (NTD) [53, 54]

[a]*Protein domain(s) responsible for the interaction with protein partner(s) is shown in brackets. Structural composition of multidomain proteins: XRCC1: NTD 1–155, XL1 156–309, BRCTa 310–405, XL2 406–528, BRCTb 529–633; [23] PARP1: ZnF1 1–96, ZnF2 97–206, NLS 207–240, ZnF3 241–366, BRCT 381–484, WGR 518–661, CD 662–1014; [55] PARP2: NTD 1–63, WGR 64–198, CD 199–559; [36] LigIIIα: ZnF 1–100, linker 101–170, DBD 171–390, CD 391–836, BRCT 837–922 [56]. Designations: NTD/CTD, N-/C-terminal domain; CD, catalytic domain; DBD, DNA-binding domain; XL1/XL2, linker 1/2 in XRCC1 protein; NLS, nuclear localization signal; ZnF, zinc finger; FHA, forkhead-associated domain. The data for human and mouse (PARP2) recombinant proteins are presented.*
[b]*Techniques used in studies: affinity coprecipitation [25, 26, 29–36, 40, 41, 44–50], two-hybrid analysis [27, 30, 31, 35, 37, 46, 51–54], gel filtration [27, 28, 41, 42], ultracentrifugation [27, 50], coimmunoprecipitation [29, 31–33, 36–39, 41, 43, 46, 47, 52–54], fluorescence titration [38], fluorescence polarization [39], surface plasmon resonance [41], small-angle X-ray scattering [42], X-ray crystallography [23, 42, 45], and NMR [48].*

Table 1.
Interactions between main proteins involved in BER.

Direct interactions between the enzymes catalyzing different, usually sequential, steps of the BER process have been demonstrated in several studies (**Table 1**). Interestingly, the enzyme of the final step of SP BER—LigIIIα has direct binding partners among the enzymes involved in both the initial and middle steps of the process (NEIL1, NEIL2, PNKP, and TDP1), utilizing the BRCT domain for the interaction. Data reported recently indicate the ability of this enzyme to control the assembly of multiprotein complexes on single-strand DNA damages similar to PARP1, thus suggesting a scaffolding function of LigIIIα in the coordination of BER [62].

Most interactions between proteins involved in BER have been detected using the affinity coprecipitation, two-hybrid analysis, and immunoprecipitation techniques (**Table 1**). These techniques provide no information on physicochemical, structural, and conformational parameters of the complexes, leaving open many questions on the mechanisms of their functioning, such as the relative contribution of the proteins to the formation of macromolecular associates and their stoichiometry, the roles of dynamic interactions, conformational changes, and DNA intermediates in the formation of functional assemblies. Information on the structural organization of these complexes is very limited. The 3D structures determined by X-ray crystallography are known for the isolated domains/fragments of the XRCC1 protein in complexes with the respective domains of its stable partners Polβ, LigIIIα, and PNKP (**Figure 3**). It is interesting to note that the specific contact region of the XRCC1 protein with LigIIIα (not involved in XRCC1 homodimerization)—a polypeptide consisting of hydrophobic amino acid residues at the N-terminus of the BRCTb domain—was revealed in the X-ray study [42]. The binding sites localized in proteins by the traditional nonequilibrium techniques participate obviously in the most stable interactions. The available structural data are not sufficient to decipher the molecular mechanisms of BER coordination.

Using quantitative equilibrium techniques—fluorescence titration and fluorescence (Förster) resonance energy transfer (FRET)—we have characterized several homo- and hetero-oligomeric complexes of various BER proteins (**Figure 4**). *N*-hydroxysuccinimide esters of 5(6)-carboxyfluorescein (FAM) and 5(6)-carboxytetramethylrhodamine (TMR) were used for N-terminal fluorescent labeling of proteins. Direct (not mediated by DNA or other proteins) interactions of APE1 with Polβ, TDP1, and PARP1 and of Polβ with TDP1 as well as homo-oligomerization of APE1 have been detected for the first time. The apparent equilibrium dissociation constant (K_d) of the complexes is in the range of 23 to 270 nM. The XRCC1-PNKP complex characterized previously by using a similar approach has a K_d value in the same range [64]. The highest stability of the XRCC1 complex with Polβ was confirmed by the nonequilibrium approach, size exclusion chromatography coupled with multi-angle laser light-scattering (SEC-MALLS) [63]. Model DNAs imitating various DNA intermediates of BER have been shown to modulate the structure of protein complexes and their stability to different extents, depending on the type of DNA damage [63]. The DNA-dependent effects on the protein affinity for each other were most pronounced for the complexes of APE1 with different proteins (Polβ, XRCC1, and PARP1). Our findings advance understanding of the mechanisms underlying coordination and regulation of the BER process. The dependence of the efficiency of APE1 interaction with Polβ on the type of DNA intermediate indicates that functions of the two key enzymes are coordinated not only due to the differences in their affinity for DNAs as proposed previously in [65] but also due to the strength of their interaction with each other, which is controlled by DNA at different steps of repair. The higher affinity of APE1 for Polβ in the presence of AP-site containing DNA than in the complex with the incision product suggests that the efficient repair is facilitated by the transfer of the DNA intermediate to Polβ immediately during the incision step. The higher affinity of APE1 and Polβ for PARP1 than for each other in the presence of SSB containing DNA suggests that the regulation of functions of the BER participants via DNA-dependent modulation of their affinity for each other represents a common mechanism for various proteins. On the contrary, the stability of the XRCC1-Polβ complex does not depend on the presence of DNA intermediates, even though the most pronounced effect of different DNAs on the FRET signal, which reflects structural rearrangement of the complex, was detected for this complex. Our data indicate that this complex revealed in [66] to protect each protein from proteasome-mediated degradation may also serve as a stable component of the multiprotein assemblies, similar to the XRCC1-LigIIIα complex. Moreover, the XRCC1 binding sites with Polβ and LigIIIα do not overlap with regions mediating interactions with most other protein partners, thus enabling participation of the preformed ternary Polβ-XRCC1-LigIIIα complex in the entire Polβ- and XRCC1-dependent BER sub-pathway. Formation of the stable ternary complex *in vivo* is evidenced by synchronous accumulation of XRCC1, Polβ, and LigIIIα at the damage sites of DNA [67, 68].

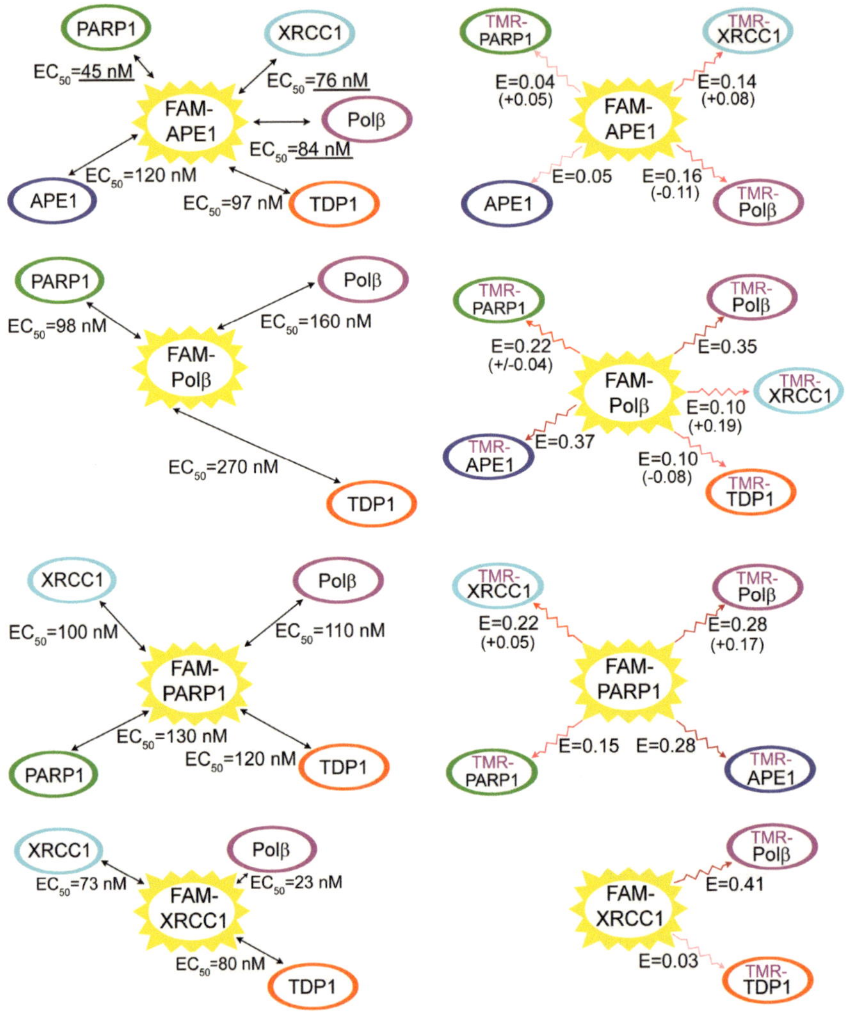

Figure 4.
Direct interactions between BER proteins detected by fluorescence titration and FRET [63]. The EC_{50} values represent apparent equilibrium dissociation constants of the complexes (determined as half-maximal effective concentrations of protein partners); the length of black arrows connecting the protein pairs is proportional to the binding affinity; the underlined EC_{50} values have changed remarkably in the presence of DNA intermediates. The interaction in each pair of FAM- (donor) and TMR-labeled (acceptor) proteins is characterized by FRET efficiency (E); the highest change of the E value induced by DNA intermediates (increase/decrease with +/− sign) is presented in brackets. Reproduced with modification from [6] with permission of Pleiades Publishing, Ltd.

Recently, the oligomeric states of BER proteins and their complexes have been estimated based on hydrodynamic sizes determined by using dynamic light scattering (DLS) technique [69]. All the proteins have been proposed to form homodimers upon their self-association. The most probable oligomerization state of the binary complexes formed by PARP1 with various proteins is a heterotetramer. The oligomerization state of the binary complexes formed by XRCC1 varies from heterodimer to heterotetramer, depending on the partner.

Interaction of PARP1 with Polβ and APE1 detected in our study [63] in both the absence and presence of DNA may contribute to regulation of the BER process. Cooperation between PARP1 and BER enzymes at different steps of DNA repair is evident from our previous studies. Interaction of PARP1, Polβ, and APE1 with the “central” DNA intermediate in BER established by photoaffinity labeling of BER proteins in the cell extract suggests interplay between these proteins during repair synthesis catalyzed by Polβ [70]. The ability of PARP1 to compete with APE1 for the binding of an AP-site containing DNA indicates possible cooperation between the proteins upon the recognition and further incision of the AP site [71]. Following the incision of AP site, PARP1 can catalyze the synthesis of poly(ADP-ribose). According to the initially proposed mechanism of its action, PARP1 dissociates from the complex with DNA after covalent attachment of the negatively charged PAR polymer. Further studies of an active role of PAR in the formation of the repair complexes have modified this hypothesis. It was established that following poly(ADP-ribosyl)ation, PARP1 was capable of covalent binding to the photoreactive DNA intermediate; the lifetime of such complexes was shown to depend on both the size of covalently bound PAR and the initial affinity of PARP1 for the DNA damage [70]. Complexes of PAR-PARP1 with damaged DNA have been detected by atomic force microscopy [72]. Recently, kinetics of poly(ADP-ribosyl)ation and PAR homeostasis (but not the PARP1 protein) have been proposed to play a primary role in protection of cells from acute DNA damage [73]. Hence, the formation of BER complexes on the damaged DNA can be regulated via either poly(ADP-ribosyl)ation of proteins or their interactions with PAR polymer synthesized by PARP1 and PARP2. Poly(ADP-ribose) is the most important cell regulator of protein-protein and protein-nucleic acid interactions. [20, 74–78].

4. Interactions of BER proteins with noncanonical factors contribute to the regulation of DNA repair

Many proteins with various cellular functions, not considered previously to be involved in BER, have been shown to regulate this process via interactions with main participants. The HMGB1 protein—a chromatin architecture factor—interacts directly with three BER enzymes (APE1, Polβ, and FEN1), modulates their catalytic activity in the process of DNA repair, and, hence, ensures regulation of the process via the SP or LP BER sub-pathway [79–81]. Human DNA-binding proteins hSSB1 and SATB1 form complexes with DNA glycosylase OGG1, thus enhancing its efficiency in recognition of DNA damage and its repair [82, 83]. The human mitochondrial single-stranded DNA binding protein (mtSSB) interacts with NEIL1 in the presence and absence of a DNA substrate revealed to modulate the oligomerization state and stability of the NEIL1-mtSSB complex [84]. Protein factors of unknown nature that are not involved in chromatin structure remodeling form complex with DNA glycosylase NTH1 and stimulate its activity in BER initiation [85]. The SSRP1 protein entailed in chromatin disassembly as a histone H2A/H2B chaperone interacts with both PAR-PARP1 and XRCC1 and facilitates repair of SSBs [86]. In general, the mechanisms of BER functioning within chromatin are largely unexplored (for example, see [87]), remaining possibility to discover new noncanonical factors of BER.

In addition to multiple enzymatic functions in DNA repair, APE1 is known to play a regulatory role in the transcription processes, RNA processing, and ribosome biogenesis [76, 88]. The activities of the multifunctional enzyme, its expression level, and intracellular localization are regulated by its interaction with the multifunctional protein nucleophosmin (NPM1) [89]. Direct interactions of APE1 and several DNA glycosylases (TDG, NEIL2, NTH1, OGG1, and UNG2) with protein factors of nucleotide excision repair (XPC, XPG, CSB, and RPA) and homologous recombination (Rad52) have been shown to play a regulatory role in the overlapping repair pathways [90].

PARP1 forms stable complexes with Ku70/Ku80 proteins, and this interaction has been proposed to be an important regulator of the Ku70/80 heterodimer function in the repair of DNA double-strand breaks (DSBs) [91, 92]. Recent studies have demonstrated the involvement of Ku70 and Ku80 proteins in different steps of BER [93]. Septin4, a member of GTP binding protein family considered to be an essential component of the cytoskeleton, is a novel PARP1 interacting protein, and the interaction is enhanced under oxidative stress [94]. PARP1 interacts with NR1D1 protein, a nuclear receptor subfamily 1 group D member 1; the interaction is enhanced under oxidative stress and inhibits the catalytic activity of PARP1 [95]. Whether the interaction of these noncanonical factors with PARP1 may contribute to regulation of BER remains to be explored. The protein DBC1 (deleted in breast cancer 1), one of the most abundant yet enigmatic proteins in mammals containing a conserved domain similar to Nudix hydrolases (hydrolyzing nucleoside diphosphates) but lacking catalytic activity, interacts directly with the BRCT domain of PARP1; the strength of the interaction shown to inhibit the catalytic activity of PARP1 is modulated by NAD+ concentration [96]. Thus, a novel function of NAD+ to directly regulate protein-protein interactions, the modulation of which may protect against cancer, radiation, and aging, has been discovered.

The multifunctional Y-box-binding protein 1 (YB-1) is another noncanonical factor of BER. The proteolytic fragment of this positively charged intrinsically disordered protein localized in the nucleus is formed in response to DNA damage [97]. We have shown that YB-1 interacts with poly(ADP-ribose) and could be an acceptor for PARP1/PARP2 catalyzed poly(ADP-ribosyl)ation *in vitro* [98]. Several proteins essential for BER—APE1, Polβ, NEIL1, PARP1, and PARP2—directly interact with YB-1, although most complexes being less stable than the complexes of BER proteins with each other (the apparent K_d values are in the range of 340 to 810 nM as compared to those presented in **Figure 4**) [99]. A strong interaction detected between APE1 and YB-1 could be an important factor for the cooperative action of these multifunctional proteins in transcription regulation [100]. Interactions of YB-1 protein with BER enzymes could be responsible for the regulation of their activities: the AP-endonuclease activity of APE1 and 5′-dRp-lyase activity of Polβ are inhibited in the presence of YB-1, while the AP-lyase activity of NEIL1 is stimulated [99]. YB-1 was found to stimulate the catalytic activity of PARP1 via strong binding with poly(ADP-ribose) linked to PARP1, which increased the lifetime of this complex in DNA [99]. Acting as a cofactor of PARP1, YB-1 decreases the efficiency of PARP1 inhibitors [101].

5. Intersection of posttranslational modifications and protein-protein interactions in BER coordination

Posttranslational modifications (PTMs) of proteins involved in BER modulate catalytic and DNA-binding activities of individual proteins, their expression, intracellular localization, structure, and stability as well as protein-protein interactions and may therefore contribute to regulation of DNA repair either directly or indirectly. Numerous studies of PTMs and their functions in BER have been reviewed previously [90, 102–106]. As mentioned above, PARP1 modifies itself and binding partners with poly(ADP-ribose). Among the targets of PARP1 catalyzed ADP-ribosylation are two key BER proteins—XRCC1 and Polβ, and XRCC1 negatively regulates PARP1 activity [35, 107]. The automodification of PARP1 has been shown to enhance its interaction with XRCC1, LigIIIα, and TDP1; the length of

PAR polymer determines the efficiency of PAR-mediated accumulation of XRCC1 on DNA damage [46, 47, 108]. Recent studies have identified other PTMs, such as phosphorylation, acetylation, and methylation, to regulate the activity of PARP1 [104, 106]. Phosphorylation of PARP1 mediated by protein kinase CDK2 represents a novel DNA-independent mechanism of PARP1 activation [106]. Modifications of PARP1 mediated by AMP-activated protein kinase (AMPK) and lysine acetyltransferase 2B (PCAF) modulate both the activity of PARP1 and ADP-ribosylation of other proteins [106]. Polyubiquitination of PARP1 by E3 ubiquitin protein ligase is promoted by the automodification of PARP1 and targets PAR-PARP1 for proteasomal degradation [106]. It has to be noted that nonproteolytic roles of protein ubiquitination in regulation of DSBs repair and NER have been demonstrated [105]. PARP1 modification (at Lys486 residue) with small ubiquitin-like protein catalyzed by SUMO E3 ligase (SUMOylation) enhances p300-dependent acetylation of PARP1, while it has no effect on its activity [106].

The most abundant evidence on PTM-mediated regulation of protein-protein interactions is available for the XRCC1 protein. XRCC1 is an extensively phosphorylated protein with more than 45 phosphorylation sites localized in the linker regions and BRCTa domain [109]. Catalyzed by p38 MAPK kinase phosphorylation of the BRCTa domain (at T358 and T367 residues) has been shown to regulate PAR-mediated recruitment of XRCC1 to DNA damage [109]. The phosphorylation of XRCC1 by checkpoint kinase 2 (CHK2) at Thr284 residue *in vivo* and *in vitro* increases the affinity of XRCC1 for DNA glycosylase MPG, facilitating thereby initiation of BER [110]. As shown recently, the same kinase interacts with PARP1 and modifies the BRCT domain; the CHK2-dependent phosphorylation of PARP1 stimulates its catalytic activity and interaction with XRCC1 [111]. Seven sites of XRCC1 phosphorylation mediated by kinase CK2 (localized in the XL2 linker) are necessary to modulate the interaction of XRCC1 with end-processing enzymes—PNKP, APTX, and PNK-like factor APLF—and the efficiency of repair of chromosomal DNA SSBs [37–39, 112, 113]. Notably, the phosphorylated and unmodified forms of XRCC1 bind different structural domains of PNKP and modulate the kinase activity of PNKP or its accumulation on DNA damage, respectively [37, 38]. The oxidized form of XRCC1 stabilized by a disulfide bridge between Cys12 and Cys20 residues forms a more stable (in comparison with the reduced form) complex with Polβ; an increase in the number of intermolecular contacts in this complex has been confirmed by X-ray analysis of the complex [23]. The existence of oxidized form of XRCC1 *in vivo* is essential to protect cells against extreme oxidative stress [114]. XRCC1 is a substrate for SUMOylation promoted by DNA damage-induced PARylation; SUMOylation of XRCC1 contributes to regulation of BER via increasing its binding affinity for Polβ [115].

The most frequent PTMs discovered for the multifunctional protein APE1 include phosphorylation, acetylation, S-nitrosylation, S-glutathionylation, formation of disulfide bonds, and ubiquitination [90, 102]. Most modifications modulate redox activity of APE1 and its regulatory function in transcription. As Cys residues are targets of different modifications, it is essential to understand the competition between these PTMs and their roles in APE1 function. Numerous studies on APE1 phosphorylation by a variety of protein kinases provide contradictory data on modulation of the repair activity of APE1 [102]. Recently, it has been shown that acetylation of APE1 (at Lys residues in the mammalian-conserved N-terminal extension) enhances both the AP-endonuclease activity and the interaction with XRCC1 and XRCC1-LigIIIα complex, ensuring cell survival in response to genotoxic stress [116].

Acetylation of DNA glycosylase TDG weakens its interaction with APE1 and produces opposite effects on the excision activity of the enzyme toward various types of base damages; repair of damage induced by the chemotherapeutic action of 5-fluorouracil is enhanced by the TDG acetylation [90]. Based on these data, the acetylation status of TDG within tumor cells was proposed to impact the chemotherapy efficacy. Phosphorylation of the flexible N-terminus of DNA glycosylase UNG2 (at Thr6 or Tyr8 residues) shown to disrupt interaction with the PCNA factor, without affecting the UNG2 catalytic activity or its RPA interaction, has been proposed to regulate the formation of the ternary PCNA-UNG2-RPA protein complex [117].

Various PTMs of Polβ (acetylation, phosphorylation, and methylation) modulate its 5′-dRp-lyase and nucleotidyl transferase activities; the only example of PTMs impacts on protein-protein interaction is inhibition of Polβ-PCNA interaction due to PRMT1-dependent methylation of Arg137 [102]. The enzymes completing BER—LigIIIα and LigI—undergo posttranslational modification *in vitro* and in *vivo*; however, the intersection of their PTMs with protein-protein interactions is yet unknown [102].

6. Conclusions

Intensive studies of DNA repair system ensuring repair of damaged bases and single-strand DNA breaks (BER) in recent decades have made impressive progress in establishing the participants of the repair process, main sub-pathways, and auxiliary mechanisms activated when the main BER sub-pathways are inefficient. In addition to the enzymes responsible for catalytic steps of BER, several proteins, such as XRCC1, PARP1, PARP2, and others, have been identified as BER participants essential for assembling and functioning of the dynamic multiprotein system. Multiprotein complexes of various compositions can be formed without the involvement of DNA, but their structure and stability are modulated by the damaged DNA and intermediates formed in different steps of BER. Interactions of individual BER enzymes with DNA substrates and products have been deciphered in detail by X-ray studies. This method is of little use to explore dynamic supramolecular structures operating in DNA repair. The next step is required to clarify how the BER system functions upon association of the multiprotein complexes with chromatin; novel methods in structural analysis, such as electron microscopy, and more complex models imitating DNA repair in chromatin structure might be helpful to apply. How protein-protein interactions and posttranslational modifications coordinate BER with other DNA repair systems requires future studies. Elucidation of molecular mechanisms underlying efficient BER and its dysregulation in pathological states will help broaden our understanding the origins of diseases and provide novel strategy of their treatment.

Acknowledgements

This work was financially supported partially under Russian State funded budget project (VI.57.1.2, 0309-2016-0001) and by the Russian Science Foundation (grant No. 14-24-00038).

Conflict of interest

The authors declare that there is no conflict of interest.

Author details

Nina Moor and Olga Lavrik*
Siberian Branch of the Russian Academy of Sciences, Institute of Chemical Biology and Fundamental Medicine, Novosibirsk, Russia

*Address all correspondence to: lavrik@niboch.nsc.ru

References

[1] Kim Y-J, Wilson DM III. Overview of base excision repair biochemistry. Current Molecular Pharmacology. 2012;**5**:3-13. DOI: 10.2174/1874467211205010003

[2] Dutta A, Yang C, Sengupta S, Mitra S, Hegde ML. New paradigms in the repair of oxidative damage in human genome: Mechanisms ensuring repair of mutagenic base lesions during replication and involvement of accessory proteins. Cellular and Molecular Life Sciences. 2015;**7**:1679-1698. DOI: 10.1007/s00018-014-1820-z

[3] Whitaker AM, Schaich MA, Smith MR, Flynn TS, Freudenthal BD. Base excision repair of oxidative DNA damage: From mechanism to disease. Frontiers in Bioscience. 2017;**22**:1493-1522

[4] Caldecott KW. DNA single-strand break repair. Experimental Cell Research. 2014;**329**:2-8. DOI: 10.1016/j.yexcr.2014.08.027

[5] Abbotts R, Wilson DM III. Coordination of DNA single strand break repair. Free Radical Biology & Medicine. 2017;**107**:228-244. DOI: 10.1016/j.freeradbiomed.2016.11.039

[6] Moor NA, Lavrik OI. Protein-protein interactions in DNA base excision repair. Biochemistry (Mosc). 2018;**83**:411-422. DOI: 10.1134/S0006297918040120

[7] Hakem R. DNA-damage repair; the good, the bad, and the ugly. The EMBO Journal. 2008;**27**:589-605. DOI: 10.1038/emboj.2008.15

[8] Pan MR, Li K, Lin SY, Hung WC. Connecting the dots: From DNA damage and repair to aging. International Journal of Molecular Sciences. 2016;**17**:E685. DOI: 10.3390/ijms17050685

[9] Gavande NS, VanderVere-Carozza PS, Hinshaw HD, Jalal SI, Sears CR, Pawelczak KS, et al. DNA repair targeted therapy: The past or future of cancer treatment? Pharmacology & Therapeutics. 2016;**160**:65-83. DOI: 10.1016/j.pharmthera.2016.02.003

[10] Dizdaroglu M, Coskun E, Jaruga P. Repair of oxidatively induced DNA damage by DNA glycosylases: Mechanisms of action, substrate specificities and excision kinetics. Mutation Research. 2017;**771**:99-127. DOI: 10.1016/j.mrrev.2017.02.001

[11] Liu Y, Beard WA, Shock DD, Prasad R, Hou EW, Wilson SH. DNA polymerase beta and flap endonuclease 1 enzymatic specificities sustain DNA synthesis for long patch base excision repair. The Journal of Biological Chemistry. 2005;**280**:3665-3674. DOI: 10.1074/jbc.M412922200

[12] Lebedeva NA, Rechkunova NI, Dezhurov SV, Khodyreva SN, Favre A, Blanco L, et al. Comparison of functional properties of mammalian DNA polymerase lambda and DNA polymerase beta in reactions of DNA synthesis related to DNA repair. Biochimica et Biophysica Acta. 2005;**1751**:150-158. DOI: 10.1016/j.bbapap.2005.05.012

[13] Woodrick J, Gupta S, Camacho S, Parvathaneni S, Choudhury S, Cheema A, et al. A new sub-pathway of long-patch base excision repair involving 5′ gap formation. The EMBO Journal. 2017;**36**:1605-1622. DOI: 10.15252/embj.201694920

[14] Amé JC, Rolli V, Schreiber V, Niedergang C, Apiou F, Decker P, et al. PARP-2, a novel mammalian DNA damage-dependent poly(ADP-ribose) polymerase. The Journal of Biological Chemistry. 1999;**274**:17860-17868. DOI: 10.1074/jbc.274.25.17860

[15] Obaji E, Haikarainen T, Lehtiö L. Structural basis for DNA break recognition by ARTD2/PARP2. Nucleic Acids Research. 2018. DOI: 10.1093/nar/gky927

[16] Ménissier-de Murcia J, Ricoul M, Tartier L, Niedergang C, Huber A, Dantzer F, et al. Functional interaction between PARP-1 and PARP-2 in chromosome stability and embryonic development in mouse. The EMBO Journal. 2003;**22**:2255-2263. DOI: 10.1093/emboj/cdg206

[17] Hanzlikova H, Gittens W, Krejcikova K, Zeng Z, Caldecott KW. Overlapping roles for PARP1 and PARP2 in the recruitment of endogenous XRCC1 and PNKP into oxidized chromatin. Nucleic Acids Research. 2017;**45**:2546-2557. DOI: 10.1093/nar/gkw1246

[18] Ronson GE, Piberger AL, Higgs MR, Olsen AL, Stewart GS, McHugh PJ, et al. PARP1 and PARP2 stabilise replication forks at base excision repair intermediates through Fbh1-dependent Rad51 regulation. Nature Communications. 2018;**9**:746. DOI: 10.1038/s41467-018-03159-2

[19] Pascal JM, Ellenberger T. The rise and fall of poly(ADP-ribose): An enzymatic perspective. DNA Repair. 2015;**32**:10-16. DOI: 10.1016/j.dnarep.2015.04.008

[20] Ray Chaudhuri A, Nussenzweig A. The multifaceted roles of PARP1 in DNA repair and chromatin remodeling. Nature Reviews. Molecular Cell Biology. 2017;**18**:610-621. DOI: 10.1038/nrm.2017.53

[21] Prasad R, Beard WA, Batra VK, Liu Y, Shock DD, Wilson SH. A review of recent experiments on step-to-step "hand-off" of the DNA intermediates in mammalian base excision repair pathways. Molecular Biology (Mosk). 2011;**45**:586-600

[22] Esadze A, Rodriguez G, Cravens SL, Stivers JT. AP-endonuclease 1 accelerates turnover of human 8-oxoguanine DNA glycosylase by preventing retrograde binding to the abasic-site product. Biochemistry. 2017;**56**:1974-1986. DOI: 10.1021/acs.biochem.7b00017

[23] London RE. The structural basis of XRCC1-mediated DNA repair. DNA Repair. 2015;**30**:90-103. DOI: 10.1016/j.dnarep.2015.02.005

[24] Gerloff DL, Woods NT, Farago AA, Monteiro AN. BRCT domains: A little more than kin, and less than kind. FEBS Letters. 2012;**586**:2711-2716. DOI: 10.1016/j.febslet.2012.05.005

[25] Breslin C, Mani RS, Fanta M, Hoch N, Weinfeld M, Caldecott KW. The Rev1 interacting region (RIR) motif in the scaffold protein XRCC1 mediates a low-affinity interaction with polynucleotide kinase/phosphatase (PNKP) during DNA single-strand break repair. The Journal of Biological Chemistry. 2017;**292**:16024-16031. DOI: 10.1074/jbc.M117.806638

[26] Kubota Y, Nash RA, Klungland A, Schär P, Barnes DE, Lindahl T. Reconstitution of DNA base excision-repair with purified human proteins: Interaction between DNA polymerase β and the XRCC1 protein. The EMBO Journal. 1996;**15**:6662-6670

[27] Marintchev A, Robertson A, Dimitriadis EK, Prasad R, Wilson SH, Mullen GP. Domain specific interaction in the XRCC1-DNA polymerase β complex. Nucleic Acids Research. 2000;**28**:2049-2059

[28] Marintchev A, Gryk MR, Mullen GP. Site-directed mutagenesis analysis of the structural interaction of the single-strand-break repair protein, X-ray cross-complementing group 1, with DNA polymerase β. Nucleic Acids Research. 2003;**31**:580-588

[29] Campalans A, Marsin S, Nakabeppu Y, O'Connor TR, Boiteux S, Radicella JP. XRCC1 interactions with multiple DNA glycosylases: A model for its recruitment to base excision repair. DNA Repair. 2005;**4**:826-835. DOI: 10.1016/j.dnarep.2005.04.014

[30] Wiederhold L, Leppard JB, Kedar P, Karimi-Busheri F, Rasouli-Nia A, Weinfeld M, et al. AP endonuclease-independent DNA base excision repair in human cells. Molecular Cell. 2004;**15**:209-220. DOI: 10.1016/j.molcel.2004.06.003

[31] Das A, Wiederhold L, Leppard JB, Kedar P, Prasad R, Wang H, et al. NEIL2-initiated, APE-independent repair of oxidized bases in DNA: Evidence for a repair complex in human cells. DNA Repair. 2006;**5**:1439-1448. DOI: 10.1016/j.dnarep.2006.07.003

[32] Fan J, Otterlei M, Wong HK, Tomkinson AE, Wilson DM III. XRCC1 co-localizes and physically interacts with PCNA. Nucleic Acids Research. 2004;**32**:2193-2201. DOI: 10.1093/nar/gkh556

[33] Akbari M, Solvang-Garten K, Hanssen-Bauer A, Lieske NV, Pettersen HS, Pettersen GK, et al. Direct interaction between XRCC1 and UNG2 facilitates rapid repair of uracil in DNA by XRCC1 complexes. DNA Repair. 2010;**9**:785-795. DOI: 10.1016/j.dnarep.2010.04.002

[34] Marsin S, Vidal AE, Sossou M, Ménissier-de Murcia J, Le Page F, Boiteux S, et al. Role of XRCC1 in the coordination and stimulation of oxidative DNA damage repair initiated by the DNA glycosylase hOGG1. The Journal of Biological Chemistry. 2003;**278**:44068-44074. DOI: 10.1074/jbc.M306160200

[35] Masson M, Niedergang C, Schreiber V, Muller S, Ménissier-de Murcia J, de Murcia G. XRCC1 is specifically associated with poly(ADP-ribose) polymerase and negatively regulates its activity following DNA damage. Molecular and Cellular Biology. 1998;**18**:3563-3571

[36] Schreiber V, Amé JC, Dollé P, Schultz I, Rinaldi B, Fraulob V, et al. Poly(ADP-ribose) polymerase-2 (PARP-2) is required for efficient base excision DNA repair in association with PARP-1 and XRCC1. The Journal of Biological Chemistry. 2002;**277**:23028-23036. DOI: 10.1074/jbc.M202390200

[37] Loizou JI, El-Khamisy SF, Zlatanou A, Moore DJ, Chan DW, Qin J, et al. The protein kinase CK2 facilitates repair of chromosomal DNA single-strand breaks. Cell. 2004;**117**:17-28

[38] Lu M, Mani RS, Karimi-Busheri F, Fanta M, Wang H, Litchfeld DW, et al. Independent mechanisms of stimulation of polynucleotide kinase/phosphatase by phosphorylated and non-phosphorylated XRCC1. Nucleic Acids Research. 2010;**38**:510-521. DOI: 10.1093/nar/gkp1023

[39] Luo H, Chan DW, Yang T, Rodriguez M, Chen BP, Leng M, et al. A new XRCC1-containing complex and its role in cellular survival of methyl methanesulfonate treatment. Molecular and Cellular Biology. 2004;**24**:8356-8365. DOI: 10.1128/MCB.24.19.8356-8365.2004

[40] Nash RA, Caldecott KW, Barnes DE, Lindahl T. XRCC1 protein interacts with one of two distinct forms of DNA ligase III. Biochemistry. 1997;**36**:5207-5211. DOI: 10.1021/bi962281m

[41] Beernink PT, Hwang M, Ramirez M, Murphy MB, Doyle SA, Thelen MP. Specificity of protein interactions mediated by BRCT domains of the XRCC1 DNA repair protein. The Journal of Biological Chemistry. 2005;**280**:30206-30213. DOI: 10.1074/jbc.M502155200

[42] Cuneo MJ, Gabel SA, Krahn JM, Ricker MA, London RE. The structural basis for partitioning of the XRCC1/DNA ligase III-α BRCT-mediated dimer complexes. Nucleic Acids Research. 2011;**39**:7816-7827. DOI: 10.1093/nar/gkr419

[43] Plo I, Liao ZY, Barceló JM, Kohlhagen G, Caldecott KW, Weinfeld M, et al. Association of XRCC1 and tyrosyl DNA phosphodiesterase (Tdp1) for the repair of topoisomerase I-mediated DNA lesions. DNA Repair. 2003;**2**:1087-1100

[44] Dantzer F, de La Rubia G, Ménissier-de Murcia J, Hostomsky Z, de Murcia G, Schreiber V. Base excision repair is impaired in mammalian cells lacking poly(ADP-ribose) polymerase-1. Biochemistry. 2000;**39**:7559-7569

[45] Ali AAE, Timinszky G, Arribas-Bosacoma R, Kozlowski M, Hassa PO, Hassler M, et al. The zinc-finger domains of PARP1 cooperate to recognize DNA strand breaks. Nature Structural & Molecular Biology. 2012;**19**:685-692. DOI: 10.1038/nsmb.2335

[46] Leppard JB, Dong Z, Mackey ZB, Tomkinson AE. Physical and functional interaction between DNA ligase IIIα and poly(ADP-ribose) polymerase 1 in DNA single-strand break repair. Molecular and Cellular Biology. 2003;**23**:5919-5927

[47] Das BB, Huang SY, Murai J, Rehman I, Amé JC, Sengupta S, et al. PARP1-TDP1 coupling for the repair of topoisomerase I-induced DNA damage. Nucleic Acids Research. 2014;**42**: 4435-4449. DOI: 10.1093/nar/gku088

[48] Luncsford PJ, Manvilla BA, Patterson DN, Malik SS, Jin J, Hwang BJ, et al. Coordination of MYH DNA glycosylase and APE1 endonuclease activities via physical interactions. DNA Repair. 2013;**12**:1043-1052. DOI: 10.1016/j.dnarep.2013.09.007

[49] Hegde PM, Dutta A, Sengupta S, Mitra J, Adhikari S, Tomkinson AE, et al. The C-terminal domain (CTD) of human DNA glycosylase NEIL1 is required for forming BERosome repair complex with DNA replication proteins at the replicating genome: Dominant negative function of the CTD. The Journal of Biological Chemistry. 2015;**290**:20919-20933. DOI: 10.1074/jbc.M115.642918

[50] Dimitriadis EK, Prasad R, Vaske MK, Chen L, Tomkinson AE, Lewis MS, et al. Thermodynamics of human DNA ligase I trimerization and association with DNA polymerase β. The Journal of Biological Chemistry. 1998;**273**:20540-20550

[51] Bennett RA, Wilson DM III, Wong D, Demple B. Interaction of human apurinic endonuclease and DNA polymerase β in the base excision repair pathway. Proceedings of the National Academy of Sciences of the United States of America. 1997;**94**:7166-7169

[52] Whitehouse CJ, Taylor RM, Thistlethwaite A, Zhang H, Karimi-Busheri F, Lasko DD, et al. XRCC1 stimulates human polynucleotide kinase activity at damaged DNA termini and accelerates DNA single-strand break repair. Cell. 2001;**104**:107-117

[53] El-Khamisy SF, Saifi GM, Weinfeld M, Johansson F, Helleday T, Lupski JR, et al. Defective DNA single-strand break repair in spinocerebellar ataxia with axonalneuropathy-1. Nature. 2005;**434**:108-113. DOI: 10.1038/nature03314

[54] Chiang SC, Carroll J, El-Khamisy SF. TDP1 serine 81 promotes interaction with DNA ligase IIIα and facilitates cell survival following DNA damage. Cell Cycle. 2010;**9**:588-595. DOI: 10.4161/cc.9.3.10598

[55] Langelier MF, Planck JL, Roy S, Pascal JM. Structural basis for DNA damage-dependent poly(ADP-ribosyl)ation by human PARP-1. Science. 2012;**336**:728-732. DOI: 10.1126/science.1216338

[56] Cotner-Gohara E, Kim IK, Tomkinson AE, Ellenberger T. Two DNA-binding and nick recognition modules in human DNA ligase III. The Journal of Biological Chemistry. 2008;**283**:10764-10772. DOI: 10.1074/jbc.M708175200

[57] Eustermann S, Wu WF, Langelier MF, Yang JC, Easton LE, Riccio AA, et al. Structural basis of detection and signaling of DNA single-strand breaks by human PARP-1. Molecular Cell. 2015;**60**:742-754. DOI: 10.1016/j.molcel.2015

[58] Gagné JP, Isabelle M, Lo KS, Bourassa S, Hendzel MJ, Dawson VL, et al. Proteome-wide identification of poly(ADP-ribose) binding proteins and poly(ADP-ribose)-associated protein complexes. Nucleic Acids Research. 2008;**36**:6959-6976. DOI: 10.1093/nar/gkn771

[59] Teloni F, Altmeyer M. Readers of poly(ADP-ribose): Designed to be fit for purpose. Nucleic Acids Research. 2016;**44**:993-1006. DOI: 10.1093/nar/gkv1383

[60] Gagné JP, Ethier C, Defoy D, Bourassa S, Langelier MF, Riccio AA, et al. Quantitative site-specific ADP-ribosylation profiling of DNA-dependent PARPs. DNA Repair. 2015;**30**:68-79. DOI: 10.1016/j.dnarep.2015.02.004

[61] Bock FJ, Chang P. New directions in poly(ADP-ribose) polymerase biology. The FEBS Journal. 2016;**28**:4017-4031. DOI: 10.1111/febs.13737

[62] Abdou I, Poirier GG, Hendzel MJ, Weinfeld M. DNA ligase III acts as a DNA strand break sensor in the cellular orchestration of DNA strand break repair. Nucleic Acids Research. 2015;**43**:875-892. DOI: 10.1093/nar/gku1307

[63] Moor NA, Vasil'eva IA, Anarbaev RO, Antson AA, Lavrik OI. Quantitative characterization of protein-protein complexes involved in base excision DNA repair. Nucleic Acids Research. 2015;**43**:6009-6022. DOI: 10.1093/nar/gkv569

[64] Mani RS, Fanta M, Karimi-Busheri F, Silver E, Virgen CA, Caldecott KW, et al. XRCC1 stimulates polynucleotide kinase by enhancing its damage discrimination and displacement from DNA repair intermediates. The Journal of Biological Chemistry. 2007;**282**:28004-28013. DOI: 10.1074/jbc.M704867200

[65] Liu Y, Prasad R, Beard WA, Kedar PS, Hou EW, Shock DD, et al. Coordination of steps in single-nucleotide base excision repair mediated by apurinic/apyrimidinic endonuclease 1 and DNA polymerase β. The Journal of Biological Chemistry. 2007;**282**:13532-13541. DOI: 10.1074/jbc.M611295200

[66] Fang Q, Inanc B, Schamus S, Wang XH, Wei L, Brown AR, et al. HSP90 regulates DNA repair via the interaction between XRCC1 and DNA polymerase β. Nature Communications. 2014;**5**:5513. DOI: 10.1038/ncomms6513

[67] Lan L, Nakajima S, Oohata Y, Takao M, Okano S, Masutani M, et al. *In situ* analysis of repair processes for oxidative DNA damage in mammalian cells. Proceedings of the National Academy of Sciences of the United States of America. 2004;**101**:13738-13743. DOI: 10.1073/pnas.0406048101

[68] Hanssen-Bauer A, Solvang-Garten K, Gilljam KM, Torseth K, Wilson DM III, Akbari M, et al. The region of XRCC1 which harbours the three most

common nonsynonymous polymorphic variants, is essential for the scaffolding function of XRCC1. DNA Repair. 2012;**11**:357-366. DOI: 10.1016/j.dnarep.2012.01.001

[69] Vasil'eva IA, Anarbaev RO, Moor NA, Lavrik OI. Dynamic light scattering study of base excision DNA repair proteins and their complexes. Biochimica et Biophysica Acta, Proteins and Proteomics. 2018. DOI: 10.1016/j.bbapap.2018.10.009

[70] Lavrik OI, Prasad R, Sobol RW, Horton JK, Ackerman EJ, Wilson SH. Photoaffinity labeling of mouse fibroblast enzymes by a base excision repair intermediate. Evidence for the role of poly(ADP-ribose) polymerase-1 in DNA repair. The Journal of Biological Chemistry. 2001;**276**:25541-25548. DOI: 10.1074/jbc.M102125200

[71] Khodyreva SN, Prasad R, Ilina ES, Sukhanova MV, Kutuzov MM, Liu Y, et al. Apurinic/apyrimidinic (AP) site recognition by the 5'-dRP/AP lyase in poly(ADP-ribose) polymerase-1 (PARP-1). Proceedings of the National Academy of Sciences of the United States of America. 2010;**107**:22090-22095. DOI: 10.1073/pnas.1009182107

[72] Sukhanova MV, Abrakhi S, Joshi V, Pastre D, Kutuzov MM, Anarbaev RO, et al. Single molecule detection of PARP1 and PARP2 interaction with DNA strand breaks and their poly(ADP-ribosyl)ation using high-resolution AFM imaging. Nucleic Acids Research. 2016;**44**:e60. DOI: 10.1093/nar/gkv1476

[73] Schuhwerk H, Bruhn C, Siniuk K, Min W, Erener S, Grigaravicius P, et al. Kinetics of poly(ADP-ribosyl)ation, but not PARP1 itself, determines the cell fate in response to DNA damage *in vitro* and *in vivo*. Nucleic Acids Research. 2017;**45**:11174-11192. DOI: 10.1093/nar/gkx717

[74] Virág L, Robaszkiewicz A, Rodriguez-Vargas JM, Oliver FJ. Poly(ADP-ribose) signaling in cell death. Molecular Aspects of Medicine. 2013;**34**:1153-1167. DOI: 10.1016/j.mam.2013.01.007

[75] Altmeyer M, Neelsen KJ, Teloni F, Pozdnyakova I, Pellegrino S, Grøfte M, et al. Liquid demixing of intrinsically disordered proteins is seeded by poly(ADP-ribose). Nature Communications. 2015;**6**:8088. DOI: 10.1038/ncomms9088

[76] Vohhodina J, Harkin DP, Savage KI. Dual roles of DNA repair enzymes in RNA biology/post-transcriptional control. Wiley Interdisciplinary Reviews: RNA. 2016;**7**:604-619. DOI: 10.1002/wrna.1353

[77] Martin-Hernandez K, Rodriguez-Vargas JM, Schreiber V, Dantzer F. Expanding functions of ADP-ribosylation in the maintenance of genome integrity. Seminars in Cell & Developmental Biology. 2017;**63**:92-101. DOI: 10.1016/j.semcdb.2016.09.009

[78] Alemasova EE, Lavrik OI. At the interface of three nucleic acids: The role of RNA-binding proteins and poly(ADP-ribose) in DNA repair. Acta Naturae. 2017;**9**:4-16

[79] Prasad R, Liu Y, Deterding LJ, Poltoratsky VP, Kedar PS, Horton JK, et al. HMGB1 is a cofactor in mammalian base excision repair. Molecular Cell. 2007;**27**:829-841. DOI: 10.1016/j.molcel.2007.06.029

[80] Liu Y, Prasad R, Wilson SH. HMGB1: Roles in base excision repair and related function. Biochimica et Biophysica Acta. 2010;**1799**:119-130. DOI: 10.1016/j.bbagrm.2009.11.008

[81] Balliano A, Hao F, Njeri C, Balakrishnan L, Hayes JJ. HMGB1 stimulates activity of polymerase β on nucleosome substrates. Biochemistry.

2017;**56**:647-656. DOI: 10.1021/acs.biochem.6b00569

[82] Kaur S, Coulombe Y, Ramdzan ZM, Leduy L, Masson JY, Nepveu A. Special AT-rich sequence-binding protein 1 (SATB1) functions as an accessory factor in base excision repair. The Journal of Biological Chemistry. 2016;**291**:22769-22780. DOI: 10.1074/jbc.M116.735696

[83] Paquet N, Adams MN, Leong V, Ashton NW, Touma C, Gamsjaeger R, et al. hSSB1 (NABP2/ OBFC2B) is required for the repair of 8-oxo-guanine by the hOGG1-mediated base excision repair pathway. Nucleic Acids Research. 2015;**43**:8817-8829. DOI: 10.1093/nar/gkv790

[84] Sharma N, Chakravarthy S, Longley MJ, Copeland WC, Prakash A. The C-terminal tail of the NEIL1 DNA glycosylase interacts with the human mitochondrial single-stranded DNA binding protein. DNA Repair. 2018;**65**:11-19. DOI: 10.1016/j.dnarep.2018.02.012

[85] Maher RL, Marsden CG, Averill AM, Wallace SS, Sweasy JB, Pederson DS. Human cells contain a factor that facilitates the DNA glycosylase-mediated excision of oxidized bases from occluded sites in nucleosomes. DNA Repair (Amst). 2017;**57**:91-97. DOI: 10.1016/j.dnarep.2017.06.029

[86] Gao Y, Li C, Wei L, Teng Y, Nakajima S, Chen X, et al. SSRP1 cooperates with PARP and XRCC1 to facilitate single-strand DNA break repair by chromatin priming. Cancer Research. 2017;**77**:2674-2685. DOI: 10.1158/0008-5472.CAN-16-3128

[87] Menoni H, Di Mascio P, Cadet J, Dimitrov S, Angelov D. Chromatin associated mechanisms in base excision repair - nucleosome remodeling and DNA transcription, two key players. Free Radical Biology & Medicine. 2017;**107**:159-169. DOI: 10.1016/j.freeradbiomed.2016.12.026

[88] Tell G, Fantini D, Quadrifoglio F. Understanding different functions of mammalian AP endonuclease (APE1) as a promising tool for cancer treatment. Cellular and Molecular Life Sciences. 2010;**67**:3589-3608. DOI: 10.1007/s00018-010-0486-4

[89] Poletto M, Lirussi L, Wilson DM III, Tell G. Nucleophosmin modulates stability, activity, and nucleolar accumulation of base excision repair proteins. Molecular Biology of the Cell. 2014;**25**:1641-1652. DOI: 10.1091/mbc.E13-12-0717

[90] Limpose KL, Corbett AH, Doetsch PW. BERing the burden of damage: Pathway crosstalk and posttranslational modification of base excision repair proteins regulate DNA damage management. DNA Repair. 2017;**56**:51-64. DOI: 10.1016/j.dnarep.2017.06.007

[91] Connelly KE, Hedrick V, Sobreira TJP, Dykhuizen EC, Aryal UK. Analysis of human nuclear protein complexes by quantitative mass spectrometry profiling. Proteomics. 2018;**14**:e1700427. DOI: 10.1002/pmic.201700427

[92] Yang G, Liu C, Chen SH, Kassab MA, Hoff JD, Walter NG, et al. Super-resolution imaging identifies PARP1 and the Ku complex acting as DNA double-strand break sensors. Nucleic Acids Research. 2018;**46**(7):3446-3457. DOI: 10.1093/nar/gky088

[93] Kosova AA, Lavrik OI, Khodyreva SN. Ku antigen interaction with apurinic/apyrimidinic sites: Nonhomologous end joining vs base excision repair. MOJ Proteomics & Bioinformatics. 2014;**1**:00018. DOI: 10.15406/mojpb.2014.01.00018

[94] Zhang N, Zhang Y, Zhao S, Sun Y. Septin4 as a novel binding partner of PARP1 contributes to oxidative

stress induced human umbilical vein endothelial cells injure. Biochemical and Biophysical Research Communications. 2018;**496**:621-627. DOI: 10.1016/j.bbrc.2018.01.105

[95] Ka NL, Na TY, Lee MO. NR1D1 enhances oxidative DNA damage by inhibiting PARP1 activity. Molecular and Cellular Endocrinology. 2017;**454**:87-92. DOI: 10.1016/j.mce.2017.06.004

[96] Li J, Bonkowski MS, Moniot S, Zhang D, Hubbard BP, Ling AJ, et al. A conserved NAD+ binding pocket that regulates protein-protein interactions during aging. Science. 2017;**355**:1312-1317. DOI: 10.1126/science.aad8242

[97] Sorokin AV, Selyutina AA, Skabkin MA, Guryanov SG, Nazimov IV, Richard C, et al. Proteasome-mediated cleavage of the Y-box-binding protein 1 is linked to DNA-damage stress response. The EMBO Journal. 2005;**24**:3602-3612

[98] Alemasova EE, Pestryakov PE, Sukhanova MV, Kretov DA, Moor NA, Curmi PA, et al. Poly(ADP-ribosyl)ation as a new posttranslational modification of YB-1. Biochimie. 2015;**19**:36-44. DOI: 10.1016/j.biochi.2015.10.008

[99] Alemasova EE, Moor NA, Naumenko KN, Kutuzov MM, Sukhanova MV, Pestryakov PE, et al. Y-box-binding protein 1 as a non-canonical factor of base excision repair. Biochimica et Biophysica Acta. 2016;**1864**:1631-1640. DOI: 10.1016/j.bbapap.2016.08.012

[100] Sengupta S, Mantha AK, Mitra S, Bhakat KK. Human AP endonuclease (APE1/ref-1) and its acetylation regulate YB-1-p300 recruitment and RNA polymerase II loading in the drug-induced activation of multidrug resistance gene MDR1. Oncogene. 2011;**30**:4482-4493. DOI: 10.1038/onc.2010.435

[101] Alemasova EE, Naumenko KN, Kurgina TA, Anarbaev RO, Lavrik OI. The multifunctional protein YB-1 potentiates PARP1 activity and decreases the efficiency of PARP1 inhibitors. Oncotarget. 2018;**9**:23349-23365. DOI: 10.18632/oncotarget.25158

[102] Almeida KH, Sobol RW. A unified view of base excision repair: Lesion-dependent protein complexes regulated by post-translational modification. DNA Repair. 2007;**6**:695-711. DOI: 10.1016/j.dnarep.2007.01.009

[103] Choi S, Joo HK, Jeon BH. Dynamic Regulation of APE1/Ref-1 as a therapeutic target protein. Chonnam Medical Journal. 2016;**52**:75-80. DOI: 10.4068/cmj.2016.52.2.75

[104] Schuhwerk H, Atteya R, Siniuk K, Wang ZQ. PARPing for balance in the homeostasis of poly(ADP-ribosyl)ation. Seminars in Cell & Developmental Biology. 2017;**63**:81-91. DOI: 10.1016/j.semcdb.2016.09.011

[105] Natarajan C, Takeda K. Regulation of various DNA repair pathways by E3 ubiquitin ligases. Journal of Cancer Research and Therapeutics. 2017;**13**:157-169. DOI: 10.4103/0973-1482.204879

[106] Piao L, Fujioka K, Nakakido M, Hamamoto R. Regulation of poly(ADP-ribose) polymerase 1 functions by post-translational modifications. Frontiers in Bioscience. 2018;**23**:13-26

[107] Ohashi Y, Itaya A, Tanaka Y, Yoshihara K, Kamiya T, Matsukage A. Poly(ADP-ribosyl)ation of DNA polymerase β *in vitro*. Biochemical and Biophysical Research Communications. 1986;**140**:666-673

[108] Kim IK, Stegeman RA, Brosey CA, Ellenberger T. A quantitative assay reveals ligand specificity of the DNA scaffold repair protein XRCC1 and efficient disassembly of complexes of XRCC1 and the poly(ADP-ribose)

polymerase 1 by poly(ADP-ribose) glycohydrolase. The Journal of Biological Chemistry. 2015;**290**:3775-3783. DOI: 10.1074/jbc.M114.624718

[109] de Sousa MML, Bjørås KØ, Hanssen-Bauer A, Solvang-Garten K, Otterlei M. p38 MAPK signaling and phosphorylations in the BRCT1 domain regulate XRCC1 recruitment to sites of DNA damage. Scientific Reports. 2017;7:6322. DOI: 10.1038/s41598-017-06770-3

[110] Chou WC, Wang HC, Wong FH, Ding SL, Wu PE, Shieh SY, et al. Chk2-dependent phosphorylation of XRCC1 in the DNA damage response promotes base excision repair. The EMBO Journal. 2008;**27**:3140-3150. DOI: 10.1038/emboj.2008.229

[111] Hsu PC, Gopinath RK, Hsueh YA, Shieh SY. CHK2-mediated regulation of PARP1 in oxidative DNA damage response. Oncogene. 2018. DOI: 10.1038/s41388-018-0506-7

[112] Kim K, Pedersen LC, Kirby TW, DeRose EF, London RE. Characterization of the APLF FHA-XRCC1 phosphopeptide interaction and its structural and functional implications. Nucleic Acids Research. 2017;**45**:12374-12387. DOI: 10.1093/nar/gkx941

[113] Horton JK, Stefanick DF, Çağlayan M, Zhao ML, Janoshazi AK, Prasad R, et al. XRCC1 phosphorylation affects aprataxin recruitment and DNA deadenylation activity. DNA Repair. 2018;**64**:26-33. DOI: 10.1016/j.dnarep.2018.02.004

[114] Horton JK, Seddon HJ, Zhao ML, Gassman NR, Janoshazi AK, Stefanick DF, et al. Role of the oxidized form of XRCC1 in protection against extreme oxidative stress. Free Radical Biology & Medicine. 2017;**107**:292-300. DOI: 10.1016/j.freeradbiomed.2017.02.005

[115] Hu LY, Chang CC, Huang YS, Chou WC, Lin YM, Ho CC, et al. SUMOylation of XRCC1 activated by poly (ADP-ribosyl)ation regulates DNA repair. Human Molecular Genetics. 2018;**27**:2306-2317. DOI: 10.1093/hmg/ddy135

[116] Roychoudhury S, Nath S, Song H, Hegde ML, Bellot LJ, Mantha AK, et al. Human apurinic/apyrimidinic endonuclease (APE1) is acetylated at DNA damage sites in chromatin, and acetylation modulates its DNA repair activity. Molecular and Cellular Biology. 2017;**37**:e00401-e00416. DOI: 10.1128/MCB.00401-16

[117] Weiser BP, Stivers JT, Cole PA. Investigation of N-terminal phospho-regulation of uracil DNA glycosylase using protein semisynthesis. Biophysical Journal. 2017;**113**:393-401. DOI: 10.1016/j.bpj.2017.06.016

Chapter 3

Mitochondrial Genome Maintenance: Damage and Repair Pathways

Ulises Omar García-Lepe and Rosa Ma Bermúdez-Cruz

Abstract

The mitochondrial genomic material (mtDNA), similarly to nuclear genome, is exposed to a plethora of exogenous and endogenous agents, as well as natural processes like replication that compromise the integrity and fidelity of the mtDNA, despite the abovementioned, the mtDNA does not contain genes involved in DNA repair, therefore mitochondria completely depend on the importation of nuclear-encoded elements to achieve genome maintenance, which implies a coordinated crosstalk between these two organelles. It has been determined that to counteract damage, mitochondria possess well-defined repair pathways quite similar to those of the nucleus, among which are: base excision repair (BER), mismatch repair (MMR), single-strand break repair (SSBR), microhomology-mediated end joining (MMEJ), and probably homology recombination dependent repair (HRR). If these repair pathways are nonfunctional and the lesions remain unrepaired, the emergence of mutations, deletions, and other insults may result in compromised cellular viability and disease.

Keywords: mitochondria, mtDNA, damage, repair, BER, MMR, SSBR, HRR, MMEJ

1. Introduction

The mitochondrion is an essential organelle involved principally in the production of ATP and other metabolites which are important to several cellular functions, besides this organelle participates in other processes as iron-sulfur cluster biogenesis, heme production, and calcium regulation [1]. The mitochondrion possesses its own circular genomic material (mtDNA), which is exposed to the same DNA lesions as nuclear genome is, however, unlike the latter, mtDNA does not encode for genes involved in DNA maintenance or repair which implies that these processes completely depend on nuclear-encoded elements translocated to mitochondria. It was first thought that mitochondria lacked the ability to repair its DNA material, and this assumption was originated due to the observation of the absence of pyrimidine dimer resolution after ultra violet light exposition in mammalian cells [2]; however, nowadays, the study of mtDNA repair pathways has evolved into a complete research area that is constantly growing, since it has been observed that mitochondria not only possess some of the nuclear-conserved mechanisms like: base excision repair (BER), mismatch repair (MMR), single-strand break repair (SSBR), microhomology-mediated end joining (MMEJ), and homologous recombination

IntechOpen

dependent repair (HRR), additionally mitochondria have evolved specific unique methods to deal with mtDNA insults based on the redundancy nature of mtDNA and mitochondrion itself, if the damage surpasses its repair capabilities, the mtDNA molecules can be destroyed and replicated again or even the whole organelle can be degraded [3]. Of importance, lesions that remain unrepaired in mtDNA such as deletions, mutations, inversions, and other rearrangements have been linked to several heritable disease syndromes [4]; further, mtDNA rearrangements and deletions have been associated with aging and cancer (www.mitomap.org/org/MITOMAP) [5]. In this chapter, we will summarize the different mechanisms by which the mammalian mtDNA can be damaged and the described pathways that are involved in maintenance of fidelity and integrity of mitochondrial genome.

2. The mitochondrial genome

One of the features of mammalian cells is that they have two DNA-containing compartments: nuclei and mitochondria. Nuclear genome is large, diploid, and linear; in contrast, mitochondrial genome is polyploid and quite small, since is formed by a 16,569 pb circular molecule that accounts for 0.0005% of the human genome and 0.1% of the total number of genes in the human; mtDNA is redundant, since a few hundred to few thousand copies can be found per cell [3], when all the copies are identical, the genotype is termed homoplasmy, instead when multiple forms exist within the same tissue or cell; the genotype is called heteroplasmy [6]. The mitochondrial genome presents 37 genes, 13 of which encode for proteins oxidative phosphorylation chain specific and the remaining are implicated in translation: 2 ribosomal RNAs (small of 12S and large of 16S) and 22 tRNAs. The grade of compaction of mtDNA is interesting since it has no introns, and the intergenic regions are almost absent, additionally there are two noncoding regions: one of approximately 1 kb known as noncoding region (NCR) and another small of 30 bp, both implicated in regulation of replication and transcription [7]. The NCR presents a triple stranded region, named D-loop, which occupies most of its extension and is related to the start of transcription [8], besides it has been observed that some genes overlap and others lack termination codons; therefore, it has been established that the promoters produce polycistronic transcripts which are further processed to generate mature RNA molecules [9]. As mentioned above, some of the proteins involved in respiratory system and ATP synthesis, which are extremely important to cellular functions, are encoded by mtDNA and not the nuclear genome, thus it is important to maintain mitochondrial genome integrity to preserve homeostasis [10].

Despite the advances made in the study of mtDNA replication mechanism, the exact machinery and steps involved in this procedure are not fully known; however, it has been determined a general head core to this process which consists of the polymerase gamma (Polγ), a DNA helicase named Twinkle, and the mitochondrial single-stranded binding protein (mtSSB) [11]. Nowadays, there are three proposed models to explain mtDNA replication: (1) the first is quite similar to nucleus DNA replication, with standard leading and lagging strand replication, (2) a strand displacement model, where the lagging strand is synthetized once the leading has advanced and synthetized a long fragment, and (3) in this model, the lagging strand is hybridized with complementary RNA, a mechanism termed RNA incorporation throughout the lagging strand (RITOL) [8]. Another interesting feature about mtDNA replication is that contrary to what occurs in nuclear genome, mitochondrial genome replication is not limited to S phase of the cell cycle [12].

Unlike the nucleus, where the DNA forms part of nucleoprotein complexes, consisting of DNA molecules wrapped around histone structures, the mitochondrial genome does not present histones. It has been thought that this lack is responsible of the high rate of mtDNA mutagenesis, which is 10-fold greater than that in nucleus; however, this hypothesis is controversial since experimental evidence has suggested that histones might provoke DNA damage instead of preventing it [3]. Despite the above, mitochondrial genome is not naked; it is packaged into protein-DNA complexes, which are termed mitochondrial nucleoids due to its similarity to bacterial chromosomes [13]. The most abundant nucleoid-associated proteins are mtSSB, transcription factor A of mitochondria (TFAM), Polγ, mitochondrial RNA polymerase (POLRMT), and Twinkle DNA helicase [14].

3. Sources of mtDNA damage

Mitochondrial genome is exposed to almost the same insults that nuclear genome is, which can be originated by internal and external sources. Six types of DNA damage have been proposed to be the more relevant in mitochondria [3].

3.1 Alkylation damage

This kind of lesion may be due to exposition to exogenous agents as chemotherapeutic drugs, diet, and tobacco smoke; however, DNA alkylation damage can also be generated from the interaction of DNA with endogenous molecules [15], such as betaine, choline, and S-adenosylmethionine (SAM); the latter is the most relevant alkylating agent in the cell; SAM is a co-substrate involved in the transfer of methyl groups, when incubated with DNA in aqueous solutions leads to base modification, forming small amounts of 7-methylguanine and 3-methyladenine nonenzymatically, therefore SAM acts as a weak DNA-alkylating agent [16]. Of interest, these DNA modifications, in specific 7-methylguanine can trigger the formation of mutagenic apurinic sites (AP) and imidazole ring opening which results in the stoppage of replication machinery [17]; moreover, 3-methylguanine itself is a cytotoxic DNA lesion that also blocks replication [15]. Interestingly, mitochondria store about 30% of total hepatic SAM [18], thus mtDNA is constantly exposed to this alkylating agent, which threats its stability and integrity.

3.2 Hydrolytic damage

There are two types of hydrolytic damage, the first is the formation of AP sites as a product of hydrolysis of the glycosidic bonds between bases and deoxyribose, and these lesions could appear due to heating, alkylation damage (previously mentioned) or by the action of N-glycosylases [19]. It has been estimated that AP is one of the most frequent lesions in the DNA, with approximately 10,000 lesions per cell, per day [20]. Interestingly, typical AP sites generate base pair modifications, since there is a preference to incorporate adenine opposite to AP by polymerases during DNA replication [21]. The other form of hydrolytic damage is the hydrolytic deamination of bases, where cytosine and its homolog 5-methylcitosine are mainly affected. It is noteworthy that the conversion of cytosine to uracil may introduce punctual mutations to the genome during replication if left unrepaired [20].

3.3 Formation of adducts

This type of lesions can be generated for exposition to ultraviolet type B and C light which produce bulky DNA adducts termed photodimers, in addition, activated metabolites of several organic contaminants, for example, polycyclic aromatic hydrocarbons and mycotoxins may bring about adducts [1]. On the other hand, adduct formation can also be stimulated by endogenous factors, for example, it has been demonstrated that reactive intermediate products of diethylstilbestrol metabolization form DNA adducts preferentially with mitochondrial genome, where these insults are suggested to avoid replication and/or transcription, thus producing mtDNA instability in vivo [22].

3.4 Mismatches

During replication, polymerases can introduce base to base mismatches as well as generate nucleotide insertions or deletions in mitochondria, which are normally known as insertion-deletion loops (IDLs). One important source of mismatches are damaged deoxyribonucleotide triphosphates (dNTPs), predominantly oxidized, which can be incorporated to DNA during synthesis [3, 10].

3.5 DNA strand breaks

These injuries are divided based on the breaking of one or both strands. Single strand breaks (SSBs) can be generated by normal cellular procedures that went wrong, such as erroneous or abortive activity of DNA topoisomerase I (Top1), which presents mitochondrial localization, and when it fails may produce protein-linked DNA breaks [23], also SSBs are produced by ineffective base excision repair (BER), or by oxidative stress [24]. One lesion related to SSBs is the formation of a covalently linked AMP to a 5′ phosphate, product of an unsuccessful DNA ligase activity [25]. On the other hand, double strand breaks (DSBs) are the most harmful, since they can provoke global cellular responses that involve many aspects of cell metabolism [26]. These lesions may occur by endogenous agents like reactive oxygen species (ROS), errors in DNA metabolism by topoisomerases, and nucleases or detention of replisome. On the other hand, lesion can be caused by exogenous insults such as ionizing radiation and chemotherapeutic drugs [1].

3.6 Oxidative damage

In living organisms, ROS are normally produced as a consequence of endogenous metabolic reactions and also by external factors. ROS include superoxide anion (O_2^-), hydrogen peroxide (H_2O_2), hydroxyl radical (OH^-), and single oxygen (O_2), all of them can oxidize DNA molecules and generate several types of damage including oxidized bases and single- and double-strand breaks [15]. Oxidative damage is by far the most prevalent and studied in mtDNA, since mitochondria are an important contributor in the creation of ROS [27], generated by the leakage of electrons from the electron transportation chain (ETC) [28], and there are at least nine sites responsible for generating the superoxide anion [29]. The importance of ROS affecting mtDNA lies in the observation that oxidative damage accumulates in several human diseases [30]. Of interest, it has also been reported that reactive nitrogen species (RNS) are able to oxidize or deaminate DNA and produce strand breaks, lesions that could be possible in mtDNA since these RNS can be found in mitochondria [31, 32].

4. Mitochondrial DNA repair machinery

Most of the repair pathways used by mitochondria to deal with its damaged DNA are quite similar to those operating in the nucleus; this observation makes sense when we realize that mitochondrion relies completely in import of DNA repair elements encoded by nuclear genome, despite that mitochondrial genome does not contain any gene implicated in repair; it appears that the mitochondrial version of the repair machinery operates with fewer proteins than the nuclear counterparts [33] (**Figure 1**).

4.1 Base excision repair (BER)

Base excision repair (BER) is the commissioned pathway to removed nonbulky lesions like alkylated, deaminated, and oxidized bases from the DNA. This pathway has been well studied in the nucleus and was the first repair mechanism reported in mitochondria and to date the best characterized in this last organelle [33, 34]. BER mechanism is highly conserved from bacteria to humans and basically comprises five stages: (1) recognition and excision of the damaged base, (2) removal of the abasic site formed, (3) DNA end processing, (4) repair synthesis, and (5) ligation [35], and at the same time, BER can be divided into two branches (both founded in mitochondria): short patch and long patch, where the difference lies in the procedure used to repair, while short patch forms a single nucleotide gap, long patch forms a bigger one of 2–10 nucleotides [36]. One of the main elements involved in BER processes are the DNA glycosylases, enzymes that catalyze the excision of the N-glycosidic bond between the altered base and its corresponding carbohydrate, thus creating an abasic site, and activity that was first observed by Lindahl et al. [37]. These glycosylases can be subdivided into monofunctional or bifunctional, depending on whether they have lyase activity or not, ability that determines the type of damage they can repair, while monofunctional glycosylases focus on nonoxidative damage, bifunctional exert their action against oxidized DNA bases [35]. In mammalian mitochondria, seven glycosylases have been reported, three monofunctional: uracil-DNA glycosylase (UNG1), *E. coli* MutY homolog (MYH), and N-methylpurine DNA glycosylase (AAG/MPG) and four bifunctional: 8-oxoguanina-DNA glycosylase (OGG1), *E. coli* endonuclease III homolog (NTH1) endonuclease VIII-like glycosylase 1 and 2 (NEIL1 and 2) [38–41]. After the action of glycosylases, the next step, DNA end processing, is catalyzed by nuclear BER enzymes that are also found in mitochondria, as apurinic-apyrimidinic endonuclease 1 (APE1) and polynucleotide kinase-3′-phosphatase (PNKP) [35], further the

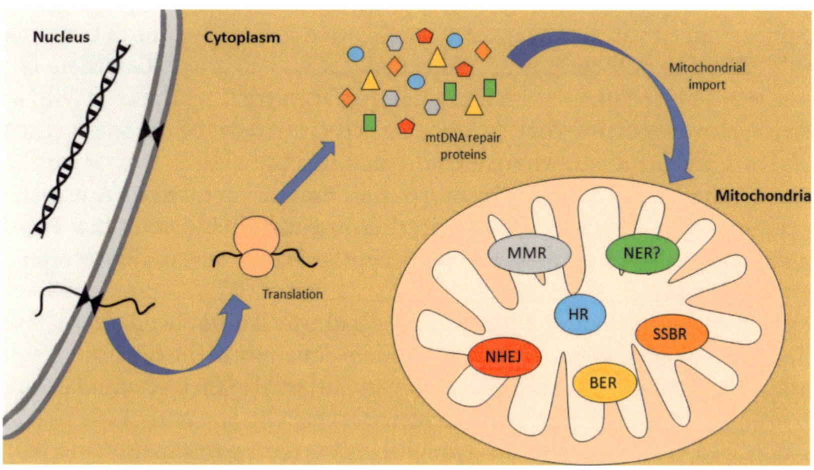

Figure 1.
Mitochondrial import and mtDNA repair pathways. The elements that participate in mitochondrial genome maintenance are nuclear encoded; therefore, mitochondria need to import these effector proteins, which are involved in different repair pathways.

synthesis is carried out by the main mitochondrial polymerase (Polγ). It was recently reported that polymerase beta (Polβ) also localizes within mitochondria, whereas similar to the nucleus, it has a relevant role in mtDNA maintenance and mitochondrial homeostasis through its participation in BER [42]. It has also been observed that FEN1, DNA2, and EXOG are involved in the removal of DNA flap generated by polymerase strand displacement synthesis [43]. Finally, the ligation activity is made by mitochondrial ligase III [44]. In conclusion, despite that BER is the most characterized pathway in mitochondria, it is still unknown whether all the nuclear elements are conserved in mitochondrial BER, or on the contrary, if this pathway have specific proteins that do not participate in nuclear version of BER, it is not well understood either which are the regulatory signals that controls the import of these elements to mitochondria.

4.2 Nucleotide excision repair (NER)

Nucleotide excision repair (NER) pathway is a complex machinery involved in recognition of lesions, adducts or structures that modifies the DNA double helix structure, having the possibility of blocking transcription, replication, and thus affecting DNA stability. One of the most important features of NER is its versatility on a wide kind of lesions since they are detected and repaired. Roughly, the process starts with damage recognition, next, the damaged strand is cleaved at both sides of the lesion to be removed later, then the missing sequence is synthesized using the complementary strand as a template, and finally the ends are ligated, thus restoring DNA sequence and integrity [45].

There is a large body of evidence reporting the absence of nucleotide excision repair activity in mitochondria. The first observation about this lack was made by Clayton et al. in 1974 [2], who reported that mitochondria were unable to remove UV-induced pyrimidine dimers. As a result, lesions that are normally repaired in nucleus by NER could persist in mitochondrial genome; this damage is not only restricted to photodimers, since NER also participates in repair of other bulky lesions and a subset of oxidative DNA damage [1]. In the nucleus, bulky lesions can also be overcome through the use of specialized translesion synthesis (TLS) polymerases; however, in mitochondria, the major polymerase (Polγ) presents a weakly thymine dimer bypass activity in vitro and at present, it is unknown whether this activity is conserved in vivo [46]. On the other hand, it was recently reported that polymerase theta (Polθ), an enzyme that acts as a translesion bypass polymerase, thus promoting the pass of replicative stalling lesions in the nucleus [47], is localized to mitochondria. Additionally, it was observed that there is an increase of Polθ localization to mitochondria after treating the cells with an oxidative agent, suggesting that the enzyme is recruited to the organelle when this kind of damage is inflicted, where it could facilitate translesion bypass synthesis. Interestingly, in POLQ KO cells, the rate of point mutation in mtDNA was significantly reduced after oxidative treatment; this observation indicates that Polθ is involved in a pathway of error-prone DNA synthesis that may facilitate replication in mitochondria [48].

Despite that the nucleotide excision repair pathway has not been clearly recognized in mitochondria, there are several proteins involved in the nuclear version of this pathway that not only localize to the organelle but also they accumulate upon oxidative damage, and when they are depleted from cells, the number of point mutation is increased, observations that strongly suggest their participation in mtDNA maintenance. Some of these proteins are: Cockayne syndrome A (CSA), Cockayne syndrome B (CSB), and Rad23A [48–50]. Therefore, further investigation is needed to completely rule out NER pathway from mitochondria, or to elucidate whether these mentioned proteins are involved in other pathways different to nucleus.

4.3 Mismatch repair (MMR)

MMR is a highly conserved pathway involved in the correction of misincorporation and slippage mistakes committed by polymerases during DNA replication, and base mismatches generated by base deamination, alkylation, and oxidation [3]. In general terms, MMR process presents the next steps: localization of the mismatch and identification of the newly synthesized strand, excision at both extremes of the mismatch lesion, DNA resynthesis, and finally ligation to complete the process [10].

The first demonstration of mammalian mitochondria capable to repair mismatch lesions was done by Mason et al. [51]. They observed that rat liver mitochondrial lysates repaired G-T and G-G mismatches; however, by using immunodetection no MSH2, a key nuclear element in MMR, was detected in these lysates, suggesting that mitochondrial MMR activity uses different elements to those of the nucleus. Posteriorly, in the pursuit of proteins responsible for the activity observed, one study reported that mismatches and small IDLs in mitochondrial genome are recognized by the Y-box binding protein 1 (YB1), which also localizes to nucleus where it exerts other functions, and its depletion in cultured cells triggers an increased mutagenesis in mtDNA. In addition, it was demonstrated that MMR activity is independent of MSH2 and that MSH3, MSH6 or MLH1 are not present in human mitochondria, at least under the experimental conditions employed [52]. In contrast to the previous observation, it was later demonstrated that MLH1 do localizes to mitochondria [53]. Through overexpression of *Mlh1* or *Msh2* in retinal endothelial cells, it was determined that MLH1 has a protective role in mtDNA after glucose-induced DNA damage, and on the other hand, this protective effect was not detected when *Msh2* was overexpressed, observation that suggests no participation in mtDNA maintenance [54], in accordance with previous studies. Additionally, it was reported that the incidence of base-mismatches in mtDNA in diabetic retina is a consequence of expression silencing of MLH1 by methylation of its promoter, activity performed by Dnmt1, enzyme overexpressed in diabetes. Thus, these observations propose that MLH1 has an important role in mtDNA maintenance, since its silencing by methylation triggers mtDNA damage [55]. In summary, MMR pathway is involved in mitochondrial genome maintenance; however, not all the elements implicated have been found. It could be possible that the proteins of mitochondrial MMR may have a different splicing or post translational versions than nuclear ones, which impairs their identification through antibody-based techniques, or in the other hand, mitochondrial MMR could not depend of all the elements involved in the canonical nuclear form, as it was seen with the participation of YB1 [52]. In any case, more research is needed to find more MMR nuclear factors within mitochondria or to discover new ones and be able to catalog the mitochondrial MMR as an original pathway.

4.4 Single strand break repair (SSBR)

The repair of SSBs in mitochondria is achieved through a BER subpathway known as base excision/SSB repair (which is also present in nucleus), since both mechanisms share common component, especially in the last steps: gap filling and DNA ligation [10, 24]. Indeed, most of the SSBs can be repaired by elements of BER pathway: APE1, PKPK, and Polγ [24]. Other members of mitochondrial SSB repair include: PARP1, a protein implicated in the detection of SSBs in the nucleus and also more recently observed in mitochondria, where not only it binds to mtDNA, but also when is depleted, this provokes accumulations of DNA damage, thus confirming its participation in mtDNA maintenance [56]. Besides, the participation of ExoG in SSB repair has been elucidated, since its depletion induces mitochondrial persisting SSBs that eventually lead to apoptosis [57].

As was previously mentioned, there are some lesions associated to SSB, like trapped topoisomerase 1 (Top1), damage that can be repaired through the action of tyrosil-DNA phosphodiesterase 1 (TDP1), an important enzyme involved in the release of covalently trapped Top1 with DNA that was first described in yeast [58]. In addition to its well characterized function, it has been observed that TDP1 also removes other types of 3′-blocking lesions, resulting oxidative damage [59–61]. A fraction of TDP1 (nuclear encoded) localizes to the mitochondria, where it has been implicated in mtDNA repair, since the treatment with chain terminator nucleotide analogs (CTNAs), which are also substrates of this enzyme, in *tdp1*$^{-/-}$ cells generate a reduction in mtDNA copy number, whereas wild type cells remain unaffected [61, 62]. These findings confirm the involvement of TDP1 in mtDNA damage repair, in this case induced by CTNAs. Another SSB-related lesion is the generation of a covalent binding of adenine monophosphate (AMP) to the 5′end of mtDNA, and this error is promoted by abortive ligase activity. The resolution of such damage relies in aprataxin (APTX) protein that is able to remove 5′-adenylate groups. APTX localizes to mitochondria, whereas its depletion generates a decline of mtDNA copy number as well as higher levels of DNA damage, observations that suggest a direct role of this enzyme in mtDNA maintenance [63]. If any of the lesions mentioned remains unrepaired, further complications may appear, since SSBs may progress to DSBs, which are more deleterious to cells.

4.5 Double strand break repair (DSBR)

In general, cells of higher eukaryotes use two main approaches to repair DSBs. The first approach is through the union of the ends in a nonhomologous dependent way, this pathway is termed nonhomologous end joining (NHEJ); it has been determined that NHEJ possesses some alternatives versions that use noncanonical elements, these sub pathways are known as alternative NHEJ (A-NHEJ); the repair with these mechanisms guarantee the restoration of DNA integrity but not sequence.

4.5.1 Nonhomologous end joining (NHEJ)

Nonhomologous end joining (NHEJ) is one of the two main pathways used by the cells to repair DNA double strand breaks. Similar to most DNA repair processes, NHEJ is based on three general steps: the action of a nuclease to resect the damaged DNA, next, the fill-in to make new DNA by a polymerase, and finally the participation of a ligase to restore the integrity of the strands. One of the most interesting features of NHEJ is the diversity of substrates that can use and convert to joined products [64]. By virtue of its template-independent operation, NHEJ is associated with insertions and deletions and hence with a lack of reliable restoration [26].

It has been observed that mammalian mitochondria do possess the capacity to bind DNA ends, activity that is retained even in Ku-deficient cells [65], additionally, the efficiency and precision of this activity apparently depend on the structure of the ends generated, since blunt-ended DNA fragment repaired are less conserved than sticky ends in comparison to the original [66]. Tadi et al. [67] demonstrated that mitochondria have a noncanonical version of NHEJ, also named alternative NHEJ (A-NHEJ). The repair by this pathway is based on microhomology and is sometimes associated with long deletions, and hence it is described as microhomology-mediated end joining (MMEJ). In this same study, using rodents and human mitochondrial extracts, a lack of end-to-end joining of nonligatable broken DNA was observed, the fact that suggests the absence of a functionally operative canonical NHEJ in mitochondria, or at least is undetected with the techniques used. In contrast, mitochondria have the ability to join oligomeric dsDNAs harboring direct repeats (microhomology) that vary in length, from 5 to 22 nt, with an efficiency that is enhanced with the increase in the length of homology. These results are supported by a previous observation, where DSBs are induced in mice through mitochondrially targeted restriction endonuclease (*Pst* I), and the repaired mtDNA presented small directed repeats (a few nucleotides) at the breakpoint [68], resolution that fits with the repair manner of MMEJ, and in addition, these repair products have also been observed in most of the mtDNA deletions associated with human diseases, which are mostly (~85%) flanked by small direct repeats [69]. Besides, it has been determined that this mitochondrial MMEJ activity involved the proteins CtIP, FEN1, Mre11, PARP1, and ligase III [67].

Therefore, MMEJ has been proposed as a central pathway in the repair of double strand breaks and maintenance of mammalian mitochondrial genome, and the use of this pathway and possibly not C-NHEJ may explain the Ku independence proteins to exert the joining activity as was previously mentioned. The possible absence of C-NHEJ activity in mitochondria is contrasting with the observation that antibodies to KU70 and KU80 cross-react with proteins from mitochondrial extracts with DNA end-binding activity [10, 70]. Furthermore, it has been determined that XRCC4, a mediator protein of nuclear DSB repair pathway, is present in mitochondrial, where it is indeed involved in mtDNA repair and possibly associated with DNA ligase III [48]. In summary, at present no NHEJ activity has been described in mitochondria; however, this organelle presents the ability to join broken DNA ends, and it appears that this action depends on the structure of the ends generated and in the presence of homology at both ends of the DSB, further, the repair by MMEJ may explain the deletions observed in the majority of mitochondrial diseases.

4.5.2 Homologous recombination (HR)

Homologous recombination (HR) is a ubiquitous process conserved from bacteriophages to humans and is one of the most important pathways used by the cells to deal with DNA double strand breaks. To achieve the restoration of molecular integrity and sequence in a free-error manner, HR needs a homologous sequence to use it as a template [26, 71].

It has been determined that HR is essential for preservation of mtDNA in plants, yeast, and fungi, and on the other hand, although there is evidence about HR in mammalian, its significance in vivo is not clear [1]. One of the first reports about mitochondrial homologous repair capabilities was made by Thyagarajan et al. [72] where they observed that mitochondrial protein extracts from mammalian cells catalyzed homologous recombination repair of plasmid DNA substrates, therefore concluding that mitochondria do possess the machinery to perform this process. Additionally, after preincubating protein extracts with anti-RecA antibodies, an inhibition of the reaction was observed, fact that suggests the participation of a mammalian mitochondrial RecA homolog. Supporting this evidence, in 2010, Sage et al. [73] demonstrated that Rad51 and the related proteins, Rad51C and XRCC3, localize to human mitochondria, and they also reported that the protein levels were enriched after stress induction and that depletion of any of these elements generates a dramatic decrease in mtDNA copy number, these results strongly suggest some type of HR participation in mitochondrial genome maintenance. Other proteins involved in HR have been observed in mitochondria, and their participation in mtDNA repair has been validated, such as Dna2 [74] and Mre11 [67, 75, 76]; moreover, it has been suggested that ExoG could supply Exo1, and therefore, many of the factors needed to perform HR process are present in mitochondria.

Recently, using biochemical assays, it was determined that HR is the major DSBR mechanism, where it has a role in maintenance of mitochondrial genome integrity, since the induction of DSBs significantly enhanced this process. Besides the participation of Rad51, Mre11 and Nibrin relevance in HR was confirmed by suppression of HR-mediated repair after immunodepletion of these proteins in the mitochondrial extracts [76]. The process of mitochondrial HR may proceed in two ways, one through intramolecular recombinant events, where a sole mtDNA molecule recombines with itself, and a second form, where a molecule can recombine with another one homologous or heterologous [77, 78]. Despite the knowledge of the elements involved in mitochondrial HR have increased over the last years, the exact mechanism about how HR is achieved in mitochondria is lacking in comparison to the nuclear models [33].

The second approach is through the use of nondamaged homologous sequences; this kind of repair restores molecular integrity as well as sequence; another pathway that uses homology sequences is single strand annealing (SSA), which needs directed repeats in both ends of the DSB, in such a way that when repairing, it restores integrity and sequence but at the expense of a variable length deletion [26].

4.6 Other pathways

As it has been previously described in this chapter, mitochondria have a repertoire of elements to deal with DNA damage, even it has been observed that mitochondria possess a mechanism to "prevent" further lesions (described below). However, if the mtDNA lesions surpass the mitochondrial repair capabilities, the cell maintains other options to avoid a higher damage, and in these circumstances, it is possible to degrade the unrepairable mtDNA, the organelle or even the whole cell [10].

4.6.1 Sanitation of the dNTP pool

The DNA is not the only molecule susceptible to chemical damage, the deoxyribonucleotide triphosphates (dNTPs) pool is also affected, being oxidative damage one of the most recurrent alterations [79]. If unrepaired, these lesions could become a source of mismatch errors during DNA synthesis [3]. To cope with this threat, mitochondria have MTH1, an specialized enzyme also found in the nucleus, which can hydrolyze oxidized dNTPs such as 8-oxo-20-deoxyguanosine triphosphate (8-oxo-dGTP), 8-oxo-20-deoxyadenosine triphosphate (8-oxo-dATP), and 2-hydroxy-20-deoxtadenosine triphosphate (2-hydroxy-ATP) to corresponding monophosphates, which cannot be assembled in the DNA by polymerases [41, 80]. In 2008, Pursell et al. [81] reported that 8-oxo-dGTP exists in some rat tissues at levels that are potentially mutagenic; therefore, these data suggest that oxidized dNTP precursors could generate mutagenesis in vivo and consequently promote mitochondrial dysfunction. In addition, it was reported that a pathogenic variant of Polγ, which is present in patients with progressive external ophthalmoplegia (PEO), increases 8-oxo-dGTP misincorporation, observation that establishes a relationship between the oxidative lesions and increased mtDNA damage observed in other models with this pathogenic version, and misincorporation of oxidized nucleotides [82]. In summary, although sanitation of premutagenic free nucleotides is not properly a DNA repair mechanism, its participation prevents the formation of mismatches in mitochondrial genome and therefore reduces the probability of mutagenesis.

4.6.2 mtDNA degradation

Compared to nuclear genome, mitochondrial genomic material has a remarkable advantage about DNA damage and repair, its redundancy, consisting of hundreds to thousands of copies per cell. Due to this characteristic, mitochondria can dispose of a considerable fraction of mtDNA, where its repair capabilities were exceeded; however, it does not compromise organelle functions, and this is not an option for nucleus, where the diploid genome cannot be submitted to degradation without affecting the cellular homeostasis [3]. It is thought that after mtDNA degradation, the lost molecules are restored by mitochondrial genome turnover, a process that was first described several decades ago [83] (**Figure 2**). There is a wide body of evidence that supports this hypothesis of mtDNA degradation after unrepairable insults; for instance, it was observed that when one of the initial steps of the BER repair pathway is inhibited by methoxyamine drug, the increase of incidence of oxidative and alkylating damage enhanced the mtDNA degradation [84]; additionally, through qPCR analysis, it has been shown a mtDNA amount decrease after persisting exposure with the oxidizing agent hydrogen peroxide [85, 86]. Furthermore, the absence of mutation fixation after persisting cell treatment with alkylating agents which have a high mutagenic potential suggests that due to the lack of mechanisms for repairing bulky lesion, the mtDNA could be selectively degraded and to prevent further modifications [87]. Nowadays, it is not completely clear how the mitochondrion degrades its damaged DNA; however, it has been recently determined that endonuclease G (EndoG) has an important role in mtDNA depletion, since it promotes cleavage of mtDNA as a response to oxidative and nitrosative stress, action that subsequently generates an upregulation of mtDNA replication as an indirect outcome [88]. This evidence is supported by the fact that endo G is the most abundant and active nuclease within mitochondria, and it has a preference on oxidized DNA harboring single-strand breaks or distorted DNA product of crosslinking agents to exert its endonuclease activity in vitro [89], also it has been reported that this nuclease preferentially cleaves 5-hydroxymethylcytosine an oxidized product of 5-methylcytosine [90]. In conclusion, despite that additional research is needed to elucidate the whole mechanisms and elements that participate in mtDNA degradation, this pathway emerges as a unique and mitochondrial specific method to maintain DNA integrity.

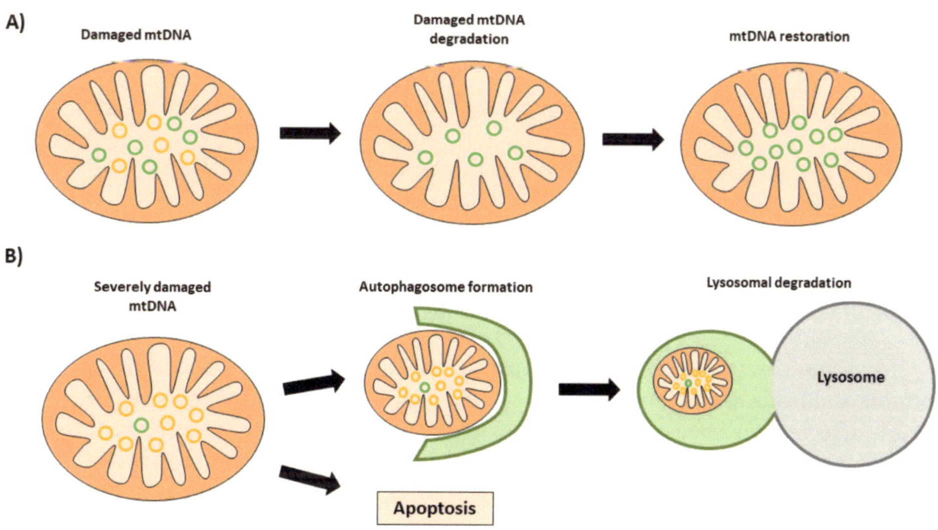

Figure 2.
mtDNA degradation and mitophagy. (A) Damaged mtDNA (yellow circles) can be selectively degraded inside mitochondria, thus keeping "healthy" mtDNA (green circles), then this can replicate to re-establish mitochondrial genome homeostasis. (B) If the mtDNA is severely damaged and the repair mechanism is surpassed, injured mitochondria can be selectively degraded by the formation of an autophagosome and subsequent fusion with lysosomes [91]. On the other hand, the mtDNA lesions can also trigger cell apoptosis.

4.6.3 Mitochondrial clearance, dynamics, and apoptosis

In general terms, autophagy is a highly conserved degradative mechanism used by cells to maintain homeostasis [92]. This is a finely regulated process that takes part in cell growth, development, and in the maintenance of an equilibrium between synthesis, degradation and recycling of cellular elements including whole organelles [11]. There is a specialized sub pathway of autophagy, which is specifically involved in degradation of damaged and dysfunctional mitochondria, and this procedure is known as mitophagy or mitochondrial clearance. Although mitophagy can emerge as a programmed cellular event, like the one that is observed during erythroblast maturation in order to generate mature red blood cells lacking mitochondria [11], it has been proposed that mitophagy could participate in the elimination of organelles harboring low levels of DNA damage stress. On the other hand, when the DNA lesions are too many to handle with mtDNA repair mechanism or by mitochondrial clearance, the cellular response could trigger apoptosis [93], therefore the choice of which pathway must be used depends on the degree of DNA damage (**Figure 2**). In accordance with the previous mechanism, Suen et al. [94] observed selectively degradation by mitophagy of organelles harboring deleterious COXI mutations after overexpressing the protein Parkin, which translocated to affected mitochondria and induced autophagic elimination, thus this selection enriched cells for nonmutated mtDNA and restoring cytochrome c oxidase activity [95].

It appears that mitophagy is closely associated with mitochondrial dynamics processes: fission and fusion [96]. Fusion is the joining of two organelles to form one, this mechanism allows mitochondria to distribute mtDNA and to replenish it when is damaged, therefore safeguarding mtDNA integrity and protecting it from mutations [97]. On the other hand, fission is the division of a single organelle to create two, this process is very important to cellular viability, it contributes to symmetrical distribution of mitochondria during mitosis, and promotes the removal of lesioned organelles by partitioning the damaged elements (like mtDNA) to a derived mitochondria that can fuse to a healthy one with the intention of recovering functionality or to be degraded by mitophagy. Therefore, mitochondrial removal by mitophagy is preceded by mitochondrial fission, which is capable of dividing the organelle into smaller pieces to be degraded easily [98]. When mitochondrial clearance, fusion, or fission are dysfunctional, the cells could be severely affected, since it has been observed that in these situations, an increase in mtDNA instability and generation of neurodegenerative, cardiovascular, and age-related diseases were obtained [99].

5. mtDNA repair, diseases, and aging

Mitochondrial diseases are a heterogeneous group of illnesses affecting multiple organs and leading to eventual degeneration and in some cases premature death. These affectations have origin in mutations on mtDNA, which are generated by errors during DNA replication, exogenous sources, and ROS; however, mitochondrial dysfunction may also arise from mutations in nuclear genes which encode proteins with mitochondrial function, involved in several processes like biogenesis, transcription, replication, mitochondrial dynamics, and mtDNA repair, among others. Of interest, neurodegeneration is a prevalent trait in mitochondrial diseases, maybe because the brain needs a higher demand of energy in comparison with other tissues [11]. On the other hand, there is a large body of evidence that underscores the relationship between mitochondrial disorders and aging; however, there is still controversy about whether these mutations in the mtDNA are the product of age-related disorders or they are themselves the cause [100].

About the genes involved in mtDNA maintenance, it has been well established that failure of the mtDNA repair pathways may promote diseases and age-related disorders in humans [11, 28]; in addition to mutations, the reduction of mtDNA copy number has also been associated with neurodegeneration, aging, diabetes, and cancer [101]. For example, it has been observed that the lack of proofreading activity of Polγ in mice generates multi-systemic disease and phenotypes resembling to premature aging [102], furthermore, over 200 mutations in POLG have been associated with mitochondrial diseases, these POLG-related disorders can be classified into five main phenotypes of neurodegeneration: Alpers-Huttenlocher syndrome (AHS), childhood myocerebrohepatopathy spectrum (MCHS), myoclonic epilepsy myopathy sensory ataxia (MEMSA), ataxia neuropathy spectrum (ANS), and PEO [28], besides, mutations in Twinkle helicase often causes infantile onset spinocerebellar ataxia (IOSCA), which usually appears in early childhood [103]. Other mtDNA repair elements, such as APTX and TDP1, implicated in SSBR, are related with the generation of ataxia with ocular motor apraxia (AOA1) when are mutated [10, 104]. Also, defects in the proteins CSA and CSB, implicated in the possibly mitochondrial DNA repair transcription coupled-NER pathway, are related with the development of progressive cerebellar pathology [105]. Furthermore, alterations in fusion, fission, or mitophagy processes due to mutations in the proteins involved generate mtDNA instability, which in turn may induce neurodegenerative, cardiovascular, and age-related diseases [99], such is the case of MFN2, which is implicated in mitochondria fusion, and its alteration lead to organelle fragmentation and causes axonal Charcot-Marie-Tooth disease (CMT2A) [106], also mutations in OPA1, lead to optic atrophy, affectation that can be accompanied with hearing loss and ophthalmoplegia [107]. Additionally, mutations in DNA2 and mitochondrial genome maintenance exonuclease 1 (MGME1) nucleases are implicated in ophthalmoplegia, myopathy, and mtDNA depletion [108, 109]. In conclusion, the importance of mtDNA maintenance lies in the observation that when the repair elements are affected, or the mechanisms exceeded, the risk of disease development increases, thus the understanding of these alterations may shed light for clinical targets to prevent diseases or treat them.

6. Concluding remarks

After decades of study, it has been concluded that like nucleus, mitochondria do possess specific mechanisms to maintain integrity of its small and polyploid genome, and although nowadays, the complete repertoire of elements participating in mtDNA repair has not been identified, it appears that these pathways resemble those of nucleus but operating with fewer elements. In addition, mitochondria have evolved organelle specific mechanisms which work as a backup when the repair pathways are surpassed by the amount of damage and that would be impossible to carry out in nuclear genome. In conclusion, the repair of mitochondrial genome is a field in continuous growth that promises new discoveries in the years to come.

Author details

Ulises Omar García-Lepe and Rosa Ma Bermúdez-Cruz*
Center for Research and Advanced Studios of National Polytechnic Institute, Mexico City, Mexico

*Address all correspondence to: roberm@cinvestav.mx

References

[1] Van Houten B, Hunter SE, Meyer JN. Mitochondrial DNA damage induced autophagy, cell death, and disease. Frontiers in Bioscience. 2016;**21**:42-54

[2] Clayton DA, Doda JN, Friedberg EC. The absence of a pyrimidine dimer repair mechanism in mammalian mitochondria. Proceedings of the National Academy of Sciences of the United States of America. 1974;**71**(7):2777-2781

[3] Alexeyev M, Shokolenko I, Wilson G, LeDoux S. The maintenance of mitochondrial DNA integrity—Critical analysis and update. Cold Spring Harbor Perspectives in Biology. 2013;**5**(5):a012641

[4] Falk MJ, Sondheimer N. Mitochondrial genetic diseases. Current Opinion in Pediatrics. 2010;**22**(6):711-716

[5] MITOMAP: A Human Mitochondrial Genome Database [Internet]. 2018. Available from: www.mitomap.org/org/MITOMAP

[6] DiMauro S, Schon EA. Mitochondrial respiratory-chain diseases. The New England Journal of Medicine. 2003;**348**(26):2656-2668

[7] Anderson S, Bankier AT, Barrell BG, de Bruijn MH, Coulson AR, Drouin J, et al. Sequence and organization of the human mitochondrial genome. Nature. 1981;**290**(5806):457-465

[8] Holt IJ, Reyes A. Human mitochondrial DNA replication. Cold Spring Harbor Perspectives in Biology. 2012;**4**(12):a012971

[9] Ojala D, Montoya J, Attardi G. tRNA punctuation model of RNA processing in human mitochondria. Nature. 1981;**290**(5806):470-474

[10] Kazak L, Reyes A, Holt IJ. Minimizing the damage: Repair pathways keep mitochondrial DNA intact. Nature Reviews Molecular Cell Biology. 2012;**13**(10):659-671

[11] Scheibye-Knudsen M, Fang EF, Croteau DL, Wilson DM 3rd, Bohr VA. Protecting the mitochondrial powerhouse. Trends in Cell Biology. 2015;**25**(3):158-170

[12] Vasileiou PVS, Mourouzis I, Pantos C. Principal aspects regarding the maintenance of mammalian mitochondrial genome integrity. International Journal of Molecular Sciences. 2017;**18**(8):1821

[13] Chen XJ, Butow RA. The organization and inheritance of the mitochondrial genome. Nature Reviews Genetics. 2005;**6**(11):815-825

[14] Marin-Garcia J. Mitochondrial DNA repair: A novel therapeutic target for heart failure. Heart Failure Reviews. 2016;**21**(5):475-487

[15] De Bont R, van Larebeke N. Endogenous DNA damage in humans: A review of quantitative data. Mutagenesis. 2004;**19**(3):169-185

[16] Rydberg B, Lindahl T. Nonenzymatic methylation of DNA by the intracellular methyl group donor S-adenosyl-L-methionine is a potentially mutagenic reaction. The EMBO Journal. 1982;**1**(2):211-216

[17] Tudek B, Boiteux S, Laval J. Biological properties of imidazole ring-opened N7-methylguanine in M13mp18 phage DNA. Nucleic Acids Research. 1992;**20**(12):3079-3084

[18] Horne DW, Holloway RS, Wagner C. Transport of S-adenosylmethionine in isolated rat liver mitochondria.

Archives of Biochemistry and Biophysics. 1997;**343**(2):201-206

[19] Lindahl T. DNA repair enzymes. Annual Review of Biochemistry. 1982;**51**:61-87

[20] Lindahl T. Instability and decay of the primary structure of DNA. Nature. 1993;**362**(6422):709-715

[21] Jackson AL, Loeb LA. The contribution of endogenous sources of DNA damage to the multiple mutations in cancer. Mutation Research. 2001;**477**(1-2):7-21

[22] Thomas RD, Roy D. Stilbene estrogen produces higher levels of mitochondrial DNA adducts than nuclear DNA adducts in the target organ of cancer (liver) of male Sprague Dawley rats. Oncology Reports. 2001;**8**(5):1035-1038

[23] Hudson JJ, Chiang SC, Wells OS, Rookyard C, El-Khamisy SF. SUMO modification of the neuroprotective protein TDP1 facilitates chromosomal single-strand break repair. Nature Communications. 2012;**3**:733

[24] Sykora P, Wilson DM 3rd, Bohr VA. Repair of persistent strand breaks in the mitochondrial genome. Mechanisms of Ageing and Development. 2012;**133**(4):169-175

[25] Ahel I, Rass U, El-Khamisy SF, Katyal S, Clements PM, McKinnon PJ, et al. The neurodegenerative disease protein aprataxin resolves abortive DNA ligation intermediates. Nature. 2006;**443**(7112):713-716

[26] Mladenov E, Magin S, Soni A, Iliakis G. DNA double-strand-break repair in higher eukaryotes and its role in genomic instability and cancer: Cell cycle and proliferation-dependent regulation. Seminars in Cancer Biology. 2016;**37-38**:51-64

[27] Meagher M, Lightowlers RN. The role of TDP1 and APTX in mitochondrial DNA repair. Biochimie. 2014;**100**:121-124

[28] Copeland WC, Longley MJ. Mitochondrial genome maintenance in health and disease. DNA Repair. 2014;**19**:190-198

[29] Andreyev AY, Kushnareva YE, Starkov AA. Mitochondrial metabolism of reactive oxygen species. Biochemistry Biokhimiia. 2005;**70**(2):200-214

[30] Muftuoglu M, Mori MP, de Souza-Pinto NC. Formation and repair of oxidative damage in the mitochondrial DNA. Mitochondrion. 2014;**17**:164-181

[31] Malinski T. Nitric oxide and nitroxidative stress in Alzheimer's disease. Journal of Alzheimer's Disease. 2007;**11**(2):207-218

[32] Mangialasche F, Polidori MC, Monastero R, Ercolani S, Camarda C, Cecchetti R, et al. Biomarkers of oxidative and nitrosative damage in Alzheimer's disease and mild cognitive impairment. Ageing Research Reviews. 2009;**8**(4):285-305

[33] Stein A, Sia EA. Mitochondrial DNA repair and damage tolerance. Frontiers in Bioscience. 2017;**22**:920-943

[34] LeDoux SP, Wilson GL, Beecham EJ, Stevnsner T, Wassermann K, Bohr VA. Repair of mitochondrial DNA after various types of DNA damage in Chinese hamster ovary cells. Carcinogenesis. 1992;**13**(11):1967-1973

[35] Prakash A, Doublie S. Base excision repair in the mitochondria. Journal of Cellular Biochemistry. 2015;**116**(8):1490-1499

[36] Krokan HE, Bjoras M. Base excision repair. Cold Spring Harbor Perspectives in Biology. 2013;5(4):a012583

[37] Lindahl T. An N-glycosidase from *Escherichia coli* that releases free uracil from DNA containing deaminated cytosine residues. Proceedings of the National Academy of Sciences of the United States of America. 1974;**71**(9):3649-3653

[38] Mandal SM, Hegde ML, Chatterjee A, Hegde PM, Szczesny B, Banerjee D, et al. Role of human DNA glycosylase Nei-like 2 (NEIL2) and single strand break repair protein polynucleotide kinase 3′-phosphatase in maintenance of mitochondrial genome. The Journal of Biological Chemistry. 2012;**287**(4):2819-2829

[39] Hu J, de Souza-Pinto NC, Haraguchi K, Hogue BA, Jaruga P, Greenberg MM, et al. Repair of formamidopyrimidines in DNA involves different glycosylases: Role of the OGG1, NTH1, and NEIL1 enzymes. The Journal of Biological Chemistry. 2005;**280**(49):40544-40551

[40] Slupphaug G, Markussen FH, Olsen LC, Aasland R, Aarsaether N, Bakke O, et al. Nuclear and mitochondrial forms of human uracil-DNA glycosylase are encoded by the same gene. Nucleic Acids Research. 1993;**21**(11):2579-2584

[41] Nakabeppu Y. Regulation of intracellular localization of human MTH1, OGG1, and MYH proteins for repair of oxidative DNA damage. Progress in Nucleic Acid Research and Molecular Biology. 2001;**68**:75-94

[42] Sykora P, Kanno S, Akbari M, Kulikowicz T, Baptiste BA, Leandro GS, et al. DNA polymerase beta participates in mitochondrial DNA repair. Molecular and Cellular Biology. 2017;**37**(16):e00237-17

[43] Saki M, Prakash A. DNA damage related crosstalk between the nucleus and mitochondria. Free Radical Biology & Medicine. 2017;**107**:216-227

[44] Gao Y, Katyal S, Lee Y, Zhao J, Rehg JE, Russell HR, et al. DNA ligase III is critical for mtDNA integrity but not Xrcc1-mediated nuclear DNA repair. Nature. 2011;**471**(7337):240-244

[45] Spivak G. Nucleotide excision repair in humans. DNA Repair. 2015;**36**:13-18

[46] Kasiviswanathan R, Gustafson MA, Copeland WC, Meyer JN. Human mitochondrial DNA polymerase gamma exhibits potential for bypass and mutagenesis at UV-induced cyclobutane thymine dimers. The Journal of Biological Chemistry. 2012;**287**(12):9222-9229

[47] Yoon JH, Roy Choudhury J, Park J, Prakash S, Prakash L. A role for DNA polymerase theta in promoting replication through oxidative DNA lesion, thymine glycol, in human cells. The Journal of Biological Chemistry. 2014;**289**(19):13177-13185

[48] Wisnovsky S, Jean SR, Kelley SO. Mitochondrial DNA repair and replication proteins revealed by targeted chemical probes. Nature Chemical Biology. 2016;**12**(7):567-573

[49] Kamenisch Y, Fousteri M, Knoch J, von Thaler AK, Fehrenbacher B, Kato H, et al. Proteins of nucleotide and base excision repair pathways interact in mitochondria to protect from loss of subcutaneous fat, a hallmark of aging. The Journal of Experimental Medicine. 2010;**207**(2):379-390

[50] Pohjoismaki JL, Boettger T, Liu Z, Goffart S, Szibor M, Braun T. Oxidative stress during mitochondrial biogenesis compromises mtDNA integrity in growing hearts and induces a global DNA repair response. Nucleic Acids Research. 2012;**40**(14):6595-6607

[51] Mason PA, Matheson EC, Hall AG, Lightowlers RN. Mismatch repair activity in mammalian mitochondria. Nucleic Acids Research. 2003;**31**(3):1052-1058

[52] de Souza-Pinto NC, Mason PA, Hashiguchi K, Weissman L, Tian J, Guay D, et al. Novel DNA mismatch-repair activity involving YB-1 in human mitochondria. DNA Repair. 2009;**8**(6):704-719

[53] Martin SA, McCabe N, Mullarkey M, Cummins R, Burgess DJ, Nakabeppu Y, et al. DNA polymerases as potential therapeutic targets for cancers deficient in the DNA mismatch repair proteins MSH2 or MLH1. Cancer Cell. 2010;**17**(3):235-248

[54] Mishra M, Kowluru RA. Retinal mitochondrial DNA mismatch repair in the development of diabetic retinopathy, and its continued progression after termination of hyperglycemia. Investigative Ophthalmology & Visual Science. 2014;**55**(10):6960-6967

[55] Mohammad. Mitochondrial DNA damage in diabetic retinopathy: Role of epigenetics. Free Radical Biology and Medicine. 2018;**128**:S139-S140

[56] Rossi MN, Carbone M, Mostocotto C, Mancone C, Tripodi M, Maione R, et al. Mitochondrial localization of PARP-1 requires interaction with mitofilin and is involved in the maintenance of mitochondrial DNA integrity. The Journal of Biological Chemistry. 2009;**284**(46):31616-31624

[57] Tann AW, Boldogh I, Meiss G, Qian W, Van Houten B, Mitra S, et al. Apoptosis induced by persistent single-strand breaks in mitochondrial genome: Critical role of EXOG (5'-EXO/endonuclease) in their repair. The Journal of Biological Chemistry. 2011;**286**(37):31975-31983

[58] Pouliot JJ, Yao KC, Robertson CA, Nash HA. Yeast gene for a Tyr-DNA phosphodiesterase that repairs topoisomerase I complexes. Science. 1999;**286**(5439):552-555

[59] Zhou T, Lee JW, Tatavarthi H, Lupski JR, Valerie K, Povirk LF. Deficiency in 3′-phosphoglycolate processing in human cells with a hereditary mutation in tyrosyl-DNA phosphodiesterase (TDP1). Nucleic Acids Research. 2005;**33**(1):28s9-28s2897

[60] Murai J, Huang SY, Das BB, Dexheimer TS, Takeda S, Pommier Y. Tyrosyl-DNA phosphodiesterase 1 (TDP1) repairs DNA damage induced by topoisomerases I and II and base alkylation in vertebrate cells. The Journal of Biological Chemistry. 2012;**287**(16):12848-12857

[61] Huang SY, Murai J, Dalla Rosa I, Dexheimer TS, Naumova A, Gmeiner WH, et al. TDP1 repairs nuclear and mitochondrial DNA damage induced by chain-terminating anticancer and antiviral nucleoside analogs. Nucleic Acids Research. 2013;**41**(16):7793-7803

[62] Das BB, Dexheimer TS, Maddali K, Pommier Y. Role of tyrosyl-DNA phosphodiesterase (TDP1) in mitochondria. Proceedings of the National Academy of Sciences of the United States of America. 2010;**107**(46):19790-19795

[63] Sykora P, Croteau DL, Bohr VA, Wilson DM 3rd. Aprataxin localizes to mitochondria and preserves mitochondrial function. Proceedings of the National Academy of Sciences of the United States of America. 2011;**108**(18):7437-7442

[64] Lieber MR. The mechanism of double-strand DNA break repair by the nonhomologous DNA end-joining pathway. Annual Review of Biochemistry. 2010;**79**:181-211

[65] Coffey G, Lakshmipathy U, Campbell C. Mammalian mitochondrial extracts possess DNA end-binding activity. Nucleic Acids Research. 1999;**27**(16):3348-3354

[66] Lakshmipathy U, Campbell C. Double strand break rejoining by mammalian mitochondrial extracts. Nucleic Acids Research. 1999;**27**(4):1198-1204

[67] Tadi SK, Sebastian R, Dahal S, Babu RK, Choudhary B, Raghavan SC. Microhomology-mediated end joining is the principal mediator of double-strand break repair during mitochondrial DNA lesions. Molecular Biology of the Cell. 2016;**27**(2):223-235

[68] Srivastava S, Moraes CT. Double-strand breaks of mouse muscle mtDNA promote large deletions similar to multiple mtDNA deletions in humans. Human Molecular Genetics. 2005;**14**(7):893-902

[69] Krishnan KJ, Reeve AK, Samuels DC, Chinnery PF, Blackwood JK, Taylor RW, et al. What causes mitochondrial DNA deletions in human cells? Nature Genetics. 2008;**40**(3):275-279

[70] Coffey G, Campbell C. An alternate form of Ku80 is required for DNA end-binding activity in mammalian mitochondria. Nucleic Acids Research. 2000;**28**(19):3793-3800

[71] Chen XJ. Mechanism of homologous recombination and implications for aging-related deletions in mitochondrial DNA. Microbiology and Molecular Biology Reviews. 2013;**77**(3):476-496

[72] Thyagarajan B, Padua RA, Campbell C. Mammalian mitochondria possess homologous DNA recombination activity. The Journal of Biological Chemistry. 1996;**271**(44):27536-27543

[73] Sage JM, Gildemeister OS, Knight KL. Discovery of a novel function for human Rad51: Maintenance of the mitochondrial genome. The Journal of Biological Chemistry. 2010;**285**(25):18984-18990

[74] Duxin JP, Dao B, Martinsson P, Rajala N, Guittat L, Campbell JL, et al. Human Dna2 is a nuclear and mitochondrial DNA maintenance protein. Molecular and Cellular Biology. 2009;**29**(15):4274-4282

[75] Dmitrieva NI, Malide D, Burg MB. Mre11 is expressed in mammalian mitochondria where it binds to mitochondrial DNA. American Journal of Physiology Regulatory, Integrative and Comparative Physiology. 2011;**301**(3):R632-R640

[76] Dahal S, Dubey S, Raghavan SC. Homologous recombination-mediated repair of DNA double-strand breaks operates in mammalian mitochondria. Cellular and Molecular Life Sciences. 2018;**75**(9):1641-1655

[77] D'Aurelio M, Gajewski CD, Lin MT, Mauck WM, Shao LZ, Lenaz G, et al. Heterologous mitochondrial DNA recombination in human cells. Human Molecular Genetics. 2004;**13**(24):3171-3179

[78] Bacman SR, Williams SL, Moraes CT. Intra- and inter-molecular recombination of mitochondrial DNA after in vivo induction of multiple double-strand breaks. Nucleic Acids Research. 2009;**37**(13):4218-4226

[79] Liu P, Demple B. DNA repair in mammalian mitochondria: Much more than we thought? Environmental and Molecular Mutagenesis. 2010;**51**(5):417-426

[80] Kang D, Nishida J, Iyama A, Nakabeppu Y, Furuichi M, Fujiwara T, et al. Intracellular localization of 8-oxo-dGTPase in human cells, with special reference to the role of the enzyme in mitochondria. The Journal of Biological Chemistry. 1995;**270**(24):14659-14665

[81] Pursell ZF, McDonald JT, Mathews CK, Kunkel TA. Trace amounts of 8-oxo-dGTP in mitochondrial dNTP

pools reduce DNA polymerase gamma replication fidelity. Nucleic Acids Research. 2008;**36**(7):2174-2181

[82] Graziewicz MA, Bienstock RJ, Copeland WC. The DNA polymerase gamma Y955C disease variant associated with PEO and parkinsonism mediates the incorporation and translesion synthesis opposite 7,8-dihydro-8-oxo-2′-deoxyguanosine. Human Molecular Genetics. 2007;**16**(22):2729-2739

[83] Gross NJ, Getz GS, Rabinowitz M. Apparent turnover of mitochondrial deoxyribonucleic acid and mitochondrial phospholipids in the tissues of the rat. The Journal of Biological Chemistry. 1969;**244**(6):1552-1562

[84] Shokolenko I, Venediktova N, Bochkareva A, Wilson GL, Alexeyev MF. Oxidative stress induces degradation of mitochondrial DNA. Nucleic Acids Research. 2009;**37**(8):2539-2548

[85] Furda AM, Marrangoni AM, Lokshin A, Van Houten B. Oxidants and not alkylating agents induce rapid mtDNA loss and mitochondrial dysfunction. DNA Repair. 2012;**11**(8):684-692

[86] Rothfuss O, Gasser T, Patenge N. Analysis of differential DNA damage in the mitochondrial genome employing a semi-long run real-time PCR approach. Nucleic Acids Research. 2010;**38**(4):e24

[87] Mita S, Monnat RJ Jr, Loeb LA. Resistance of HeLa cell mitochondrial DNA to mutagenesis by chemical carcinogens. Cancer Research. 1988;**48**(16):4578-4583

[88] Wiehe RS, Gole B, Chatre L, Walther P, Calzia E, Ricchetti M, et al. Endonuclease G promotess mitochondrial genome cleavage and replication. Oncotarget. 2018;**9**(26):18309-18326

[89] Ikeda S, Ozaki K. Action of mitochondrial endonuclease G on DNA damaged by L-ascorbic acid, peplomycin, and cis-diamminedichloroplatinum (II). Biochemical and Biophysical Research Communications. 1997;**235**(2):291-294

[90] Robertson AB, Robertson J, Fusser M, Klungland A. Endonuclease G preferentially cleaves 5-hydroxymethylcytosine-modified DNA creating a substrate for recombination. Nucleic Acids Research. 2014;**42**(21):13280-13293

[91] Youle RJ, Narendra DP. Mechanisms of mitophagy. Nature reviews Molecular Cell Biology. 2011;**12**(1):9-14

[92] Rabinowitz JD, White E. Autophagy and metabolism. Science. 2010;**330**(6009):1344-1348

[93] Fang EF, Scheibye-Knudsen M, Chua KF, Mattson MP, Croteau DL, Bohr VA. Nuclear DNA damage signalling to mitochondria in ageing. Nature Reviews Molecular Cell Biology. 2016;**17**(5):308-321

[94] Suen DF, Narendra DP, Tanaka A, Manfredi G, Youle RJ. Parkin overexpression selects against a deleterious mtDNA mutation in heteroplasmic cybrid cells. Proceedings of the National Academy of Sciences of the United States of America. 2010;**107**(26):11835-11840

[95] Fan W, Waymire KG, Narula N, Li P, Rocher C, Coskun PE, et al. A mouse model of mitochondrial disease reveals germline selection against severe mtDNA mutations. Science. 2008;**319**(5865):958-962

[96] Youle RJ, van der Bliek AM. Mitochondrial fission,

fusion, and stress. Science. 2012;**337**(6098):1062-1065

[97] Chen H, Vermulst M, Wang YE, Chomyn A, Prolla TA, McCaffery JM, et al. Mitochondrial fusion is required for mtDNA stability in skeletal muscle and tolerance of mtDNA mutations. Cell. 2010;**141**(2):280-289

[98] Westermann B. Mitochondrial fusion and fission in cell life and death. Nature Reviews Molecular Cell Biology. 2010;**11**(12):872-884

[99] Liesa M, Palacin M, Zorzano A. Mitochondrial dynamics in mammalian health and disease. Physiological Reviews. 2009;**89**(3):799-845

[100] Kauppila TES, Kauppila JHK, Larsson NG. Mammalian mitochondria and aging: An update. Cell Metabolism. 2017;**25**(1):57-71

[101] Clay Montier LL, Deng JJ, Bai Y. Number matters: Control of mammalian mitochondrial DNA copy number. Journal of Genetics and Genomics = Yi chuan xue bao. 2009;**36**(3):125-131

[102] Trifunovic A, Wredenberg A, Falkenberg M, Spelbrink JN, Rovio AT, Bruder CE, et al. Premature ageing in mice expressing defective mitochondrial DNA polymerase. Nature. 2004;**429**(6990):417-423

[103] Palin EJ, Paetau A, Suomalainen A. Mesencephalic complex I deficiency does not correlate with parkinsonism in mitochondrial DNA maintenance disorders. Brain. 2013;**136**(Pt 8): 2379-2392

[104] Katyal S, El-Khamisy SF, Russell HR, Li Y, Ju L, Caldecott KW, et al. TDP1 facilitates chromosomal single-strand break repair in neurons and is neuroprotective in vivo. Embo Journal. 2007;**26**(22):4720-4731

[105] Scheibye-Knudsen M, Croteau DL, Bohr VA. Mitochondrial deficiency in Cockayne syndrome. Mechanisms of Ageing and Development. 2013;**134**(5-6):275-283

[106] Rouzier C, Bannwarth S, Chaussenot A, Chevrollier A, Verschueren A, Bonello-Palot N, et al. The MFN2 gene is responsible for mitochondrial DNA instability and optic atrophy 'plus' phenotype. Brain. 2012;**135**:23-34

[107] Yu-Wai-Man P, Griffiths PG, Gorman GS, Lourenco CM, Wright AF, Auer-Grumbach M, et al. Multi-system neurological disease is common in patients with OPA1 mutations. Brain. 2010;**133**(Pt 3):771-786

[108] Kornblum C, Nicholls TJ, Haack TB, Scholer S, Peeva V, Danhauser K, et al. Loss-of-function mutations in MGME1 impair mtDNA replication and cause multisystemic mitochondrial disease. Nature Genetics. 2013;**45**(2):214-219

[109] Ronchi D, Di Fonzo A, Lin W, Bordoni A, Liu C, Fassone E, et al. Mutations in DNA2 link progressive myopathy to mitochondrial DNA instability. American Journal of Human Genetics. 2013;**92**(2):293-300

Chapter 4

Cellular Responses to Aflatoxin-Associated DNA Adducts

Michael Fasullo

Abstract

Aflatoxin B1 (AFB1) is the most potent known hepatocarcinogen. The signature p53 mutation (p53 249^{ser}) that is found in AFB1-associated liver cancer suggests that AFB1 is a potent genotoxin. AFB1 is not genotoxic *per se* but is metabolically activated by cytochrome P450 enzymes that convert the promutagen into a highly reactive epoxide, which primarily reacts with the N^7 group of guanine, forming 8,9-dihydro-8-(N^7-guanyl)-9-hydroxyaflatoxin B1 (AFB1-N^7-dG). While this primary adduct is unstable, the subsequent trans-8,9-dihydro-8-(2,6-diamino-4-oxo-3,4-dihydropyrimid-5-yl-formamido)-9-hydroxy aflatoxin B1 (AFB1-Fapy)-derived adducts are stable and are mutagenic. Studies have revealed that nucleotide excision repair (NER), base excision repair (BER), recombinational repair, and DNA replication bypass are all involved in conferring AFB1 resistance. To minimize the genotoxicity of AFB1, pathways function to detoxify the metabolically active intermediate, excise resulting DNA adducts, bypass unrepaired adducts, and repair secondary DNA breaks. How these repair pathways functionally cooperate to minimize AFB1-associated genetic instability phenotypes is not well understood. Insights can be gained from epidemiological research and model organisms. Gene profiling and next-generation sequencing are facilitating how pathways and tissue-specific differences are induced. This review will encompass studies concerning human genetic susceptibility to AFB1 and pathways that repair and tolerate AFB1-associated DNA damage.

Keywords: aflatoxin B1, liver carcinogenesis, DNA damage tolerance, oncogenes, p53

1. Introduction

The mycotoxin aflatoxin B1 (AFB1) is the most potent known liver carcinogen [1] and is also a lung [2] and esophageal carcinogen [3]. The International Agency for Research and Cancer (IARC) has classified AFB1 as a Group 1 human carcinogen [1]. AFB1 was discovered as the causative chemical agent in Turkey X disease, so named after a 1960 occurrence where 100,000 turkeys in Great Britain died after feeding on contaminated peanut meal imported from Brazil [4]. Its notoriety is underscored by its persistence in grain supplies, ground nuts and animal feed, which must be continually monitored [5]. Produced by aspergillus parasiticus and aspergillus flavis, the mycotoxin is a particular problem in subtropical areas of China, and in tropical areas of Southeast Asia and Africa [6, 7]. In temperate climates, such as in North America, high levels of AFB1 contamination have been found in corn and nuts, such as almonds and pistachios [8]. To minimize health risks in humans, the Food and Drug Administration (FDA) mandates that the human food supply contain no more than 20 ppb AFB1 [5]. While human food supply is relatively protected in developed countries, outbreaks of acute mycotoxin contamination have been noted in third world countries and among animals, as recently as 2006 [5]. Although the incidence of acute aflatoxicosis is rare, it is estimated that a large fraction of the population in the developing world are chronically exposed to AFB1 and thus at a higher risk for aflatoxin-associated cancer, especially liver cancer [6].

Liver cancer ranks third in all worldwide cancer mortalities [9–11] and ninth in cancer mortalities in the United States [12, 13]. 4–28% of cancer cases are related to AFB1 exposure [2]. Most liver cancer is characterized as hepatocellular carcinoma (HCC). HCC is highest where there is both a high rate of hepatitis B (HBV) [14, 15] and C virus (HCV) infection [15–17] and high levels of AFB1 contamination in the human food supply, especially in areas of Southeast Asia, China and Africa [6]. Interestingly, the incidence for liver cancer is higher in men than women, regardless of whether the cancer is associated with AFB1 exposure [18]. Because diagnosis is often late and there is no effective treatment for late-stage cancer, the five year survival rate is low in both men and women [12, 13]. The carcinogenic potency of AFB1 is correlated with AFB1 being a strong genotoxin, the signature p53 mutation, p53 249^{ser} [19, 20], is found in 40–60% of all liver cancer derived from patients in heavily contaminated areas [2]. Animal studies have further strengthened the idea that AFB1 carcinogenicity is associated with its genotoxicity; AFB1-associated DNA adduct levels are directly proportional to the number of the animals stricken with liver cancer [21, 22].

Observations that HCC incidence is correlated to AFB1 exposure continues to motivate biomedical researchers to study the repair and toleration of AFB1-associated DNA adducts, the cellular response to these DNA adducts, and associated factors that may enhance or mitigate the high mutagenicity of the DNA adducts in humans. This review will address (1) associated risk factors that enhance or synergize with AFB-associated DNA adducts that increase liver cancer incidence, (2) genetic instability phenotypes associated with AFB1-associated DNA adducts, and (3) repair mechanisms that have been elucidated in model organisms and conserved in humans, (4) cellular responses that enhance repair mechanisms, and (5) future directions in understanding the contributions of genes in AFB1-associated DNA repair. In particular, novel research that addresses epigenetic factors that can alter the repair of AFB1-associated genotoxic damage will be addressed.

2. Progression of HCC

Liver cancer progression is slow and the median age of onset is 60–65 years [11]; populations in areas that are at high risk for environmental and life-style factors are exceptions. For example, the incidence of liver cancer in the Qidong province of China peaks at 45 years [9, 11]. HCC generally develops as a consequence of liver injury, whether caused by chronic hepatitis or cirrhosis, which leads to chronic inflammation and deposition of connective tissue. Chronic hepatitis leads to upregulation of mitogenic pathways, partially through epigenetic mechanisms [23]. Monoclonal populations of dysplastic hepatocytes may exhibit telomere erosion and re-expression of telomerase to maintain viability. Eventual malignant cells accumulate irreversible genetic alterations [23]. As the transformed phenotype advances, the rate in the accumulation of genetic alterations increases [24]. The exact threshold for the number of mutations or alterations present in liver cancer has not been established. Thus, the progression of liver cancer is associated and is accelerated with the accumulation of genetic mutations and altered gene expression patterns.

2.1 Mutations that contribute to liver cancer

Understanding which HCC-associated genetic changes are associated with AFB1 exposure requires a comparison of the genomic alterations that occur in sporadic HCC or HCC associated with other causes. For sporadic HCC, similar to solid tumors, there is both a multiplicity and heterogeneity in genetic alterations in HCC [23–25]. In general, these genetic alterations can be grouped into those that result in loss of function and those that result in gain of function. Genetic alterations that result in loss of function include dominant negative mutations and recessive mutations, which are expressed after loss of heterozygosity (LOH).

Among sporadic tumors, both loss of heterozygosity (LOH) and mutations have been found in HCC tumors. Among 363 patients, The Cancer Genome Atlas Research Network [25], report that the most heavily mutated gene was TP53 (31%), encoding p53, followed by WNT pathway member CTNNB1 (27%), encoding β-catenin, and AXIN (8%), encoding a WNT signaling scaffolding protein, and chromatin remodeling genes (12%) [25]. In greater than 10% of HCC, mutations are found in CDH1, TP53, IGF2H, RB1, CDKN2A, PTEN, KLC, TP73, EXT, MLH1, THRB, THRA, E2F5, and CTNNB1 [23]. Whether these mutations occur early or late in the etiology of liver cancer is still not understood. While the p53 gene functions in controlling the DNA damage response and apoptosis, the WNT pathway is important in controlling cell proliferation [23]. Many of the mutagenic events result from G to T transversions, unlike events found other tumors. The strong bias for G to T transversions suggests that these genetic alterations likely result from chemical DNA damaging agents, rather than spontaneous events, such as cytosine deamination [23]. While the heterogeneity in genetic mutations may reflect multiple mechanisms for liver cell transformation, identifying alterations in HCC are informative in understanding the etiology and possible treatment of individual cancer cases. For example, β-catenin defective liver cancer may be easier to treat than liver cancer resulting from multiple mutations [23–25].

In addition to mutation and LOH events, gain-of-function genetic alterations may confer higher levels of oncogene expression and thereby accelerate carcinogenesis [26–29]. Such alterations could include gene amplification events, such as c-N-methyl-N′-nitro-N-nitroso-guanidine HOS transforming gene (c-MET) and cyclin D (CCND1) [27]. Other gains of function mutations include mutations in the promoter for telomerases reverse transcriptase (TERT) promoter. TERT mutations frequently were shown to be among the earliest and most prevalent neoplastic events in HCC [28, 30].

Both epidemiological and molecular pathology studies have facilitated the identification of which genetic alterations are likely to be associated AFB1 exposure. Mutated genes found in HCC from areas with high AFB1 exposure include p53 and β-catenin [30]. The p53 249^{ser} mutation shows a strong correlation with HCC associated with AFB1 exposure, while is less frequent or absent in HCC from localities where there is little AFB1 exposure [19, 20]. For example, among have HCCs from southern Guangxi province of China, an area of high AFB1 exposure, the p53 249^{ser} mutation was found in 36% of tumors [30]. *CTNNB1* mutations and β-catenin protein accumulation in human hepatocellular carcinomas is also associated with high exposure to AFB1, although it is less clear whether these mutations directly result from AFB1-associated DNA adducts [30]. Whether these mutations must occur early or late in cancer progression is still unclear. One hypothesis is that initial mutations confer a higher level genetic instability that is aggravated by further exposure to genotoxic agents.

To determine whether mutations found in HCC confer higher levels of genetic instability and a higher probability of liver cancer when present in a non-cancerous liver, scientists have constructed transgenic mice that exhibit similar genotypes found in human cancer. Ghebranious and Sell [31] constructed transgenic mice that were both homozygous and heterozygous for the p53ser246 gene, equivalent to the human p53 249^{ser} mutations. Male mice expressing p53ser246 increased the incidence of AFB1-associated high-grade tumors to 14%, compared to 0% exhibited by p53+ (wild type) mice [31]. These studies indicate that the mutant p53 249^{ser} may also be a driver of AFB1-associated liver cancer.

The role of inflammation in liver cancer has led to insights into the gender bias of its incidence. Men are afflicted more than women in nearly all age groups; however the prognosis of liver cancer in either sex is about the same [9]. Naugler et al. [18], have shown that inflammatory cytokines, such as IL-6, are more prevalent in men than women, estrogen having a negative effect on IL-6 production. This gender difference is not only true for humans [32, 33] but also for rodents, including mice and rats [31]. The gender bias underscores the notion that inflammatory responses play a role in liver cancer etiology.

2.2 Associated risk factors that accelerate AFB1-associated liver cancer: role of HBV and HCC virus

The incidence of HCC synergistically increases when individuals are both exposed to AFB1 and infected with either HBV or HCV virus. Interestingly, the incidence of high grade tumors in p53ser246 transgenic mice that are HBsAg-positive is 100% [31]. The common molecular mechanisms by which HBV and HCV infection stimulates AFB1-associated genetic instability phenotypes are still not completely understood; HBV is a DNA virus that replicates by reverse transcription while HCC is a RNA virus that replicates by RNA replication and encodes a single polycistronic message [34, 35]. While 257 million individuals are estimated to be infected with HBV, 140 million individuals are estimated to be infected with HCV; and chronic HBV and HCV infection is the leading cause for 60–70% of HCC [35, 36]. Although HCC contains no oncogenes *per se*, HCV-associated carcinogenesis is associated with increase in reactive oxygen species (ROS), ROS-associated genetic instability, inflammation, and hepatocyte proliferations [36]. Similarly, HBV-associated HCC is associated with inflammation and necro-inflammatory liver damage [16, 36]. Both viruses are not cytopathic *per se*; liver damage caused by HCV and HBV is likely induced by viral-specific $CD8^+$ T and natural killer cells (NK) [35, 36]. Thus, both HCV and HBV create an inflammatory cellular environment that stimulates repopulation of hepatocytes, enhancing AFB1-associated genetic instability.

However, different pathologies of HBV and HCV infection may accelerate HCC progression at different rates. While the median onset age for HBV-associated HCC is 55 years that of HCV is 65 years [11]. HBV can chronically infect children after transmission from the mother [11, 36]. Once HBV is stably integrated into the host genome, HBV can promote chromosomal rearrangements and mutations in cancer-associated genes and interfere with checkpoint controls [37, 38]. For example, HBV integration can occur in TERT promoters, stimulating expression of telomerase, and near LINE sequences [39]. The HBV-encoded oncogene HBx can activate both Src and Ras signaling and is essential for viral DNA (cccDNA) replication. To facilitate replication, HBx mediates chromatin changes by recruiting histone acetyltransferases to acetylate histone H3. HBx is also thought to interact with p53 249^{ser}, and attenuate DNA repair and apoptosis [20].

Besides stimulating host cell replication, HBx may also interfere with the host cell's DNA repair pathways and promote genetic instability and replication [38, 40–44]. HBx binds to DNA damage binding protein 1 (DDB1) and cullin-4 (Cul4), which form a ubiquitinase complex, and can perturb the stability of structural maintenance of chromosome proteins 5 and 6 (Smc5/6) and thus affect DNA replication and DNA damage tolerance [35]. HBx may also interfere with nucleotide excision repair (NER) of AFB1-associated DNA adducts [40–42, 44]. Although less substantiated, HBx is also thought to interfere with PARP1 and decrease excision repair of DNA adducts. Thus HBx drives carcinogenesis by multiple mechanisms that accelerate carcinogenesis.

2.3 Gene polymorphisms associated with AFB1-associated liver cancer

While HBV and HCV infections are the primary factors that aggravate the risk for AFB1-associated HCC, genetic risk factors have also been postulated [45]. With the advent of technologies that accelerate genome sequencing, such as next generation sequencing (NGS), epidemiologists have identified candidate polymorphic genes that increase the risk for aflatoxin-associated liver cancer. Single nucleotide polymorphisms (SNPs) may be located in the amino acid coding region, the introns, or the promoter regions of the candidate genes. Risk factors generally can be grouped into those that (1) are associated with AFB1 metabolic activation and detoxification and (2) that function in DNA repair or DNA damage tolerance genes.

To understand genetic risk factors that affect metabolic activation and detoxification of AFB1 it is necessary to identify genes involved in these pathways. AFB1 is activated by cytochrome P450 enzymes that hydroxylate AFB1 so that the metabolized carcinogen can be rendered hydrophilic and effectively excreted; for review, see [46–48]. Referred to as phase I enzymes and monooxygenases, the cytochrome P450 enzymes contain a heme group at their active sites and catalyze the transfer of single oxygen to specific sites on the target molecule [46]. Cytochrome P450 enzymes require NADPH oxidoreductase (POR) to maintain activity [46]. The P450 enzymes are located in the endoplasmic reticulum in the vicinity of the POR [46]. Of the characterized enzymes expressed by 57 CYP450 genes, CYP1A2 is liver specific and has a high affinity for AFB1, while CYP3A4 constitutes approximately 50% of the hepatic P450 activity. While there have been disagreements over which cytochrome P450 enzymes is chiefly responsible for AFB1 activation in the liver [46, 49, 50], several reports favored CYP3A4 [50, 51], while another report suggested that CYP3A5 has the highest catalytic activity [52]. Among extrahepatic CYPs, CYP2A13 activates AFB1 in the lung, while CYP1A1 catalyzes the formation of AFM1, a hydroxylated AFB1 derivative that can be excreted in milk, which is still carcinogenic [2]. A transient intermediate in the hydroxylation pathway is a highly reactive epoxide, referred to as AFB_1-8,9-exo-epoxide (AFBO) (**Figure 1**). This epoxide can be effectively detoxified by either epoxide hydrolases (EHs) or glutathione S-transferases (GSTs), referred to as phase II enzymes [47, 48]. While multiple cytochrome P450s can activate AFB1, the highly reactive epoxide is thought to be the predominant reactive intermediate in all P450 reactions. Thus, gene polymorphisms that increase the risk of HCC could: (1) increase P450 enzyme levels or activation, (2) downregulate phase II enzymes, (3) decrease the repair of DNA existing lesions, and (4) channel the repair of the DNA lesions into mutagenic pathways.

One source of polymorphic enzymes that can influence the fate of AFB1 is glutathione S-transferases that are present in the liver [53]. In the mouse, knock-out of GSTa3 confers extreme AFB1-associated toxicity [54] and GSTa3 expression levels correlate with AFB1-associated liver cancer in young mice [55]. In humans, HCC risk is dramatically increased by SNPs in glutathione S transferase mu1 (GSTMI) and (glutathione-S-transferase theta1) (GSTT1) [56]. Expression of epoxide hydrolase in yeast also leads to detoxification of AFBO [57]; however, polymorphisms associated with epoxide hydrolase only have a weak association with liver

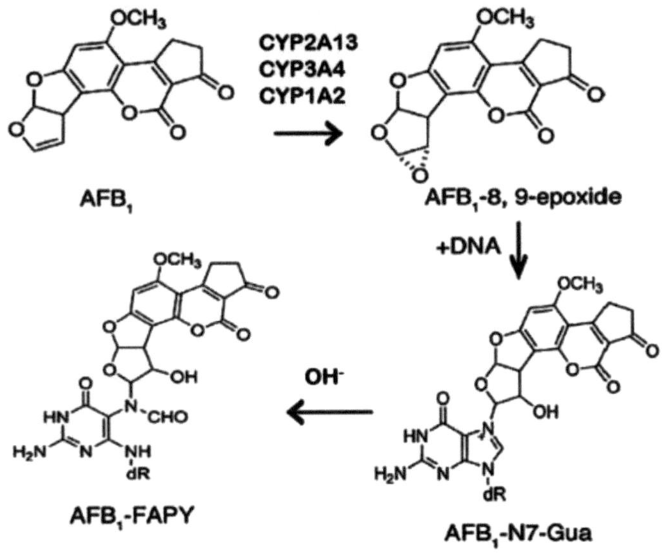

Figure 1.
CYP-mediated metabolic activation of AFB1 to the activated AFB1-8,9 epoxide and adduct formation and conversion to AFB1-Fapy. Adapted from Ref. [130].

cancer [45]. These studies support the idea that detoxification of the highly reactive epoxide is critical in reducing AFB1 toxicity.

While diminished ability to detoxify AFBO is a risk factor for AFB1-associated liver cancer, higher or altered P450 activity could also increase HCC risk. HBx activates the pregnane receptor (PXR) and stimulates expression of CYP3A4 [58]. Particular CYP3A5 alleles, such as CYP3A5*3, are correlated with higher levels of expression and aflatoxin-protein adducts in individuals from Gambia, Africa [59]. CYP3A5*3 is present in a high percentage of individuals in Gambia but not in the Caucasian population [59]; the allele found in the Caucasian population confers an altered spliced mRNA, which is poorly expressed [60]. However, establishing correlations between HCC and increased expression of other P450 genes is complicated by the multiple interactions between P450 enzymes.

Genetic risk factors have also been identified among polymorphic alleles of DNA repair and cell cycle checkpoint genes, which may increase chromosomal instability in cells chronically exposed to AFB1. These risk factors have been found in p53, XRCC1, XRCC3, and ERCC1. The combination of p53 codon 72 Arg72Pro and MDM2 (mouse double minute 2 homolog) SNP309 (T>G) increases the risk of HCC in individuals infected with HBV [61]; p53 codon 72 Arg72Pro affects the frequency of double strand breaks and is associated with hyper-methylation of promoters in tumor suppressor genes [61]. XRCC3 (X-ray complementing defective repair in Chinese hamster cells) encodes a Rad51 paralog which is involved in double-strand break repair and could be involved in error-free by pass of AFB1-associated DNA lesions. The XRCC3 rs861539 allele (codon Thr241Met polymorphism) is a risk factor for HCC, and the risk is aggravated if individuals are exposed to AFB1 [62–64]. Other alleles that have been associated with higher risk for HCC include those participating in the base excision repair (BER) and NER pathways, such as XRCC1 rs25487 polymorphism (codon Arg399Gln polymorphism) [65, 66] and XPD rs25487 polymorphism, respectively [67]. These studies reinforce the idea that AFB1-associated genotoxicity can accelerate HCC progression. To understand the genotoxicity in more detail it is important to understand the nature of the AFB1-associated DNA adducts.

2.4 AFB1-associated DNA adducts and cellular targets

AFB1-associated DNA adducts have been characterized *in vitro* and isolated from organisms that were exposed *in vivo*. DNA exposed to synthesized AFBO reacts predominately with the N^7 group of guanine bases forming 8,9-dihydro-8-(N^7-guanyl)-9-hydroxyaflatoxin B1 (AFB1-N^7-Gua), as identified by mass spectrometry analysis. In the presence of hydroxyl ions (base), N^7-guanine DNA adduct is unstable and decays into an apurinic site and a AFB_1 formamidopyrimidine (Fapy, **Figure 2**) DNA adduct; for review, see [68]. It is unclear whether both apurinic sites and AFB1-Fapy DNA adducts are equally generated; based on mutations generated by DNA lesions constructed *in vitro*, it has been suggested that AFB1-Fapy DNA adducts are the primary source of genetic mutations [69, 70], especially G to T transversion mutations that are found in AFB1-associated liver cancer [71, 72]. The AFB1-Fapy adduct is stable and can be present in two anomer forms; the alpha and the beta forms. While the beta form is highly mutagenic in *Escherichia coli* [69], the alpha form can stabilize the duplex helix and interfere with DNA replication [70]. In the rat liver, the half-life for AFB1-N^7-Gua is 7.5 h, while that for AFB1-Fapy is at least 24 h [68]. While the AFB1-N^7-Gua is unstable, the accumulation of AFB1-Fapy in the rat liver may also result from differential repair of the two types of DNA adducts.

AFB1 exposure also generates oxidative stress (ROS) in exposed cultured cells *in vitro* and in the liver and lung *in vivo* [73]. Multiple factors may contribute to

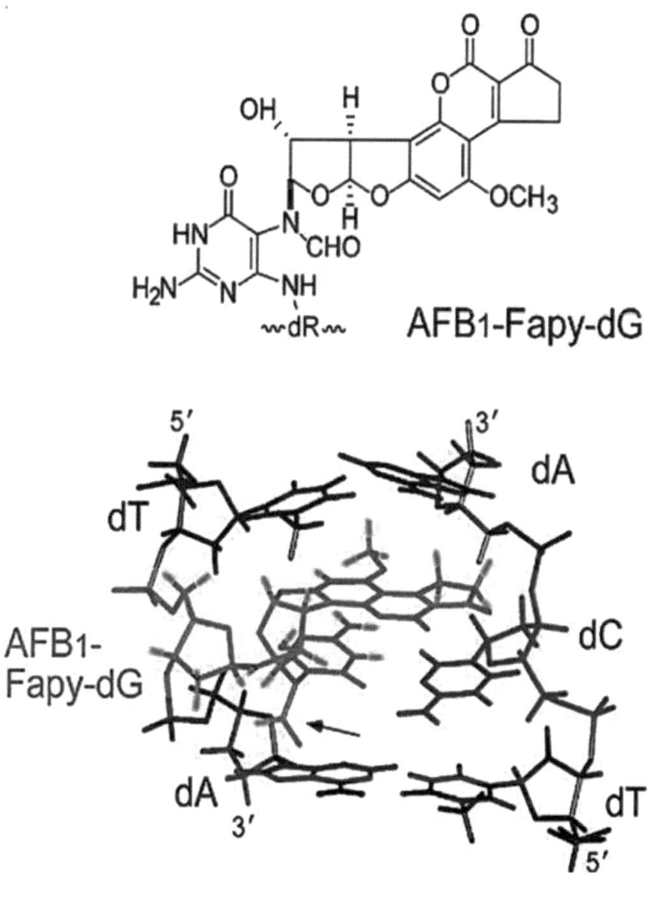

Figure 2.
Intercalation of the AFB1-Fapy-dG in duplex DNA. The adduct is in lighter tone; adapted from Ref. [121].

AFB1-associated oxidative stress including cytochrome P450 activity that involves iron-catalyzed reactions and Kupffer cells [68]. Oxidative stress generates hydroxyl radicals that form 8′-hydroxy-2′-deoxyguanosine (8oxodG) DNA damage. AFB1 exposure increases the 8OH-dG in the livers of ducks [74] and rats [75] and cultured woodchuck hepatocytes [68].

Interestingly, Niranjan et al. [76] observed that in rats, AFB1 bound to mitochondria l DNA exceeded the amount that was bound to the nuclear DNA and persisted for a longer period of time [76]. Furthermore, the persistence of mitochondrial DNA adducts correlated with a longer delay in expression of mitochondrial proteins, compared to that of nuclear-encoded proteins. The authors speculated that the persistence of AFB1 in the mitochondria may result from the lack of NER in the mitochondria. These studies support the notion that mitochondria are a prime target for acute effects of AFB1 exposure, and oxidative stress associated with AFB1-exposure could be indirect due to damage to mitochondria and the generation of superoxide.

To further elucidate the pathological consequences of AFB1-associated mitochondrial DNA lesions, Liu and Wang [77] measured AFB1-associated mitochondrial damage in primary broiler hepatocytes by monitoring mitochondrial membrane potential (MMP), ROS generation, apoptosis, and nuclear factor erythroid 2-like factor 2 (Nrf2)-related signal pathway. They observed mitochondrial ROS generation, decreased MMP and induced apoptosis. The increase in apoptotic cells correlated with an increase expression of caspase-9 and caspase-3. They concluded that AFB1 exposure results in a disruption of mitochondrial functions, generating more ROS, and consequently inducing apoptosis while triggering the Nrf2 signaling pathway [77].

2.5 Epigenetic changes associated with AFB1-associated damage

While genetic instability associated with AFB1 have been described, less well known are epigenetic changes. Epigenetic changes are inheritable changes that result in phenotypic changes without affecting the DNA sequence. Epigenetic changes can result from DNA methylation (hypermethylation) or demethylation (hypomethylation), histone modifications, and changes in microRNA (miRNA) expression [78]. AFB1-associated epigenetic changes have been observed in cell cultures, animal studies, and human tumors (**Table 1**). Hypomethylation has been observed to increase the expression of oncogenes and repetitive sequences, while hypermethylation may decrease expression of DNA repair and tumor suppressor genes (**Table 1**). Zhang et al. [79] observed global hypomethylation in AFB1-associated cancers, where particular genomic repetitive elements, such as LINE-1 elements, were hypomethylated; correlating with increased retro transposition and genetic instability [80]. Hypomethylation also correlated with increased expression of the oncogene c-MET, which is associated with accelerated liver cancer progression and poor prognosis [81]. Hyper-methylated genes include the DNA repair gene methylguanine methyl transferase (MGMT) and p16, which have a negative effect on DNA repair and apoptosis [82]. Thus, methylation patterns may possibly serve as biomarker that can indicate increased risk for HCC [83–85].

Additional biomarkers that indicate AFB1 exposure include alterations in miRNA expression. miRNAs are small noncoding RNAs that are generally 19–25 nucleotides in length and regulate gene express at the post-transcriptional level. They are important factors in regulating HCC development in mammalian organisms [87, 88], and a list of miRNAs that correlate with AFB1 exposure is shown in **Table 1**. This comprises a partial group of total miRNAs that have been associated with HCC. Several miRNAs upregulated after rats or liver cell lines are exposed to

Epigenetic change	Gene functions affected	Consequence	Context/ref.
DNA methylation			
DNA hyper methylation	MGMT expression decreased	DNA Repair downregulated	Human tumor tissue [82]
DNA hypo methylation	c-MET, RAB27A, TXNRD1 expression increased LINE 1	Growth and metastasis increased, decreased expression of GSTs, LINE1 transposition increased	Human tumor tissue [79, 81, 82]
miRNA expression			
miR-429 ⬇	Downregulates Rab23	Metastasis increased when miR-429 decreased	HCC tumor tissue [83, 85]
miR-4-34a ⬆	Downregulation of WNT/β-catenin pathway	Tumor suppressor effect; p53 enhances its expression	HepG2 cell lines [83]
miR-33a ⬆	Downregulation of WNT/β-catenin pathway	Tumor suppressor effect; p53 enhances its expression	HepG2 and normal cell lines [83]
miR-24 ⬆	Inhibition of apoptosis	Larger tumor size	HCC tumor tissue [83]
miR-34a-5p ⬆	c-MET, CCND1, CCNE2 suppressed	Cell cycle arrest	*In vivo* rat livers [83]
miR-122 ⬇	CUTL1 suppressed in mice	Required for tumor differentiation	Human studies [83, 88]
miR-138-1* ⬇	PDK1 and indirectly PI3K/PDK/Akt	Inhibits colony formation, migration, invasiveness	P450-B-2A13 human cell culture [83]
Histone modification			
H3K9me3 ⬆	Repression of gene expression (multiple)	Reprogramming of pluripotency	Porcine oocytes [83]
H3K27me3 ⬇	Repression of gene expression (multiple)	Developmental gene programing in stem cell differentiation	Porcine oocytes [83]
H3K4me2 ⬇	Activating gene expression (multiple)	Developmental gene programing in stem cell differentiation	Porcine oocytes [83]

⬆, *up arrow designates upregulation;* ⬇, *down arrow designates down regulation.*

Table 1.
Epigenetic changes associated with AFB1 exposure.

AFB1 may be protective by downregulating cell proliferation, while upregulated miRNAs found in AFB1-associated HCC may promote tumor size or carcinogenesis. While an individual microRNA may target multiple genes, the expression of individual microRNA can be influenced by multiple transcriptional and epigenetic factors, as well as by genomic changes. These factors include CpG methylation, c-Met signaling, and gene copy number.

Among HCC tumor cells associated with AFB1 exposure, upregulation of several miRNAs, such as miR-429 and miR-24 [86], are associated with larger tumor size [83]. In human bronchial epithelial cells that express CYP2A13 (P50-B-2a13 CELLS), AFB1 exposure induces malignant transformation of immortalized cells [89]. Among transformed cells, one downregulated miRNA was miR-138-1, observed to inhibit proliferation, colony formation, and transformation of P50-B-2a13 CELLS [89]. This miRNA preferentially inhibits 3-phosphoinositide dependent protein kinase-1 (PDK1), which lowers the expression of the P13K/PDK/Akt pathway [89]. These studies indicate that changes in miRNA expression in AFB1-associated HCC may promote carcinogenesis.

HBV infection also upregulates the expression of miRNAs in hepatocytes and may promote HBV-associated HCC. The expression of miR106b-25 is upregulated in HCC patients in general, and in HCC patients infected with HBV [90]. Hep 3B cells transformed with an HBx expression plasmid also express higher levels of miR106b-25, compared to cells that do not express HBx. The miR106b-25 is a member of a cluster of miRNAs in MCM7 that downregulate the expression of several tumor suppressors, including p21, E2F, BIM, and pTEN [91]. Thus, HBV infection may not only interfere with DNA repair mechanisms but also epigenetically silence tumor suppressor genes and accelerate HCC progression.

2.6 Mutagenic signatures associated with AFB1-associated DNA adducts

Mutation signatures are useful biomarkers to determine AFB1 exposure and HCC progression. AFB1 is known to induce mutations in *E. coli*, *Saccharomyces cerevisiae* (budding yeast), and in mammalian cells. AFB1 was one of the original carcinogens published in the Ames assay [92, 93]. While G to T transversions are considered associated with chronic AFB1 exposure in humans [19, 20, 68, 71], in *E. coli*, carcinogen-induced transversion mutations require over-expression of expression of MucAB, which encodes the polV error-prone polymerase [94]. In budding yeast expressing either human CYP1A2 or CYP1A1, AFB1 has been shown to increase mutation frequencies at a *CAN1*, *LYS2*, and *URA3*; however the mutagenic signature of AFB1 in yeast has yet to be identified [95, 96]. The mutagenicity of AFB1 in yeast, however, is low compared to many alkylating agents, such as ethyl methane sulfonate (EMS) [95].

While AFB1 is well-known to cause G to T transversion mutation in mammalian cells, other nucleotide substitutions occur, some of which are in the vicinity of the AFB1-DNA adduct. Investigators have used two approaches to determine the DNA sequence context of AFB1-associated mutations; one technique utilizes PCR (QPCR) and ligation-mediated PCR (LMPCR), and the second technique utilizes whole genome sequencing. Using the first technique, Denissenko et al. [97] mapped total AFB1 adducts in genomic DNA treated with AFB_1-8,9-epoxide. In a second experiment, Denissenko et al. [97] mapped total AFB adducts in hepatocytes exposed to either AFB1 activated by rat liver microsomes or AFB1 activated by human liver microsomal preparations. The p53 gene-specific adduct frequencies in DNA, modified in cells with 40–400 μM AFB1, were 0.07–0.74 adducts per kilobase (kb). *In vitro* modification with 1–4 ng AFB_1-8,9-epoxide per microgram DNA produced 0.03–0.58 lesions per kb. The adduct patterns obtained with the epoxide and the different microsomal systems were virtually identical indicating that AFB1 adducts share similar sequence-specificity whether occurring *in vitro* and *in vivo*.

With the advent of next generation sequencing (NGS) [98], investigators have studied the entire genome and determine whether particular mutation signatures. Huang et al. [99] determine whole genome sequencing data to determine the position of >40,000 mutations in two human cell lines, and in liver tumors from wild type mice and a transgenic mouse carrying the hepatitis B surface antigen. The mutational signature from all four experimental systems was remarkably similar and compared well with experimental mutational signatures derived from sequenced HCCs form Qidong County in China, an area of high AFB1 exposure [100]. The Catalog of Somatic Mutations in Cancer (COSMIC) mutational signature 24 [101], previously associated with AFB1-associated liver cancer, was confirmed and also shown to be present in a high proportion (16%) in HCC from Hong Kong, but in 1% or less from HCC from Japan or North America. The COSMIC mutation signature 24 indicates guanine damage with a very strong transcriptional strand bias for C>A mutations. Additional studies being performed by multiple research groups [25, 102] confirm the presence of signature 24 in human HCC tumors and in tumors induced by AFB1 in mice. In addition to signature 24, investigators have also noted the presence of transition mutations that might also occur in the context of oxidative stress. It has not been determined which of these minor mutation classes drive HCC.

2.7 AFB1 is a potent recombinagen

In budding yeast expressing CYP1A2, AFB1 is potent recombinagen but a poor mutagen [95]. Exposure to AFB1 stimulates homologous recombination between sister chromatids (sister chromatid exchange or SCE), chromosome homologs, and repeated sequences located on non-homologous chromosomes. Using a recombination assay involving truncated fragments of *his3* [103] positioned on non-homologous chromosomes, Sengstag et al. [95] showed that homologous recombination could be stimulated 50-fold in contrast to a less than 10-fold stimulation of mutations. AFB1 concentrations as low as 5 μM were shown to be effective at stimulating the formation of reciprocal translocations, and the karyotypes were confirmed by pulse field gel electrophoresis [103]. AFB1 is also a recombinagen in human and Chinese hamster ovary (CHO) cells and can increase the frequencies of SCE [104–107]. It is unclear whether the same AFB1-associated DNA lesions can stimulate both mutations and recombination. For example, it could be possible that particular lesions that stall DNA replication and generate breaks generate more recombination events while other lesions that can be bypassed by DNA polymerases generate more mutagenic events. These studies thus demonstrate that the genotoxicity of AFB1 extends beyond making mutations and involves stimulating chromosomal rearrangements in model eukaryotic organisms and in humans.

2.8 Repair of AFB1-associated DNA damage

Considering the genotoxicity of AFB1-associated DNA adducts and possible hindrance of DNA replication, it is important to identify which DNA repair pathways and which replication bypass mechanisms are used to tolerate the most persistent AFB1-associated DNA adducts. There are several pathways that are involved in repairing AFB1-associated DNA damage. Among these repair pathways are nucleotide excision repair NER, BER, and recombinational repair; for a general review see [108]. Post-replication repair pathways to bypass DNA adducts involve (1) either error-prone or error-free DNA polymerases, or (2) template switch mechanisms. The later mechanism involves DNA recombination mechanisms, which are utilized in tolerating UV-induced DNA damage and alkylated DNA bases. While in some organisms there are preferred pathways, a general theme in DNA repair is that organisms have evolved redundant DNA repair mechanisms. A prediction of redundant DNA repair pathways is that eliminating genes in two or more repair pathways should effectively lead to a synergistic decrease in AFB1 resistance, while eliminating genes in the same pathway should confer no greater sensitivity than the most sensitive mutant.

Nucleotide excision repair (NER) involves the recognition of the DNA adduct, the opening of the helix at the DNA damage site, the excision of the DNA adduct and the re-synthesis of DNA using the non-damaged DNA strand as a template. In general, 12–13 nucleotides are excised in prokaryotes (for review see [109]) while 24–32 nucleotides are excised in eukaryotes. Global genome repair (GGR) can occur on either the transcribed or non-transcribed strand. Transcription-coupled repair (TCR) does discriminate and preferentially repairs the transcribed strand. The mechanistic difference between the two pathways is how the DNA adduct is recognized; in GGR specific proteins recognize the DNA helical distortion while in TCR, the RNA polymerase stalled complex is recognized; for general review see [110]. In eukaryotes and prokaryotes, both mechanisms are used. While the mechanism is widely conserved among eukaryotes, the mechanism differs between prokaryotes and eukaryotes in the amount of DNA that is excised.

NER is likely to be the predominant mechanism for the repair of AFB1-associated DNA damage in many eukaryotic and prokaryotic organisms [68]. The AFB1-N^7-guanine adduct is fairly unstable while the AFB1-Fapy DNA adduct can insert between the base pairs of the DNA double helix [111]. UvrABC from *E. coli* can effectively excise both DNA adducts, although the AFB1-Fapy adduct appears to be more chemically stable [68, 112]. The excision of the DNA adducts does not depend on the SOS response; thus, basal levels of the DNA repair enzymes appear to be adequate in repairing the DNA lesions. In *E. coli*, both AFB1-N^7-Gua and AFB1-Fapy adduct appear to be excised at a similar rate. One explanation is that the UvrABC complex does not rely on helix distortion to repair the DNA adduct, but rather size and structure of the aromatic rings [68, 112].

Other insights from model organism yeast revealed that the NER genes are required to excise AFB1-associated DNA adducts [96, 113, 114]. *RAD14* (XPA) and *RAD1-RAD10* (XPF-ERCC1) are required for AFB1 resistance. Failure to repair the DNA adducts in a *rad4* (XPC) haploid mutant results in S phase arrest, supporting the notion that particular AFB1-associated DNA adducts interfere with DNA replication [113, 114]. In addition, in *rad4* mutants the level of AFB1-N^7-Gua DNA adducts was reported to increase three fold [114]. These studies support the notion that the yeast NER pathway recognizes and repairs AFB1-N^7-Gua DNA adducts.

In mammalian cells, the NER pathway preferential repairs AFB1-N^7-Gua DNA adducts but still participates in the repair of AFB1-Fapy DNA adducts [115, 116]. In XPA human fibroblast cells, the loss of AFB1-N^7-Gua DNA is much slower and the accumulation of the AFB1-Fapy DNA adducts is greater compared to wild type cells [116]. $XPA^{-/-}$ deficient mice are also more susceptible to AFB1-associated tumorigenesis compared to wild-type mice [117]. Since the accumulation of DNA adducts correlate with the increased carcinogenicity of the DNA adducts [71, 72, 118], it is likely that the burden of AFB1-associated DNA adducts increases the frequencies of carcinogen-associated mutations in the XPA deficient mice.

The second major pathway to repair DNA involves the BER pathway (for review, see Fortini and Dogliotti [119]). As in NER, the DNA damage base is excised and new DNA is synthesized using the undamaged DNA as template for repair (**Figure 3**). In BER, the modified DNA base is recognized and excised by a specific enzyme that generally referred to as a glycosylase. Subsequently, a apurinic endonuclease (APE1)

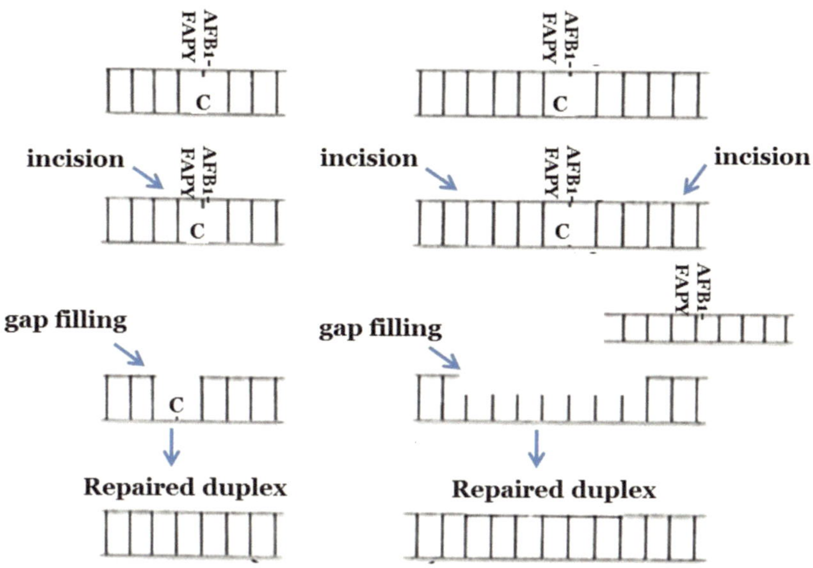

Figure 3.
BER (left) and NER (right) mechanisms to repair the AFB1-Fapy adduct. Both mechanisms involve incision and excision of the damage base, followed by unscheduled DNA synthesis.

generates a 3′OH for primer recognition and new DNA synthesis. In mammalian cells, polymerase β synthesizes new DNA across the gap and removes the deoxyribose residue, and XRCC1/Ligase III cooperate to seal the nick An alternative pathway that does not involve APE1, employs endonuclease VIII like-1 (NEIL1). Following excision of the damaged base by a βδ excision mechanism, the 3′ phosphate is excised by polynucleotide kinase (PNK) to yield a 3′OH for primer recognition and new DNA synthesis. For long patch repair, DNA polymerase δ/PCNA/RFC synthesizes across the gap, the displaced oligonucleotide is excised by FEN1, and the nick is sealed by Ligase I [119]. Poly(ADP-ribose) polymerase PARP1 generally protects the single-strand gap from being subjected to further cleavage or from serving as a substrate for recombinational repair proteins although additional pathways have been proposed [120].

Interestingly, while BER mechanisms have been thought to play a minor role for DNA repair of some AFB1-associated DNA adducts in yeast, BER mechanisms for AFB1-associated DNA adducts can occur in mammalian cells. In budding yeast, the *apn1/apn2* haploid double mutant is no more AFB1 sensitive than the haploid wild type [96]. However, AFB1-associated mutagenesis is lower in the *apn1/apn2* haploid double mutant compared to wild type [96], suggesting that either Apn1 or Apn2 still function in processing the AFB1-associated adducts for post-replication repair. One interpretation of these results is that there is redundancy in both NER and BER mechanisms for conferring AFB1 resistance, while another interpretation is that budding yeast lack the BER enzymes, such as NEIL1, which may actively participate in the repair of AFB1-associated DNA adducts.

In mice, the NEIL1 gene has been isolated and knock-out of the gene leads to higher levels of AFB1-associated DNA adducts and AFB1-associated HCC [121]. The NEIL1 enzyme recognizes and excises AFB1-Fapy-dG adducts in “bubble” DNA structures, such as the one described by Brown et al. [70, 111]. One idea is that AFB1-Fapy-dG adducts may stably intercalate in the helix and be recognized by NEIL1-dependent BER pathway but not by the NER pathway; the repair pathway may thus depend on the DNA sequence context of the AFB1-Fapy-dG adduct. Knock-out of NEIL1 in mice leads to an increase of AFB1-associated tumors and an accumulation of Fapy-adducts [121]. Vartanian et al. [121] assert that the AFB1-associated carcinogenicity in *Neil1*$^{-/-}$ mice is as high if not higher than that observed in *Xpa*$^{-/-}$ mice, noting that both the size and number of tumors are greater in the *Neil1*$^{-/-}$ mice compared to the *Xpa*$^{-/-}$ mice. However, the investigators indicate that spontaneous tumors arise at a much higher frequency in *Xpa*$^{-/-}$ mice, so that the increase in AFB1-associated tumors were measured until the mice were 11 months in age and not when the mice were 15 months in age.

AFB1 exposure is also associated with oxidative stress, as evident by the accumulation of 8-oxodG lesions. It is particularly interesting whether 8-oxodG accumulates in particular DNA repair mutants and contributes to genotoxicity and the etiology of liver cancer. The contribution of 8-oxodG to overall AFB1-associated genotoxicity is unclear; *Ogg1*$^{-}$/*Ogg1*$^{-}$ transgenic mice do not exhibit more AFB1-associated lung tumors than those that are wild type, but do exhibit increased weight loss and mortality [122]. However, *Ogg1*$^{-/-}$ null mice succumb to other cancers after being exposed to oxidizing agents and carcinogens [123]. These studies suggest that AFB1-associated 8-oxodG lesions are not the causative lesions in liver or lung cancer.

The third major pathway in cells that function in AFB1-associated DNA damage is recombination repair. Knocking out *RAD51* in either *rad14* or *rad4* cells leads to a synergistic increase in AFB1 sensitivity in yeast [96, 113]. There are two different explanations. One explanation is that some AFB1-associated DNA lesions that accumulate in *rad4* cells are converted into single or double-strand breaks and require recombinational repair. A single double-strand break has previously been shown to be lethal in strains defective in homologous recombination [124]. An alternative explanation is that cells require *RAD51* to bypass the DNA lesions and accumulate stalled replication forks. Studies have shown that *RAD51* is required for DNA damage-associated SCE [125], which likely occur by replication bypass mechanisms. This second reason is also supported by the notion that *rad4* cells tend to arrest in a small budded stage upon entry into the cell cycle.

2.9 DNA damage tolerance and AFB1-associated DNA damage

DNA damage tolerance pathways allow cellular replication mechanisms to bypass blocking DNA adducts, such as the AFB1-Fapy DNA adduct, resulting in persistence of the DNA adduct in the divided cells. These mechanisms are divided into error-free mechanisms where the original "correct" base is opposite the modified base and error-prone mechanisms where an "incorrect" base is inserted opposite the damaged base, thereby generating mutations. The insertion of the "incorrect" base is generally accomplished by substituting a "high fidelity" polymerase with a lower fidelity polymerase that also has lower processivity. The polymerase switch mechanism is accomplished by a series of ubiquitination reactions on PCNA, which is the processivity factor for DNA polymerase on the DNA template; for review, see [126, 127]. The first ubiquitination reaction of PCNA is a monoubiquitination reaction catalyzed by Rad18/Rad6. Subsequent polyubiquitination of PCNA by Rad5/Ubc13/Mms2 is required for error-free by-pass mechanisms, which includes template-switch mechanisms. Both *RAD18/RAD6* and *RAD5* genes are well conserved in eukaryotes.

The function of replication bypass in conferring AFB1 resistance has been validated in model organisms. In budding yeast, *RAD18*, *RAD5*, *REV1*, and *REV7/REV3* are required for AFB1 resistance [96]. These genes are also required for AFB1-associated mutagenesis [96]. These results indicate that all three translesion polymerases are required for AFB1 resistance, while it is unclear which gene is required for replication bypass of individual AFB1-associated DNA adduct.

While there are only three translesion DNA polymerases in budding yeast, in humans, there are at least 11 translesion polymerases, forming the majority of the 15 DNA template-dependent DNA polymerases [128]. Both the AFB1-N7-Guanine and the AFB1-Fapy DNA adducts can be bypassed by translesion polymerases [129, 130]. Of the translesion polymerases, DNA polymerase ζ, also referred to as Rev3L the Rev3 homolog in humans, limits chromosomal damage and promotes cell survival following AFB1 exposure [131]. The authors suggest that Rev3 is required for progression through S phase since mouse embryonic fibroblasts, derived from *Rev3L*$^{-/-}$ knock down mice, arrest in S/G2 after AFB1 exposure [131]. These cells also exhibit an increase in gamma-H2AX foci, micronuclei, and chromosomal aberrations; the kinetics of micronuclei formation support a replication-dependent mechanism that results in the accumulation of unrepaired DSBs in. The Rev3 requirement for DNA replication of an AFB1-associated DNA adduct was also demonstrated for a single lesion present on a replicating plasmid in HEK239 cells [131]. Considering the number of mammalian translesion polymerases [128], the Rev3 requirement for replication bypass may reflect the efficiency by which AFB1-associated DNA adducts block other polymerases or Rev3's ability to minimize detrimental chromosomal damage [132].

2.10 Template-switch mechanisms as an alternative mechanism for tolerating DNA damage

Exposure to AFB1 stimulates SCE in multiple organisms. One possible mechanism is that in post-replication repair, processing of AFB1-associated DNA damage generates apurinic sites and/or subsequent DNA single-strand gaps, which initiate SCE by serving as substrates for DNA recombination proteins. Template switch mechanisms are another mechanism (**Figure 4**) that avoid the necessity of using error-prone polymerase for replication bypass. In support of the role of template switching in AFB1-associated SCE, studies have been performed in budding yeast indicating that *rad51* null mutants, deficient in DNA damage-associated SCE [125], exhibit higher frequencies of AFB1-associated mutations [96, 133]. In addition, Rad51 foci appear as cells enter S phase [114] and not in G2, suggesting that the appearance of Rad51 foci are replication-dependent and not associated with double- or single-strand breaks after replication. However, it is possible that multiple mechanisms are involved.

AFB1-associated SCE are also observed in human and mammalian cells. SCEs have been detected in human lymphocytes, Chinese hamster V79 cells, rat and mouse hepatocyte cell lines [104–107]. It has not yet been determined whether mammalian cells defective in homologous recombination exhibit more AFB1-associated mutations. Nonetheless, it is interesting that polymorphisms of XRCC3 [62–64], which functions in homologous recombination, are a risk factor for HCC.

2.11 Tissue specificity of DNA damage repair of AFB1-associated DNA adducts

Since AFB1-associated DNA adducts are found in different tissues, the question can be asked whether there are tissue-specific differences in repair mechanisms. Mudler et al. [134] addressed the question whether oxidative damage caused by AFB1, 8-oxodG, was repaired more efficiently in the mouse lung compared to the mouse liver. They exposed mice to a low chronic amount of AFB1 (0.2 or 1.0 ppm AFB1) and then assayed for the amount of dGTP incorporation. Interestingly, they found that although Ogg1 was present in both the lung and the liver, there was a lower repair efficiency in the liver after exposure to 1.0 ppm AFB1. The lower efficiency of the repair in the liver did not correspond to AFB1-associated cytotoxic effects, and they speculated that the differences could result from AFB1 directly inhibiting Ogg1 [134].

Bedard et al. [135] asked the question whether AFB1-N^7-Gua and AFB1-Fapy DNA adducts were repaired more efficiently in the mouse liver or lung. They also compared the efficiency of repair in the rat liver and the mouse liver. After exposing mice to 50 mg/kg AFB1, extracts were obtained from the various tissues and used to determine the repair of plasmid DNA AFB1-N^7-guanine or AFB1-Fapy adducts as

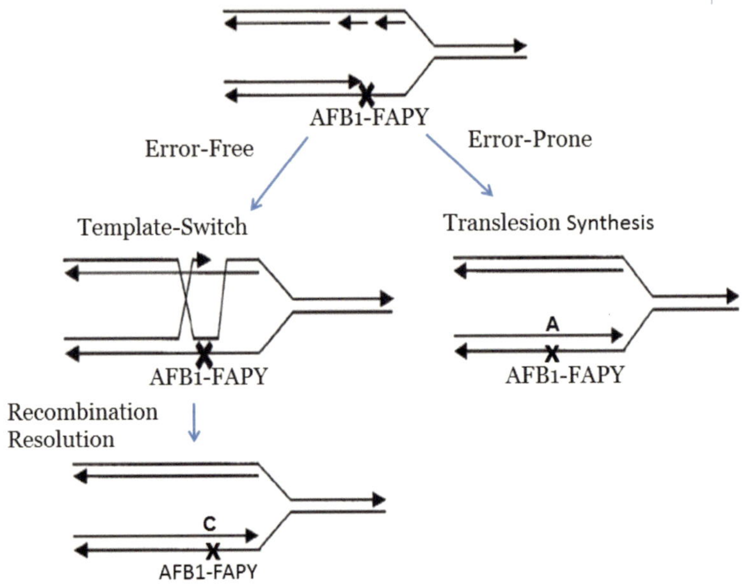

Figure 4.
DNA damage tolerance mechanisms used to bypass a AFB1-Fapy DNA adduct blocking the leading strand polymerase on a growing replication fork. Error-free (left) bypass uses a template switch mechanism while error-prone (right) bypass uses a low fidelity DNA polymerase, resulting in the insertion of an A opposite the DNA adduct.

substrates. Mouse liver extracts repaired AFB1-N^7-guanine and AFB1-Fapy adducts 5- and 30-fold more effectively, respectively, than did extracts from the mouse lung. Mouse liver extracts also repaired the adducts 6-fold and 4-fold more effectively, respectively, than did liver extracts from rats. They conclude that there is a tissue-specific induction in repair in the mouse liver that renders the mouse liver more resistant to AFB1-associated carcinogenesis. However, further studies are needed to determine which NER and BER enzymes are preferentially induced in the liver.

2.12 AFB1-induction of DNA repair and protective mechanisms

The redundancy in repair mechanisms for DNA adducts in yeast and in mammalian organisms provokes the question of which genes are transcriptionally induced after the exposure of AFB1. Two complementary studies have been performed using budding yeast and several studies have been performed in mammalian cells. While studies in yeast utilized microarrays, more recent studies in mammalian cells have used RNAseq and NGS technology. The common genes that are induced have provided clues into which pathways are shared among eukaryotic organisms.

Keller-Seitz et al. [113] determined which budding yeast genes were induced after exposure to AFB1. Essentially, an exponentially grown culture was concentrated to 4 × 10e8 cells/ml and then exposed to 25 μM AFB1 in phosphate buffer (pH 7.5). After RNA was extracted, cDNA was synthesized and labeled for analysis on microarrays. Fourteen DNA repair genes were upregulated more than two-fold, with *RAD51* being upregulated more than seven-fold. Among NER genes, *RAD16*, *RAD3*, and *RAD1* were AFB1-inducible. The upregulation of selected genes was verified by RT-PCR. Additional genes that were induced included those involved in mismatch repair and DNA synthesis, while genes participating in NHEJ were downregulated.

A similar study was done by Guo et al. [136], except AFB1-inducible genes were identified in actively growing cultures. Similar to the Keller-Seitz study [113], *RAD51* was upregulated over seven-fold. However, additional genes involved in regulating dNTP levels were also upregulated including *DUN1*, which encodes a DNA damage-signaling kinase, and *RNR2* and *RNR4*, which are subunits of ribonucleotide reductase. Although the functional significance of the AFB1-associated inducibility is unknown, there is good overlap with a cluster of genes identified as DNA damage-inducible but not generally stress-inducible [137]; DNA damage-inducible genes from multiple studies include *DUN1*, *RAD51*, *RNR2*, and *RNR4*. In contrast to the previous study by Keller-Seitz, NER genes were not upregulated. In both studies, the DNA damage-inducibility of *RAD51* is *MEC1*-dependent; *MEC1* is the ATM/ATR orthologue of yeast. The functional significance of the upregulation was illustrated by showing that the recombination deficiency exhibited by *mec1* mutants could be partially suppressed by over-expression of *RAD51* [113]. Thus, upregulation of particular DNA repair genes could enhance AFB1 genotoxic effects.

Additional genes that were upregulated in both studies included genes involved in cell cycle control, protein transport, DNA metabolism, and ion homeostasis [113, 136]. Although the functional significance of the upregulation of each of these genes is unknown, many of these genes are involved cell cycle regulation. Interestingly, genes involved in histone biosynthesis were downregulated, reflecting a delay in S phase [136]. The delay in S phase may result from the stability of the AFB1-Fapy DNA adduct during the exposure time.

Identification of AFB1-inducible genes in mammalian cells revealed broader classes of upregulated genes, compared to the yeast studies, reflecting the hepatic cell's ability to metabolize and neutralize xenobiotic agents. Merrick et al. [138] performed RNA seq analysis on liver cells after the rat was injected with AFB1. In brief, RNA was obtained from male rats exposed 1 ppm AFB1 in feed for 90 days, and RNA seq analysis was performed using the appropriate number of unexposed rats as controls. 1026 differentially induced transcripts were identified. Genes upregulated more than five-fold relevant to hepatocellular proliferation include follistatin (442-fold), Aldh3a1 (302-fold), Mybl2 (21-fold), Mybl1 (6-fold), and Sox9 (6-fold). Genes upregulated and involving the E2f1 transcription factor included Cdk1, Mdm2, Ect2, Mad2L1, and Nuf2. Of those genes that were upregulated, of particular interest are those involved in DNA damage tolerance and repair. A two to four-fold increase was observed for Mgmt, Top2a, Rad51, Rad18, Xrcc6, Mnd1, and Tynns [138]. These studies indicate that chronic AFB1 exposure in animals can also induce DNA repair genes that are involved in cell cycle regulation and DNA replication bypass.

2.13 Signal transduction and checkpoint activation

Both studies in yeast and in mammalian cells indicate that AFB1 triggers a checkpoint response that delays cell cycle progression so that DNA damage can be repaired. The mechanism by which the AFB1 DNA adducts are sensed is unknown. However, it is likely that DNA replication stress triggers S phase delay that is associated with Rad53 (Chk2 orthologue) phosphorylation [133]. In budding yeast, exposure to 50 μM AFB1 is sufficient to delay S phase [133, 135]. The Rad53 phosphorylation is dependent on MEC1, the ATM/ATR orthologue. Fasullo et al. [133] observed that the downstream effector of Rad53, DUN1, was required for both AFB1-associated mutation and AFB1-associated recombination. However, the substrates for the signaling cascade that affect AFB1-associated recombination and mutation are unknown. One possibility is that Rad55 phosphorylation is important in triggering AFB1-associated recombination.

In mammalian cells, the DNA damage response to AFB1-associated DNA adducts has been addressed by only a few studies. After exposure to AFB1, HepG2 cells exhibit 53BP1 foci and H2AX foci but not Chk1 or Chk2 activation [139]. However, other studies [140] in other cell lines suggest a robust stimulation of the checkpoint response. In human bronchial epithelial cells (BEAS-2B) expressing CYP2A13 and exposed to low concentrations of AFB1, AFB1-DNA adducts and 8oxodG significantly increased, along with phosphorylation of ATR and BRCA1. In addition, Mre11, Rad50 and Rad51 were significantly increased. These studies suggest that similar to yeast, checkpoint activation leads to higher expression of DNA recombination genes in3BEAS-2B cells.

3. Conclusions

Liver cancer is the third leading cause of cancer deaths, and unfortunately the incidence of liver cancer is increasing in the USA. Environmental and lifestyle factors include AFB1 exposure and infection with HCV and HBV viruses. AFB1 is a potent liver carcinogen because it is a potent genotoxin and AFB1 exposure is correlated to signature mutations found in HCC. Liver injury and inflammation set the stage for regenerative cell proliferation that enhances AFB1-associated genetic instability. As liver cancer progresses, multiple genetic mutations and epigenetic changes accumulate that eventually accelerate an irreversible path toward malignancy and poor prognosis.

Nonetheless, cellular defense mechanisms have evolved to diminish the AFB1 genotoxicity and repair or tolerate AFB1 DNA adducts so that mutations and chromosomal instability are avoided. First, there are multiple pathways to repair AFB1-associated DNA adducts. These include BER repair involving NEIL1 and NER pathways that excise AFB1-associated DNA adducts. However, it is still unclear which pathway is favored in humans and whether they are redundant. Second, there are common repair and checkpoint pathways that are upregulated in both model organisms and in mammalian organisms; these include ATR signaling pathways and recombinational repair pathways. These pathways may suppress chromosomal instability by error-free mechanisms by which DNA adducts can be bypassed by the DNA replication machinery. One error free mechanism involves recombination-mediated template switch mechanisms. Supporting this idea, RAD51 expression is enhanced in yeast and particular polymorphisms XRCC3, a RAD51 paralogue, may be risk factors for HCC. Nonetheless the DNA repair process can be thwarted by HBV virus, where Hepatitis B virus may directly interfere with NER and perpetuate the replication of cells containing damaged DNA.

The studies presented in this chapter point to future directions in elucidating repair mechanisms of AFB1-associated DNA damage and genetic susceptibility to AFB1-associated cancer. The advent of NGS technology has made it possible to profile the yeast and mammalian genomes for AFB1 resistance which will facilitate identifying the most prominent AFB1 resistant genes. This will facilitate epidemiological studies in determining potential gene polymorphisms that may pose the greatest risk for HCC. NGS technology can facilitate characterizing the DNA sequence contexts where AFB1-associated mutations occur. With the advent of NGS it may be possible to determine the temporal and sequence contexts by with AFB1-associated mutations occur. With the accumulation of genetic information, new biomarkers may be available to aid clinicians and epidemiologists to detect individuals most of risk for HCC and to take appropriate prophylactic actions at earl signs of HCC progression.

Acknowledgements

The author was supported by NIH grants R21ES015954, F33ES021133, and R15E023685.

Conflict of interest

The author declares no conflict of interest.

Author details

Michael Fasullo
State University of New York Polytechnic Institute, Albany, New York, United States

*Address all correspondence to: mfasullo@sunypoly.edu

References

[1] World Health Organization; International Agency for Research on Cancer. Aflatoxins. In: IARC Monographs on the Evaluation of Carcinogenic Risks to Humans. Vol. 56. Lyon, France: IARC Press; 1993. pp. 245-395

[2] Marchese S, Polo A, Ariano A, Velotto S, Costantini S, Severino L. Aflatoxin B1 and M1: Biological properties and their involvement in cancer development. Toxins (Basel). 2018;**10**(6). pii: E214. DOI: 10.3390/toxins10060214

[3] Ghasemi-Kebria F, Joshaghani H, Taheri NS, Semnani S, Aarabi M, Salamat F, et al. Aflatoxin contamination of wheat flour and the risk of esophageal cancer in a high risk area in Iran. Cancer Epidemiology. 2013;**37**:290-293. DOI: 10.1016/j.canep.2013.01.010

[4] Blount WP. Turkey "X" disease. Turkeys. 1961;**9m**:52-54

[5] Strosnider H, Azziz-Baumgartner E, Banziger M, et al. Workgroup report: Public health strategies for reducing aflatoxin exposure in developing countries. Environmental Health Perspectives. 2006;**114**:1898-1903. DOI: 10.1289/ehp.9302

[6] McGlynn KA, London WT. Epidemiology and natural history of hepatocellular carcinoma. Best Practice & Research. Clinical Gastroenterology. 2005;**19**:3-23

[7] Liu Y, Wu F. Global burden of aflatoxin-induced hepatocellular carcinoma: A risk assessment. Environmental Health Perspectives. 2010;**118**:818-824

[8] Bui-Klimke TR, Guclu H, Kensler TW, Yuan JM, Wu F. Aflatoxin regulations and global pistachio trade: Insights from social network analysis. PLoS One. 2014;**9**(3):e92149. DOI: 10.1371/journal.pone.0092149. eCollection 2014

[9] Torre LA, Siegel RL, Ward EM, Jemal A. Global cancer incidence and mortality rates and trends—An update. Cancer Epidemiology, Biomarkers & Prevention. 2016;**25**(1):16-27. DOI: 10.1158/1055-9965.EPI-15-0578

[10] Lamarca A, Mendiola M, Barriuso J. Hepatocellular carcinoma: Exploring the impact of ethnicity on molecular biology. Critical Reviews in Oncology/Hematology. 2016;**105**:65-72. DOI: 10.1016/j.critrevonc.2016.06.007

[11] Bosch FX, Ribes J, Díaz M, Cléries R. Primary liver cancer: Worldwide incidence and trends. Gastroenterology. 2004;**127**:S5-S16

[12] Centers for Disease Control and Prevention (CDC). Hepatocellular carcinoma—United States, 2001-2006. MMWR. Morbidity and Mortality Weekly Report. 2010;**59**:517-520

[13] Balogh J, Victor DIII, Asham EH, Burroughs SG, Boktour M, Saharia A, et al. Hepatocellular carcinoma: A review. Journal of Hepatocellular Carcinoma. 2016;**3**:41-53. DOI: 10.2147/JHC.S61146

[14] Kew MC. Synergistic interaction between aflatoxin B1 and hepatitis B virus and hepatocarcinogenesis. Liver Internation. 2003;**23**:405-409

[15] Wild CP, Montesano R. A model of interaction: Aflatoxins and hepatitis viruses in liver cancer aetiology and prevention. Cancer Letters. 2009;**286**:22-28. DOI: 10.1016/j.canlet.2009.02.053

[16] Anwar WA, Khaled HM, Amra HA, El-Nezami H, Loffredo CA. Changing pattern of hepatocellular carcinoma (HCC) and its risk factors in Egypt:

Possibilities for prevention. Mutation Research. 2008;**659**:176-184. DOI: 10.1016/j.mrrev.2008.01.005

[17] Chu YJ, Yang HI, Wu HC, Lee MH, Liu J, Wang LY, et al. Aflatoxin B(1) exposure increases the risk of hepatocellular carcinoma associated with hepatitis C virus infection or alcohol consumption. European Journal of Cancer. 2018;**94**:37-46. DOI: 10.1016/j.ejca.2018.02.010

[18] Naugler WE, Sakurai T, Kim S, Maeda S, Kim K, Elsharkawy AM, et al. Gender disparity in liver cancer due to sex differences in MyD88-dependent IL-6 production. Science. 2007;**317**:121-124

[19] Hsu IC, Metcalf RA, Sun T, Welsh JA, Wang NJ, Harris CC. Mutational hotspot in the p53 gene in human hepatocellular carcinomas. Nature. 1991;**350**: 427-428

[20] Hussain SP, Schwank J, Staib F, Wang XW, Harris CC. TP53 mutations and hepatocellular carcinoma: Insights into the etiology and pathogenesis of liver cancer. Oncogene. 2007;**26**:2166-2176

[21] Bechtel DH. Molecular dosimetry of hepatic aflatoxin B1-DNA adducts: Linear correlation with hepatic cancer risk. Regulatory Toxicology and Pharmacology. 1989;**10**:74-81

[22] Bailey GS, Dashwood R, Loveland PM, Pereira C, Hendricks JD. Molecular dosimetry in fish: Quantitative target organ DNA adduction and hepatocarcinogenicity for four aflatoxins by two exposure routes in rainbow trout. Mutation Research. 1998;**399**:233-244

[23] Thorgeirsson SS, Grisham JW. Molecular pathogenesis of human hepatocellular carcinoma. Nature Genetics. 2002;**31**:339-346

[24] Niu Z-S, Niu X-J, Wang W-H. Genetic alterations in hepatocellular carcinoma: An update. World Journal of Gastroenterology. 2016;**22**:9069-9095. DOI: 10.3748/wjg.v22.i41.9069

[25] Cancer Genome Atlas Research Network. Electronic address: wheeler@bcm.edu; Cancer Genome Atlas Research Network. Comprehensive and integrative genomic characterization of hepatocellular carcinoma. Cell. 2017;**169**:1327-1341.e23. DOI: 10.1016/j.cell.2017.05.046

[26] Nault JC, Rebouissou S, Zucman Rossi J. NRF2/KEAP1 and Wnt/β-catenin in the multistep process of liver carcinogenesis in humans and rats. Hepatology. 2015;**62**(3):677-679. DOI: 10.1002/hep.27828

[27] Kondo S, Ojima H, Tsuda H, Hashimoto J, Morizane C, Ikeda M, et al. Clinical impact of c-Met expression and its gene amplification in hepatocellular carcinoma. International Journal of Clinical Oncology. 2013;**18**:207-213. DOI: 10.1007/s10147-011-0361-9

[28] Zucman-Rossi J, Villanueva A, Nault JC, Llovet JM. Genetic landscape and biomarkers of hepatocellular carcinoma. Gastroenterology. 2015;**149**(5):1226-1239.e4. DOI: 10.1053/j.gastro.2015.05.061

[29] Devereux TR, Stern MC, Flake GP, Yu MC, Zhang ZQ, London SJ, et al. CTNNB1 mutations and beta-catenin protein accumulation in human hepatocellular carcinomas associated with high exposure to aflatoxin B1. Molecular Carcinogenesis. 2001;**31**:68-73

[30] Stern MC, Umbach DM, Yu MC, London SJ, Zhang ZQ, Taylor JA. Hepatitis B, aflatoxin B(1), and p53 codon 249 mutation in hepatocellular carcinomas from Guangxi, People's Republic of China,

and a meta-analysis of existing studies. Cancer Epidemiology, Biomarkers & Prevention. 2001;**10**(6):617-253

[31] Ghebranious N, Sell S. The mouse equivalent of the human p53ser249 mutation p53ser246 enhances aflatoxin hepatocarcinogenesis in hepatitis B surface antigen transgenic and p53 heterozygous null mice. Hepatology. 1998;**27**:967-973

[32] Prieto J. Inflammation, HCC and sex: IL-6 in the centre of the triangle. Journal of Hepatology. 2008;**48**:380-381

[33] Shimizu I, Kohno N, Tamaki K, et al. Female hepatology: Favorable role of estrogen in chronic liver disease with hepatitis B virus infection. World Journal of Gastroenterology: WJG. 2007;**13**:4295-4305. DOI: 10.3748/wjg.v13.i32.4295

[34] Schietroma I, Scheri GC, Pinacchio C, Statzu M, Petruzziello A, Vullo V. Hepatitis C virus and hepatocellular carcinoma: Pathogenetic mechanisms and impact of direct-acting antivirals. Open Virology Journal. 2018;**12**:16-25. DOI: 10.2174/1874357901812010016

[35] Ringehan M, McKeating J, Protzer U. Viral hepatitis and cancer. Philosophical Transactions of the Royal Society B. 2017;**372**:20160274. DOI: 10.1098/rstb.2016.0274

[36] Szabó E, Páska C, Kaposi Novák P, Schaff Z, Kiss A. Similarities and differences in hepatitis B and C virus induced hepatocarcinogenesis. Pathology Oncology Research. 2004;**10**:5-11

[37] Benn J, Schneider RJ. Hepatitis B virus HBx protein deregulates cell cycle checkpoint controls. Proceedings of the National Academy of Sciences of the United States of America. 1995;**92**:11215-11219. DOI: 10.1073/pnas.92.24.11215

[38] Kew MC. Hepatitis B virus x protein in the pathogenesis of hepatitis Bvirus-induced hepatocellular carcinoma. Journal of Gastroenterology and Hepatology. 2011;**26**(Suppl 1):144-152. DOI: 10.1111/j.1440-1746. 2010.06546

[39] Toh ST, Jin Y, Liu L, Wang J, Babrzadeh F, Gharizadeh B, et al. Deep sequencing of the hepatitis B virus inhepatocellular carcinoma patients reveals enriched integration events, structuralalterations and sequence variations. Carcinogenesis. 2013;**34**(4):787-798. DOI: 10.1093/carcin/bgs406

[40] Becker SA, Lee TH, Butel JS, Slagle BL. Hepatitis B virus X protein interferes with cellular DNA repair. Journal of Virology. 1998;**72**:266-272

[41] Jia L, Wang XW, Harris CC. Hepatitis B virus X protein inhibits nucleotide excision repair. International Journal of Cancer. 1999;**80**:875-879

[42] Lee AT, Ren J, Wong ET, Ban KH, Lee LA, Lee CG. The hepatitis B virus X protein sensitizes HepG2 cells to UV light-induced DNA damage. The Journal of Biological Chemistry. 2005;**280**:33525-33535

[43] Na TY, Ka NL, Rhee H, Kyeong D, Kim MH, Seong JK, et al. Interaction of hepatitis B virus X protein with PARP1 results in inhibition of DNA repair in hepatocellular carcinoma. Oncogene. 2016;**35**(41):5435-5445. DOI: 10.1038/onc.2016.82

[44] Qadri I, Fatima K, AbdeL-Hafiz H. Hepatitis B virus X protein impedes the DNA repair via its association with transcription factor, TFIIH. BMC Microbiology. 2011;**11**:48. DOI: 10.1186/1471-2180-11-48

[45] Kirk GD, Turner PC, Gong Y, Lesi OA, Mendy M, Goedert JJ, et al. Hepatocellular carcinoma and polymorphisms in

carcinogen-metabolizing and DNA repair enzymes in a population with aflatoxin exposure and hepatitis B virus endemicity. Cancer Epidemiology, Biomarkers & Prevention. 2005;**14**:373-379

[46] Nebert DW, Dalton TP. The role of cytochrome P450 enzymes in endogenous signalling pathways and environmental carcinogenesis. Nature Reviews. Cancer. 2006;**6**:947-960

[47] Guengerich FP, Johnson WW, Shimada T, Ueng YF, Yamazaki H, Langouët S. Activation and detoxication of aflatoxin B1. Mutation Research. 1998;**402**:121-128. Review. PubMed PMID: 9675258

[48] Guengerich FP, Johnson WW, Ueng YF, Yamazaki H, Shimada T. Involvement of cytochrome P450, glutathione S-transferase, and epoxide hydrolase in the metabolism of aflatoxin B1 and relevance to risk of human liver cancer. Environmental Health Perspectives. 1996;**104**:557-562

[49] Eaton DL, Gallagher EP. Mechanisms of aflatoxin carcinogenesis. Annual Review of Pharmacology and Toxicology. 1994;**34**:135-172

[50] Gallagher EP, Kunze KL, Stapleton PL, Eaton DL. The kinetics of aflatoxin B1 oxidation by human cDNA-expressed and human liver microsomal cytochromes P450 1A2and 3A4. Toxicology and Applied Pharmacology. 1996;**141**:595-606

[51] Kamdem LK, Meineke I, Gödtel-Armbrust U, Brockmöller J, Wojnowski L. Dominant contribution of P450 3A4 to the hepatic carcinogenic activation of aflatoxin B1. Chemical Research in Toxicology. 2006;**19**:577-586

[52] Pelkonen P, Lang MA, Negishi M, Wild CP, Juvonen RO. Interaction of aflatoxin B1 with cytochrome P450 2A5 and its mutants: Correlation with metabolic activation and toxicity. Chemical Research in Toxicology. 1997;**10**:85-90

[53] Gross-Steinmeyer K, Stapleton PL, Tracy JH, Bammler TK, Strom SC, Eaton DL. Sulforaphane- and phenethyl isothiocyanate-induced inhibition of aflatoxin B1-mediated genotoxicity in human hepatocytes: Role of GSTM1 genotype and CYP3A4 gene expression. Toxicological Sciences. 2010;**116**:422-432. DOI: 10.1093/toxsci/kfq135

[54] Ilic Z, Crawford D, Vakharia D, Egner PA, Sell S. Glutathione-S-transferase A3 knockout mice are sensitive to acute cytotoxic and genotoxic effects of aflatoxin B1. Toxicology and Applied Pharmacology. 2010;**242**:241-246. DOI: 10.1016/j.taap.2009.10.008

[55] Shupe T, Sell S. Low hepatic glutathione S-transferase and increased hepatic DNA adduction contribute to increased tumorigenicity of aflatoxin B1 in newborn and partially hepatectomized mice. Toxicology Letters. 2004;**148**:1-9

[56] Shen YH, Chen S, Peng YF, Shi YH, Huang XW, Yang GH, et al. Quantitative assessment of the effect of glutathione S-transferase genes GSTM1 and GSTT1 on hepatocellular carcinoma risk. Tumour Biology. 2014;**35**:4007-4015. DOI: 10.1007/s13277-013-1524-2

[57] Kelly EJ, Erickson KE, Sengstag C, Eaton DL. Expression of human microsomal epoxide hydrolase in Saccharomyces cerevisiae reveals a functional role in aflatoxin B1 detoxification. Toxicological Sciences. 2002;**65**(1):35-42

[58] Niu Y, Wu Z, Shen Q, Song J, Luo Q, You H, et al. Hepatitis B virus X protein co-activates pregnane X receptor to induce the cytochrome P450 3A4 enzyme, a potential implication in

hepatocarcinogenesis. Digestive and Liver Disease. 2013;**45**:1041-1048. DOI: 10.1016/j.dld.2013.06.004

[59] Wojnowski L, Turner PC, Pedersen B, Hustert E, Brockmöller J, Mendy M, et al. Increased levels of aflatoxin-albumin adducts are associated with CYP3A5 polymorphisms in the Gambia, West Africa. Pharmacogenetics. 2004;**14**(10):691-700

[60] Kuehl P, Zhang J, Lin Y, Lamba J, Assem M, Schuetz J, et al. Sequence diversity in CYP3A promoters and characterization of the genetic basis of polymorphic CYP3A5 expression. Nature Genetics. 2001;**27**:383-391

[61] Yang Y, Xia T, Li N, Zhang J, Yang Y, Cong W, et al. Combined effects of p53 and MDM2 polymorphisms on susceptibility and surgical prognosis in hepatitis B virus-related hepatocellular carcinoma. Protein & Cell. 2013;**4**:71-81. DOI: 10.1007/s13238-012-2067-9

[62] Avadanei ER, Giusca SE, Negura L, Caruntu ID. Single nucleotide polymorphisms of XRCC3 gene in hepatocellular carcinoma-relationship with clinicopathological features. Polish Journal of Pathology. 2018;**69**:73-81. DOI: 10.5114/pjp.2018.75340

[63] Ji RB, Qian YS, Hu AR, Hu YR. DNA repair gene XRCC3 T241M polymorphism and susceptibility to hepatocellular carcinoma in a Chinese population: A meta-analysis. Genetics and Molecular Research. 2015;**14**:15988-15996. DOI: 10.4238/2015.December.7.11

[64] Long XD, Ma Y, Qu de Y, Liu YG, Huang ZQ, Huang YZ, et al. The polymorphism of XRCC3 codon 241 and AFB1-related hepatocellular carcinoma in Guangxi population, China. Annals of Epidemiology. 2008;**18**:572-578

[65] Liu F, Li B, Wei Y, Yan L, Wen T, Zhao J, et al. XRCC1 genetic polymorphism Arg399Gln and hepatocellular carcinoma risk: A meta-analysis. Liver International. 2011;**31**:802-809. DOI: 10.1111/j.1478-3231.2011.02508

[66] Qi Y, Cui L, Song Y, Li N. XRCC1 Arg399Gln genetic polymorphism and the risk of hepatocellular carcinoma: A meta-analysis. Molecular Biology Reports. 2014;**41**:879-887. DOI: 10.1007/s11033-013-2929-2930

[67] Long XD, Ma Y, Zhou YF, Yao JG, Ban FZ, Huang YZ, et al. XPD codon 312 and 751 polymorphisms, and AFB1 exposure, and hepatocellular carcinoma risk. BMC Cancer. 2009;**9**:400

[68] Bedard LL, Massey TE. Aflatoxin B1-induced DNA damage and its repair. Cancer Letters. 2006;**241**:174-183

[69] Smela ME, Hamm ML, Henderson PT, Harris CM, Harris TM, Essigmann JM. The aflatoxin B(1) formamidopyrimidine adduct plays a major role in causing the types of mutations observed in human hepatocellular carcinoma. Proceedings of the National Academy of Sciences of the United States of America. 2002;**99**:6655-6660

[70] Brown KL, Deng JZ, Iyer RS, Iyer LG, Voehler MW, Stone MP, et al. Unraveling the aflatoxin-FAPY conundrum: Structural basis for differential replicative processing of isomeric forms of the formamidopyrimidine-type DNA adduct of aflatoxin B1. Journal of the American Chemical Society. 2006;**128**:15188-15199

[71] Wang JS, Groopman JD. DNA damage by mycotoxins. Mutation Research. 1999;**42**:167-181

[72] Croy RG, Wogan GN. Temporal patterns of covalent DNA adducts in rat liver after single and multiple doses of aflatoxin B1. Cancer Research. 1981;**41**:197-203

[73] Guindon-Kezis KA, Mulder JE, Massey TE. In vivo treatment with aflatoxin B1 increases DNA oxidation, base excision repair activity and 8-oxoguanine DNA glycosylase 1 levels in mouse lung. Toxicology. 2014;**321**:21-26. DOI: 10.1016/j.tox.2014.03.004

[74] Barraud L, Douki T, Guerret S, Chevallier M, Jamard C, Trepo C, et al. The role of duck hepatitis B virus and aflatoxin B1 in the inductionof oxidative stress in the liver. Cancer Detection and Prevention. 2001;**25**(2):192-201

[75] Shen HM, Shi CY, Shen Y, Ong CN. Detection of elevated reactive oxygen species level in cultured rat hepatocytes treated with aflatoxin B1. Free Radical Biology & Medicine. 1996;**21**:139-146

[76] Niranjan BG, Bhat NK, Avadhani NG. Preferential attack of mitochondrial DNA by aflatoxin B1 during hepatocarcinogenesis. Science. 1982;**215**:73-75

[77] Liu Y, Wang W. Aflatoxin B1 impairs mitochondrial functions, activates ROS generation, induces apoptosis and involves Nrf2 signal pathway in primary broiler hepatocytes. Animal Science Journal. 2016;**87**:1490-1500. DOI: 10.1111/asj.12550

[78] Taby R, Issa JP. Cancer epigenetics. CA: A Cancer Journal for Clinicians. 2010;**60**:376-392. DOI: 10.3322/caac.20085

[79] Zhang YJ, Wu HC, Yazici H, Yu MW, Lee PH, Santella RM. Global hypomethylation in hepatocellular carcinoma and its relationship to aflatoxin B(1) exposure. World Journal of Hepatology. 2012;**4**:169-175. DOI: 10.4254/wjh.v4.i5.169

[80] Kim MJ, White-Cross JA, Shen L, Issa JP, Rashid A. Hypomethylation of long interspersed nuclear element-1 in hepatocellular carcinomas. Modern Pathology. 2009;**22**:442-449. DOI: 10.1038/modpathol.2008.203

[81] Zhu C, Utsunomiya T, Ikemoto T, Yamada S, Morine Y, Imura S, et al. Hypomethylation of long interspersed nuclear element-1 (LINE-1) is associated with poor prognosis via activation of c-MET in hepatocellular carcinoma. Annals of Surgical Oncology. 2014;**21**(Suppl 4):S729-S735. DOI: 10.1245/s10434-014-3874-4

[82] Zhang YJ, Chen Y, Ahsan H, Lunn RM, Lee PH, Chen CJ, et al. Inactivation of the DNA repair gene O6-methylguanine-DNA methyltransferase by promoter hypermethylation and its relationship to aflatoxin B1-DNA adducts and p53 mutation in hepatocellular carcinoma. International Journal of Cancer. 2003;**103**:440-444

[83] Dai Y, Huang K, Zhang B, Zhu L, Xu W. Aflatoxin B1-induced epigenetic alterations: An overview. Food and Chemical Toxicology. 2017;**109**:683-689. DOI: 10.1016/j.fct.2017.06.034

[84] Huang S, He X. The role of microRNAs in liver cancer progression. British Journal of Cancer. 2011;**104**:235-240. DOI: 10.1038/sj.bjc.6606010

[85] Xue H, Tian GY. MiR-429 regulates the metastasis and EMT of HCC cells through targeting RAB23. Archives of Biochemistry and Biophysics. 2018;**637**:48-55. DOI: 10.1016/j.abb.2017.11.011

[86] Liu YX, Long XD, Xi ZF, Ma Y, Huang XY, Yao JG, et al. Micro RNA-24 modulates aflatoxin B1-related hepatocellular carcinoma prognosis and tumorigenesis. BioMed Research International. 2014;**2014**:482926. DOI: 10.1155/2014/482926

[87] Livingstone MC, Johnson NM, Roebuck BD, Kensler TW, Groopman JD. Profound changes in miRNA

expression during cancer initiation by aflatoxin B(1) and their abrogation by the chemopreventive triterpenoid CDDO-Im. Molecular Carcinogenesis. 2017;**56**:2382-2390. DOI: 10.1002/mc.22635

[88] Bandiera S, Pfeffer S, Baumert TF, Zeisel MB. miR-122—A key factor and therapeutic target in liver disease. Journal of Hepatology. 2015;**62**:448-457. DOI: 10.1016/j.jhep.2014.10.004

[89] Wang Y, Zhang Z, Wang H, Zhang Y, Ji M, Xu H, et al. miR-138-1* regulates aflatoxin B1-induced malignant transformation of BEAS-2B cells by targeting PDK1. Archives of Toxicology. 2016;**90**:1239-1249. DOI: 10.1007/s00204-015-1551-4

[90] Yen CS, Su ZR, Lee YP, Liu IT, Yen CJ. miR-106b promotes cancer progression in hepatitis B virus-associated hepatocellular carcinoma. World Journal of Gastroenterology. 2016;**22**(22):5183-5192. DOI: 10.3748/wjg.v22.i22.5183

[91] Luo J-H. Oncogenic activity of MCM7 transforming cluster. World Journal of Clinical Oncology. 2011;**2**:120-124. DOI: 10.5306/wjco.v2.i2.120

[92] Ames BN, Durston WE, Yamasaki E, Lee FD. Carcinogens are mutagens: A simple test system combining liver homogenates for activation and bacteria for detection. Proceedings of the National Academy of Sciences of the United States of America. 1973;**70**(8):2281-2285

[93] McCann J, Spingarn NE, Kobori J, Ames BN. Detection of carcinogens as mutagens: Bacterial tester strains with R factor plasmids. Proceedings of the National Academy of Sciences of the United States of America. 1975;**72**:979-983

[94] Foster PL, Groopman JD, Eisenstadt E. Induction of base substitution mutations by aflatoxin B1 is mucAB dependent in *Escherichia coli*. Journal of Bacteriology. 1988;**170**:3415-3420

[95] Sengstag C, Weibel B, Fasullo M. Genotoxicity of aflatoxin B1: Evidence for a recombination-mediated mechanism in Saccharomyces cerevisiae. Cancer Research. 1996;**56**:5457-5465

[96] Guo Y, Breeden LL, Zarbl H, Preston BD, Eaton DL. Expression of a human cytochrome p450 in yeast permits analysis of pathways for response to and repair of aflatoxin-induced DNA damage. Molecular and Cellular Biology. 2005;**25**:5823-5833

[97] Denissenko MF, Cahill J, Koudriakova TB, Gerber N, Pfeifer GP. Quantitation and mapping of aflatoxin B1-induced DNA damage in genomic DNA using aflatoxin B1-8,9-epoxide and microsomal activation systems. Mutation Research. 1999;**425**:205-211

[98] Bahassi el M, Stambrook PJ. Next-generation sequencing technologies: Breaking the sound barrier of human genetics. Mutagenesis. 2014;**29**:303-310. DOI: 10.1093/mutage/geu031. Review. PubMed PMID: 25150023

[99] Huang MN, Yu W, Teoh WW, Ardin M, Jusakul A, Ng AWT, et al. Genome-scale mutational signatures of aflatoxin in cells, mice, and human tumors. Genome Research. 2017;**27**:1475-1486. DOI: 10.1101/gr.220038.116

[100] Aguilar F, Harris CC, Sun T, Hollstein M, Cerutti P. Geographic variation of p53 mutational profile in nonmalignant human liver. Science. 1994;**26**:1317-1319

[101] https://cancer.sanger.ac.uk/cosmic/signatures

[102] Chawanthayatham S, Valentine CC 3rd, Fedeles BI, Fox EJ, Loeb LA, Levine SS, et al. Mutational spectra

of aflatoxin B(1) in vivo establish biomarkers of exposure for human hepatocellular carcinoma. Proceedings of the National Academy of Sciences of the United States of America. 2017;**114**(15):E3101-E3109. DOI: 10.1073/pnas.1700759114

[103] Fasullo MT, Davis RW. Recombinational substrates designed to study recombination between unique and repetitive sequences in vivo. Proceedings of the National Academy of Sciences of the United States of America. 1987;**84**:6215-6219

[104] Stettler PM, Sengstag C. Liver carcinogen aflatoxin B1 as an inducer of mitotic recombination in a human cell line. Molecular Carcinogenesis. 2001;**31**:125-138

[105] Turkez H, Geyikoğlu F, Dirican E, Tatar A. In vitro studies on chemoprotective effect of borax against aflatoxin B1-induced genetic damage in human lymphocytes. Cytotechnology. 2012;**64**:607-612. DOI: 10.1007/s10616-012-9454-1

[106] Thomson VE, Evans HJ. Induction of sister-chromatid exchanges in human lymphocytes and Chinese hamster cells exposed to aflatoxin B1 and N-methyl-N-nitrosourea. Mutation Research. 1979;**67**(1):47-53

[107] Batt TR, Hsueh JL, Chen HH, Huang CC. Sister chromatid exchanges and chromosome aberrations in V79 cells induced by aflatoxin B1, B2, G1 and G2 with or without metabolic activation. Carcinogenesis. 1980;**1**:759-763

[108] Iyama T, Wilson DM 3rd. DNA repair mechanisms in dividing and non-dividing cells. DNA Repair (Amst). 2013;**12**:620-636. DOI: 10.1016/j.dnarep.2013.04.015

[109] Kisker C, Kuper J, Van Houten B. Prokaryotic nucleotide excision repair. Cold Spring Harbor Perspectives in Biology. 2013;**5**(3):a012591. DOI: 10.1101/cshperspect.a012591

[110] Kuper J, Kisker C. Damage recognition in nucleotide excision DNA repair. Current Opinion in Structural Biology. 2012;**22**:88-93. DOI: 10.1016/j.sbi.2011.12.002

[111] Brown KL, Voehler MW, Magee SM, Harris CM, Harris TM, Stone MP. Structural perturbations induced by the alpha-anomer of the aflatoxin B(1) formamidopyrimidine adduct in duplex and single-strand DNA. Journal of the American Chemical Society. 2009;**131**:16096-16107. DOI: 10.1021/ja902052v

[112] Oleykowski CA, Mayernik JA, Lim SE, Groopman JD, Grossman L, Wogan GN, et al. Repair of aflatoxin B1 DNA adducts by the UvrABC endonuclease of *Escherichia coli*. The Journal of Biological Chemistry. 1993;**268**(11):7990-8002

[113] Keller-Seitz MU, Certa U, Sengstag C, Würgler FE, Sun M, Fasullo M. Transcriptional response of yeast to aflatoxin B1: Recombinational repair involving RAD51 and RAD1. Molecular Biology of the Cell. 2004;**15**:4321-4336

[114] Fasullo M, Chen Y, Bortcosh W, Sun M, Egner PA. Aflatoxin B(1)-associated DNA adducts stall S phase and stimulate Rad51 foci in *Saccharomyces cerevisiae*. Journal of Nucleic Acids. 2010;**2010**:456487. DOI: 10.4061/2010/456487

[115] Leadon SA, Tyrrell RM, Cerutti PA. Excision repair of aflatoxin B1-DNA adducts in human fibroblasts. Cancer Research. 1981;**41**(12, Pt 1):5125-5129

[116] Alekseyev YO, Hamm ML, Essigmann JM. Aflatoxin B1 formamidopyrimidine adducts are preferentially repaired by the nucleotide excision repair pathway in vivo. Carcinogenesis. 2004;**25**:1045-1051

[117] Takahashi Y, Nakatsuru Y, Zhang S, Shimizu Y, Kume H, Tanaka K, et al. Enhanced spontaneous and aflatoxin-induced liver tumorigenesis in xeroderma pigmentosum group A gene-deficient mice. Carcinogenesis. 2002;**23**(4):627-633

[118] Croy RG, Wogan GN. Quantitative comparison of covalent aflatoxin-DNA adducts formed in rat and mouse livers and kidneys. Journal of the National Cancer Institute. 1981;**66**:761-768

[119] Fortini P, Dogliotti E. Base damage and single-strand break repair: Mechanisms and functional significance of short- and long-patch repair subpathways. DNA Repair (Amst). 2007;**6**:398-409

[120] Helleday T. The underlying mechanism for the PARP and BRCA synthetic lethality: Clearing up the misunderstandings. Molecular Oncology. 2011;**5**:387-393. DOI: 10.1016/j.molonc.2011.07.001

[121] Vartanian V, Minko IG, Chawanthayatham S, Egner PA, Lin YC, Earley LF, et al. NEIL1 protects against aflatoxin-induced hepatocellular carcinoma in mice. Proceedings of the National Academy of Sciences of the United States of America. 2017;**114**:4207-4212. DOI: 10.1073/pnas.1620932114

[122] Mulder JE, Turner PV, Massey TE. Effect of 8-oxoguanine glycosylase deficiency on aflatoxin B1 tumourigenicity in mice. Mutagenesis. 2015;**30**:401-409. DOI: 10.1093/mutage/geu087

[123] Kakehashi A, Ishii N, Okuno T, Fujioka M, Gi M, Wanibuchi H. Enhanced susceptibility of Ogg1 mutant mice to multiorgan carcinogenesis. International Journal of Molecular Sciences. 2017;**18**(8). pii: E1801. DOI: 10.3390/ijms18081801

[124] Bennett CB, Lewis AL, Baldwin KK, Resnick MA. Lethality induced by a single site-specific double-strand break in a dispensable yeast plasmid. Proceedings of the National Academy of Sciences of the United States of America. 1993;**90**:5613-5617

[125] Fasullo M, Giallanza P, Dong Z, Cera C, Bennett T. *Saccharomyces cerevisiae* rad51 mutants are defective in DNA damage-associated sister chromatid exchanges but exhibit increased rates of homology-directed translocations. Genetics. 2001;**158**:959-972

[126] Boiteux S, Jinks-Robertson S. DNA repair mechanisms and the bypass of DNA damage in *Saccharomyces cerevisiae*. Genetics. 2013;**193**(4):1025-1064. DOI: 10.1534/genetics.112.145219

[127] Chatterjee N, Siede W. Replicating damaged DNA in eukaryotes. Cold Spring Harbor Perspectives in Biology. 2013;**5**(12):a019836. DOI: 10.1101/cshperspect.a019836

[128] Vaisman A, Woodgate R. Translesion DNA polymerases in eukaryotes: What makes them tick? Critical Reviews in Biochemistry and Molecular Biology. 2017;**52**(3):274-303. DOI: 10.1080/10409238.2017.1291576

[129] Lin YC, Li L, Makarova AV, Burgers PM, Stone MP, Lloyd RS. Molecular basis of aflatoxin-induced mutagenesis-role of the aflatoxin B1-formamidopyrimidine adduct. Carcinogenesis. 2014;**35**:1461-1468. DOI: 10.1093/carcin/bgu003

[130] Lin YC, Li L, Makarova AV, Burgers PM, Stone MP, Lloyd RS. Error-prone replication bypass of the primary aflatoxin B1 DNA adduct, AFB1-N7-Gua. The Journal of Biological Chemistry. 2014;**289**(26):18497-18506. DOI: 10.1074/jbc.M114.561563

[131] Lin YC, Owen N, Minko IG, Lange SS, Tomida J, Li L, et al. DNA

polymerase ζ limits chromosomal damage and promotes cell survival following aflatoxin exposure. Proceedings of the National Academy of Sciences of the United States of America. 2016;**113**:13774-13779

[132] Sharma S, Helchowski CM, Canman CE. The roles of DNA polymerase ζ and the Y family DNA polymerases in promoting or preventing genome instability. Mutation Research. 2013;**743-744**:97-110. DOI: 10.1016/j.mrfmmm.2012.11.002

[133] Fasullo M, Sun M, Egner P. Stimulation of sister chromatid exchanges and mutation by aflatoxin B1-DNA adducts in *Saccharomyces cerevisiae* requires MEC1(ATR), RAD53, and DUN1. Molecular Carcinogenesis. 2008;**47**:608-615. DOI: 10.1002/mc.20417

[134] Mulder JE, Bondy GS, Mehta R, Massey TE. The impact of chronic Aflatoxin B1 exposure and p53 genotype on base excision repair in mouse lung and liver. Mutation Research. 2015;**773**:63-68. DOI: 10.1016/j.mrfmmm.2015.01.015

[135] Bedard LL, Alessi M, Davey S, Massey TE. Susceptibility to aflatoxin B1-induced carcinogenesis correlates with tissue-specific differences in DNA repair activity in mouse and in rat. Cancer Research. 2005;**65**:1265-1270

[136] Guo Y, Breeden LL, Fan W, Zhao LP, Eaton DL, Zarbl H. Analysis of cellular responses to aflatoxin B(1) in yeast expressing human cytochrome P450 1A2 using cDNA microarrays. Mutation Research. 2006;**593**:121-142

[137] Gasch AP, Spellman PT, Kao CM, Carmel-Harel O, Eisen MB, Storz G, et al. Genomic expression programs in the response of yeast cells to environmental changes. Molecular Biology of the Cell. 2000;**11**:4241-4257

[138] Merrick BA, Phadke DP, Auerbach SS, Mav D, Stiegelmeyer SM, Shah RR, et al. RNA-Seq profiling reveals novel hepatic gene expression pattern in aflatoxin B1 treated rats. PLoS One. 2013;**8**:e61768. DOI: 10.1371/journal.pone.0061768

[139] Gursoy-Yuzugullu O, Yuzugullu H, Yilmaz M, Ozturk M. Aflatoxin genotoxicity is associated with a defective DNA damage response bypassing p53 activation. Liver International. 2011;**31**(4):561-571. DOI: 10.1111/j.1478-3231.2011.02474

[140] Zhang Z, Lu H, Huan F, Meghan C, Yang X, Wang Y, et al. Cytochrome P450 2A13 mediates the neoplastic transformation of human bronchial epithelial cells at a low concentration of aflatoxin B1. International Journal of Cancer. 2014;**134**(7):1539-1548. DOI: 10.1002/ijc.28489

Section 3

Epigenetics Insight

Chapter 5

Epigenetics: Dissecting Gene Expression Alteration in PDAC

Alia Abukiwan and Martin R. Berger

Abstract

Pancreatic cancer is the fourth leading cause of cancer deaths, with a low 5-year survival rate of about 7% due to its highly invasive nature. Pancreatic ductal adenocarcinoma (PDAC) comprises more than 90% of all pancreatic cancer cases. At the time of detection, around 80% of cases harbor metastases due to the lack of early diagnosis. For decades, scientists have primarily focused on dissecting the origin of pancreatic cancer through genetic alterations and their contribution to diagnosis. Recently, PDAC research has turned into epigenetics to revolutionize our understanding about the silencing of critical regulatory genes. Epigenetic events can be divided mechanistically into various components, including DNA methylation, histone posttranslational modification, nucleosome remodeling, and regulation of transcription or translation by microRNA. The identified epigenetic processes in PDAC contribute to its specific epigenotype and are correlated phenotypic features. Strikingly, some of them have been suggested to have potential as cancer biomarkers, for disease monitoring, prognosis, and risk validation. As epigenetic aberrations are reversible, their correction will become as a promising therapeutic target.

Keywords: PDAC, epigenetics, DNA methylation, histone modification, microRNA, 3' UTR

1. Introduction

Pancreatic ductal adenocarcinoma (PDAC) comprises more than 90% of all pancreatic cancer cases. It is highly aggressive, extremely lethal and shows resistance to chemotherapy [1–3]. At diagnosis, around 80% of PDAC cases have already metastasized, thus rendering the current therapeutic options practically ineffective. In line with this, potentially curative surgical resection is limited to a very small portion of patients [4].

On the other hand, cancer metastasis is associated not only with simple gene/protein expression models but also with the existence of epigenetic mechanisms [5], which complicates this process through DNA methylation, histone modifications, and microRNA regulation (see **Figure 1**). Recent studies uncovered the regulatory mechanisms of each process and their key role in EMT and cancer metastasis [6].

2. PDAC from genetics to epigenetics

Historically, the development of PDAC was attributed to DNA mutations, which are classified into three main types: oncogenes (KRAS, BRAF, AKT2, MYB, and AIBI),

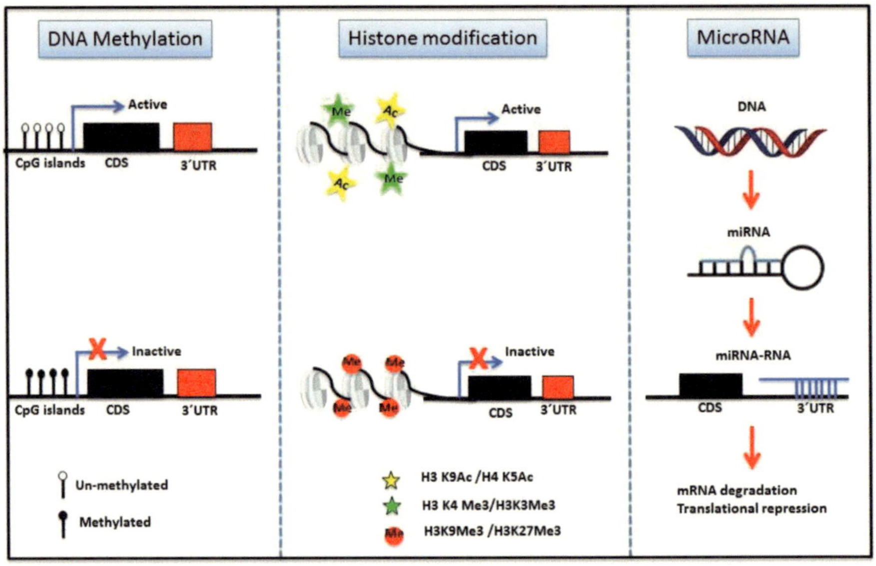

Figure 1.
Schematic diagram of epigenetic mechanisms influencing gene expression. DNA methylation is an epigenetic mechanism through which cytosine residues within CpG regions are covalently modified (left). In addition, the modification of histones has two consequences on genes, which pending on the type of modification and the target residues can either activate or repress the target gene (middle). The epigenetic mechanism is also influenced by microRNAs (miRNAs). These are small noncoding RNAs, which have a proximal length of 22 nucleotides. Functionally, the miRNAs influence gene expression through base pairing with 3' UTRs of messenger RNAs (right).

tumor suppressor genes (p16, CDKN2A, p53, p21, BRCA2, and SMAD4), and genome maintenance and repair genes (MLH, MSH2, and BRCA2) [1, 2]. Several studies explained the complexity of genetic aberrations and their regulatory signaling pathways [3]. Although a large variety of signal transduction pathways have already been studied in PDAC, much less is known about the cross talk between epigenetic mechanism and signaling pathways typical for PDAC [1]. Strikingly, there are also particular cases where signaling pathways are altered, which directly affect important components of the epigenetic machinery. Therefore, a clear understanding of the epigenetic mechanisms and their implication in PDAC development will open new avenues of therapy. This approach will exploit the intricate process through which cells induce changes at transcription level [4–6].

Epigenetic mechanisms are defined in a way that they can both silence or activate genes without alteration to the DNA sequence itself. Mechanistically, epigenetic changes represent DNA hypermethylation or hypomethylation, histone-based mechanisms that include posttranslational modifications and nucleosome remodeling, as well as aberrant expression of microRNAs [5, 7]. These modifications affect chromatin structure and promoter accessibility, which contribute to genetic alterations [8].

In PDAC, the famous mutant gene KRAS and its downstream signaling cascade are an example for the low therapeutic effect, which is accomplished by current therapies against this gene and its downstream effectors. Interestingly, recent studies demonstrate that dysregulation of epigenetic regulators is essential for PDAC progression as well as for that of many other tumors [9]. Genomic deletions, mutations, and rearrangements frequently target genes encoding components of the chromatin remodeling complex (SWI/SNF), which have been identified in 10–15% of PDAC patients [10].

In general, the discovery of the involvement of the epigenetic effect in cancer added a new concept of gene therapy and informative markers for the diagnosis and prognosis for many malignancies [11]. Whole genomic sequencing studies have revealed driver mutations in epigenetic regulators in various cancer types such as IDH1/2, DNMT3A, KDM6A, DNMT3B, SMARCB1, and CREBBP/EP300 [12]. In PDAC, the sequencing experiments showed more pathogenic mutations in genes encoding multiple components of the SWI/SNF complexes, including ARID1A, ARID1B, PBRM1, SMARCA2, and SMARCA4 [13]. Additionally, recent studies found mutations in important epigenetic regulators like histone methyltransferase enzymes MLL1, MLL2, and MLL3 and histone demethylase KDM6A [13, 14]. Specifically, KDM6A has been found mutated in 5–10% of PDAC patients [15].

Several studies on familial PDAC have shown an association between DNA repair genes' dysfunction and those genes that are responsible for this inheritance (BRCA2, BRCA1, CDKN2A/p16, STK11/LKB1) [13, 16]. Strikingly, the altered DNA repair system is a hallmark of cancer, which causes genome instability and DNA damage [17]. Each cell contains a specific enzymatic system termed the DNA mismatch repair (MMR), which is responsible for detecting and correcting DNA replication errors [18, 19]. Loss or silencing of any protein in this system leads to the accumulation of gene mutations. In this regard, studies reported that MMR inactivation was caused by the epigenetic silencing of the hMLH1 and hMLH2 genes [20, 21]. The hMLH1 protein is one component of a family of seven members of MMR proteins that work coordinately to regulate DNA replication error in humans [20]. In this context, hypermethylation of the hMLH1 promoter has been shown to be an early detection marker of esophageal cancer and also a prognostic marker in colorectal and pancreatic cancers. On the other hand, this mechanism cannot be generalized, as methylation of the hMLH2 gene results less clear into gene inactivation, because the respective promoter is a weak target for CpG island methylation [16, 17, 20–22].

Another example of an affected DNA repair gene is the O^6-methylguanine-DNA transferase (MGMT), which is most intensively regulated by CpG promoter methylation [23]. MGMT is responsible for removing alkyl groups from O^6 in guanine and thus prevents mismatch errors during DNA replication. The silencing of the MGMT activity in human colorectal adenomas has been linked to K-ras GC → AT transition mutations [24, 25]. Interestingly, the epigenetic silencing of MGMT has two main effects in human cancer. First, it reveals a new mutator pathway that causes the accumulation of G-to-A transition mutations. Second, there is a strong and significant positive association between MGMT promoter hypermethylation and enhanced tumor sensitivity to alkylating drugs. These findings highlight the significance of MGMT promoter hypermethylation in translational cancer research [17, 26, 27].

3. DNA methylation

The first epigenetic modification to be identified was DNA methylation [28], which is based on stable and heritable changes in gene structure without a change in DNA sequence [12]. Methylation refers to the addition of a methyl group to the fifth carbon in cytosine forming 5-methylcytosine (5-mC), which is mediated by DNMTs [29]. Generally, methylation occurs in intergenic regions and repetitive sequences such as satellite repeats, and long and short interspersed nuclear elements, while CpG islands of gene promoters often are unmethylated [5, 7, 30]. Interestingly, the global effects of epigenetic alterations in gene regulatory sequences from over 100 cancer cell lines have been identified by the ENCODE project [31]. Normally, DNA methylation is critical for maintaining pluripotency, X chromosome inactivation, and genome imprinting [12]. Aberrant DNA methylation is one of the hallmarks of cancer [32].

Methylation of DNA is catalyzed by the enzymes DNMT3A and DNMT3B and is then maintained by the major DNA methyltransferase DNMT1, which is also assisted by DNMT3A and DNMT3B [9, 12]. A recent study found that DNMT1, DNMT3A, and DNMT3B are themselves differentially methylated in PDAC [33]. Besides, a very recent finding suggests that the interactions between TP53 and H3K4, MLL3 and MOZ genes play a major role in chromatin regulation [34]. The methylation of tumor suppressor genes is the best-characterized epigenetic event in several malignancies, including PDAC [11]. In fact, several genes such as APC, BRCA1, P16INK4a, P15INK4b, RARβ, and p73 are frequently methylated [10]. Recent studies have revealed that apparent DNA methylation occurred in critical signaling pathways in PDAC such as TGFβ, WNT, integrin, cell adhesion, and axon guidance signaling pathways [35]. Likewise, TGFβ induces epithelial-mesenchymal transition (EMT) by enhancing hypermethylation of CpG islands in the VAV1 gene promoter [36] (see **Figure 2**). Furthermore, the WNT signaling pathway is a target of hypermethylation in PDAC. This has been found for WNT ligands WNT5A, WNT7A, and WNT9A, or the cell surface receptor FZD9, or the cytoplasmic transducer APC2, the nuclear factors SOX1, SOX7, SOX14, and SOX17, and the pathway inhibitors FRZB, SFRP1, SFRP2, KREMEN2, NKD2, and WIF1. Strikingly, the tumor suppressor candidate HIC1 is hypermethylated, which is acting as a transcriptional repressor for abnormal survival circuits of the transcription factors involved in the WNT signaling pathway [33, 37].

Furthermore, several studies demonstrated that promoter DNA hypermethylation is associated with the transcriptional repression of multiple microRNAs (miRNAs). This results into upregulation of oncogenic target genes of the microRNAs, such as observed for the downregulation of miR-181b, which promotes the

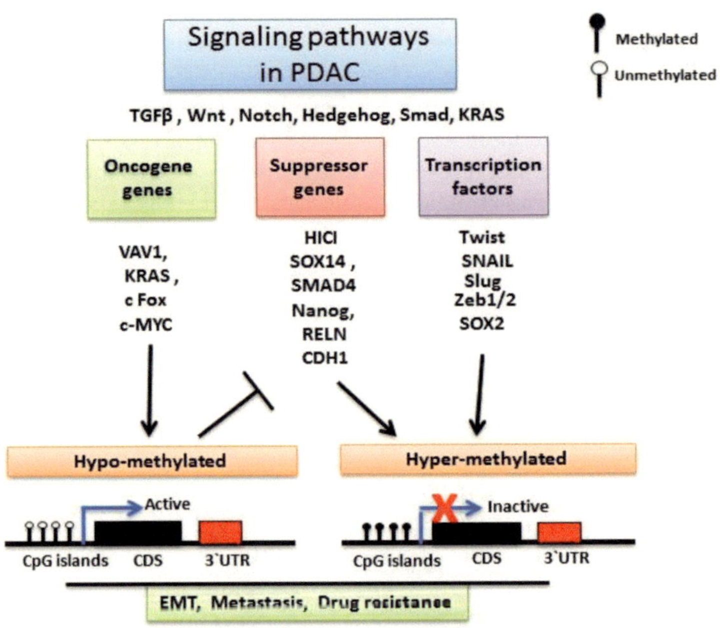

Figure 2.
Schematic diagram of signaling pathways in PDAC, which are deregulated by DNA methylation. Critical tumor suppressors and transcription factors are silenced, whereas oncogenes are activated. This deregulation promotes EMT and metastasis.

Gene	Gene name	Epigenetic alteration	Function	References
CADM1	Cell adhesion molecule 1	Hypermethylation	Cell-cell interaction	[41]
CDH1	Epithelial cadherin	Hypermethylation	Cell adhesion and invasion	[42]
DKK3	Dickkopf-related protein 3	Hypermethylation	Tumor suppressor	[43]
S100A4	S100 calcium-binding protein A4	Hypermethylation	Invasion, motility, and tubulin polymerization	[44]
P16	Cyclin-dependent kinase inhibitor 2A	Hypermethylation	Multiple tumor suppressor	[45]
DNMT3A	DNA (cytosine-5-)-methyltransferase 3 alpha	Hypermethylation	Enzyme	[33]
BMP3	Bone morphogenetic protein 3	Hypermethylation	Growth factor	[33]
ST6GAL2	ST6 beta-galactosamide alpha-2,6-sialyltranferase 2	Hypermethylation	Generation of the cell surface carbohydrate determinants and differentiation antigens	[42]
ST8SIA5	ST8 alpha-N-acetyl-neuraminide α-2,8-sialyltransferase 5	Hypermethylation	A member of glycosyltransferase family	[42]
ST8SIA2	ST8 α-N-acetyl-neuraminide alpha-2,8-sialyltransferase 2	Hypermethylation	A member of glycosyltransferase family	[42]
ST8SIA3	ST8 α-N-acetyl-neuraminideα-2,8-sialyltransferase 3	Hypermethylation	A member of glycosyltransferase family	[42]
AKT1	v-Akt murine thymoma viral oncogene homolog 1	Hypermethylation	Kinases	[30]
LCN2	Lipocalin 2	Hypomethylation	Epithelial differentiation	[33]
CCND2	Cyclin D2	Hypermethylation	Cell cycle control	[33]
CLDN4	Claudin-4	Hypomethylation	Cell adhesion	[44]
miR-9-1	MicroRNA-9	Hypomethylation	miRNA translation control	[40]
P59	Cyclin-dependent kinase inhibitor 1C	Hypermethylation	Cyclin-dependent kinase inhibitor	[34]
P16	Cyclin-dependent kinase inhibitor 2A	Hypermethylation	Cyclin-dependent kinase inhibitor	[33]
RARB	Retinoic acid receptor	Hypermethylation	Cell growth control	[33]
SFN	Stratifin (14-3-3sigma)	Hypomethylation	P53-induced G2/M cell cycle arrest	[9]
LCN2	Tissue factor pathway inhibitor	Hypomethylation	Epithelial differentiation	[9]

Gene	Gene name	Epigenetic alteration	Function	References
CDKN1C/ P57	Cyclin-dependent kinase inhibitor 1C	Hypomethylation	Cyclin-dependent kinase inhibitor	[42]
FOXE1	Forkhead box E1	Hypomethylation	Thyroid transcription factor	[42]

Table 1.
A series of methylated genes in PDAC.

expression of BCL 2 [38]. Moreover, downregulation of the miR-29 family was associated with the overexpression of the DNA methyltransferases DNMT3A and DNM3B [39]. The noncoding RNAs and antisense RNA sequences are strongly involved in the respective DNA hypermethylation process, which silences important genes such as polycomb group (PcGs), which in turn may expose these regions to DNA methylation changes [40]. More examples are listed in **Table 1**, all of which are related to PDAC.

4. Histone modification

Nucleosomes are considered to be the basic constituents of chromatin. Each nucleosome is an octamer of histones, which consist of two copies each of histone proteins H2A, H2B, H3, and H4 [46]. The most interesting epigenetic events in PDAC are histone modifications, since several studies revealed that the most frequently mutated epigenetic genes occurred in the histone family [13]. The posttranslational modifications include methylation, acetylation, citrullination, phosphorylation, SUMOylation, and ADP ribosylation. However, the most studied histone modifications in cancer are lysine alterations, including lysine methylation, acetylation, and phosphorylation [47–49]. In normal cell development, histone modifications regulate critical cell processes such as DNA replication and transcription or repair [46], while in cancer, histone modifications contribute to the maintenance of malignant phenotypes. In PDAC, the most common modification includes methylation and acetylation of lysine residues within the N terminal tails of histone proteins [11].

In the context of epithelial-mesenchymal transition (EMT) in PDAC, SNAIL is a critical transcription repressor of E-cadherin in EMT process. It plays a significant role in embryonic development and tumorigenesis [50]. Moreover, SNAIL has an essential function in histone modifications. This includes the activation of a set of chromatin modifiers such as lysine-specific demethylase, euchromatic histone lysine methyltransferase 2 (G 9a), suppressor of variegation 3–9 homolog 1 histone methyltransferases (Suv39H1), SIN3 transcription regulator family member A (SIN3A), and histone deacetylases (HDAC1 and HDAC2) [51, 52].

4.1 Histone methylation

Methylation of histones is coordinated by histone methyltransferases (HMTs) and histone demethylases (HDMs). There are at least 17 different HMTs, all of which share the conserved (Su (var) 3–9, enhancer-of-zeste, trithorax) motif. The lysine methylation residue is most common and is mediated by histone lysine methyltransferases (HKMTs) [53]. Particularly, methylation at H3K9, H3K27, and H3K20 is associated with transcriptional repression, while methylation of H3K4, H3K36, and H3K79 causes transcriptional activation [47]. The silencing of tumor suppressor genes in cancer is caused by the corresponding activities of the HMT and HDMT enzymes. On the other hand, the H3K27me3-specific HMT EZH2 (enhancer of zeste homolog 2), the catalytic subunit of PRC2, is overexpressed in a broad range of solid tumors, including prostate, lung, breast, colon, skin, and pancreatic cancers [54, 55].

The most frequently altered histone methylated genes in PDAC are KDM6A and MLL2 [33]. KDM6A is an H3K27me3 demethylase, which has a role in endoderm differentiation by regulating the expression of WNT signaling and HOX genes [56]. Other studies found that the loss of trimethylation at K27 of histone H3, which causes nuclear accumulation of EZH2, is strongly correlated with a poor PDAC outcome [57]. Various interactions have been shown to occur between DNA methylation and histone methylation. For example, the interaction between EZH2 and DNMTs renders the EZH2 gene a potential therapeutic target. Mucins (MUCs) are also known to play essential roles in tumor growth and invasion in pancreatic neoplasms. MUC1 and MUC4 are high-molecular-weight transmembrane mucins. Overexpression of mucins in cancer is associated with poor prognosis. It has been shown that mucin expression changes in PDAC are due to DNA methylation of H3 at the lysine9 residue [58, 59].

4.2 Histone acetylation

Histone acetylation is the first discovered histone modification. The acetylation of lysine residues neutralizes their positive charge, which induces chromatin relaxation and activates a set of genes associated with transcription. On the other hand, removal of the acetyl groups is associated with gene silencing. Histone acetylases (HATs) and deacetylases (HDAC) are the required enzymes for this process [60, 61] (see **Figure 3a**).

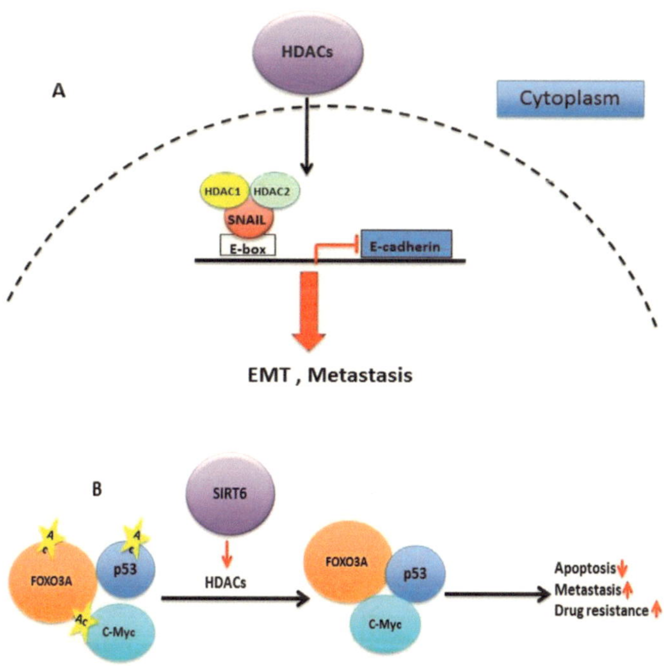

Figure 3.
Schematic diagram on the role of HDACs in PDAC. (A) HDACs mediate E-cadherin translational repression by activating the binding of EMT transcription factors to the E-boxes present in the E-cadherin promoter. (B) SIRT6 mediates the deacetylation of p53, FOXO3A, and C-Myc, which leads to increased metastasis and drug resistance.

Recent studies show a series of significant alterations of the acetylation process in PDAC, as well as mutations in the histone acetylase EP300 [33]. Furthermore, the SIRT6 gene is associated with the deacetylation of histone H3 at lysine residues 9 and 56, thus increasing the expression of the SIRT6 gene associated with PDAC metastasis by deacetylation of p53 and FOXOA3 [62] (see **Figure 3b**). For instance, the activation of KRAS and increased expression of the c-Myc transcription factor promote PDAC metastasis [13]. Also, expression of HDAC7 and HDAC2 has been found increased in PDAC [63]. In addition, HDACs/HATs play important roles in the activation of several tumor suppressor genes in PDAC, such as p53 and EP300 [11, 14, 53, 64].

A recent study identified the acetylation of glutamate oxaloacetate transaminases 2 (GOT2) at three lysine residues (K159, K185, and K404) in PDAC. This promotes the transfer of NADH from the cytoplasm into mitochondria, enhancing PDAC cell proliferation and tumor growth in vivo. On the other hand, the acetylation of GOT2 at only K159 is correlated with downregulation of SIRT3 expression [65].

4.3 Histone phosphorylation

Histone phosphorylation has been associated with different cell processes, including apoptosis, cell cycle, DNA transcription, DNA repair, chromosome condensation, gene regulation, cell signaling pathways, energy, and metabolic pathways [66]. Phosphorylation of histones occurs on serine, threonine, and tyrosine residues, a process mediated by different kinases and phosphatases [46]. In cell development, the most important site for histone phosphorylation is the serine 10 of histone H3 (H3S10P), which is mediated by the Aurora-B kinase. This modification is a critical event in cell mitosis and meiosis [67].

Several studies identified histone phosphorylation changes during DNA damage, such as the phosphorylation of serine 139 on the histone H2A(X). On the other hand, phosphorylation of serines, e.g., 10 and 28 on H3, and serine 32 on H2B have been contributed by the activation of the epidermal growth factor (EGF). Moreover, H3ser28p mediated the expression of c-fos and α-globin [68–70].

It has been shown that H2A T120 is phosphorylated in PDAC by VRK1 on the promoter region of CCND1, which consequently activates the transcription of cyclin D1 [71]. Besides, KRAS is most well-studied and known activated oncogene in PDAC [72]. Other studies have implicated the activation of the Ras-MAPK pathway with the upregulation of phospho-ERK1/2 and their downstream levels of H3 S10ph [73].

5. MicroRNA

MicroRNAs (miRNAs) are small (20–23 nucleotides), endogenous, noncoding, single-stranded RNA molecules, which control the expression of around 60% of the protein-coding genes [74]. Moreover, they can control both physiological and pathological processes, such as development and cancer [75]. In addition, the miRNA machinery is of great importance for drug development, since a functional miRNA machinery is a compulsory prerequisite for any RNA interference (RNAi)-based therapy approach. A total of 700 miRNAs have been discovered in human diseases, and more than 1000 predicted miRNA genes are yet to be experimentally validated [76].

Mature microRNAs require several steps of preprocessing before they can become functional. After they are transcribed by RNA polymerase II/III from intragenic regions or from regions that code for introns, the primary transcript (pri-miRNA) is processed by the ribonuclease Drosha and DGCR8 in the nucleus. The process produces pre-microRNAs, hairpin-shaped intermediates of 70–100 nucleotides. Exportin-5, a Ran-GTP-dependent dsRNA-binding protein, transports pre-microRNAs into the cytoplasm where they are further processed by the ribonuclease Dicer and TRBP (Tar RNA-binding protein) into a double-stranded miRNA. The strands separate and a mature single-stranded molecule join an RNA-induced silencing complex (RISC). The double miRNA strands are required to interact with RISC complex or to be degraded. Ordinarily, one miRNA strand can give rise to two individual mature miRNA sequences with different targets due to complementary seed sequence [74, 77, 78]. The single-stranded mature microRNA remains stable on the miRISC and induces posttranscriptional silencing of one or more target genes, usually through imperfect pairing with a target sequence in the 3' UTR [74]. However, this is not the only binding region for miRNAs, as there are also binding sites located in 5' UTR or even within the coding DNA sequence of mRNAs [77]. The seed sequence or seed region is a conserved heptametrical sequence, which is mostly situated at positions 2–7 from the miRNA 5' end [79, 80]. Furthermore, degradation of mature miRNAs appears to depend on their activity; in the absence of complementary targets, the miRNA could be released from miRNA-RISC complex, and then its 5′ end becomes accessible to the 5′ → 3′ exonuclease XRN2, which degrades the miRNA [81].

Cancer represents a heterogeneous group of diseases characterized by uncontrolled growth of cells, high proliferation rates, and apoptosis resistance. All of these features result from a complex of structural and expression abnormalities of genes, including those encoding microRNAs [75, 82]. The classification of cancer is more accurately defined with microRNA profiling than with mRNA profiling because of the strong correlation between microRNA expression signatures and tumor origin [75]. In general, microRNAs have two main functions in cancer; they can act as tumor suppressors (TSmiRs) or oncogenes (OncomiRs) [75, 76, 82, 83].

One of the first indications that miRNAs serve as tumor suppressors (TSmiRs) came from Calin and colleagues when they discovered that miR-15a and miR-16-1 were deleted or downregulated in about 68% of chronic lymphocytic leukemia (CLL) samples. MiR-15a and miR-16-1 have been shown to control the expression of VEGF, a key proangiogenic factor involved in tumor angiogenesis. Furthermore, both of them induce the apoptosis of leukemic cells by affecting the antiapoptotic protein BCL2 [75, 84]. Another prominent TSmiR is the let-7 family, located at a chromosomal region, which is usually deleted in human cancers. It has been reported as a TSmiR in lung, breast [84], urothelial, and cervical cancers [85]. Recent studies found that let-7 was able to regulate the RAS oncogene in lung cancer. In addition, let-7 regulates late embryonic development by suppressing a number of genes such as c-Myc, RAS, and HAMGA2 [76, 82]. Taken together, reduced expression of TSmiRs in cancer releases oncogenic genes and promotes tumor initiation and progression.

In contrast, oncogenic miRNAs (OncomiRs) promote tumorigenesis by inhibiting tumor suppressor genes that play roles within other functions, such as cell differentiation and apoptosis. The first OncomiR that was discovered is the miR-17-92 cluster, which encodes miR-17-5p, miR-17-3p, miR-18a, miR-19a, miR-20a, miR19b-1, and miR-92-1. This cluster is located on chromosome 13 and is commonly found to be amplified in human B-cell lymphomas, lung cancer, and anaplastic thyroid cancer cells [86]. Another oncogenic miRNA, miR-21, has been validated in nine solid tumor types (lung, breast, head and neck, prostate, colon, pancreas, esophagus, stomach, and brain). Experimental data confirmed that miR-21 plays a significant role in cancer cell proliferation, apoptosis, and invasion. Accordingly, inhibition of miR-21 induces cell cycle arrest, increased apoptosis, and increased chemosensitivity to anticancer agents [87].

The important emerging role of miRNAs in many cancer types, together with the fact that they can function as TSmiRs or OncomiRs, supports the potential of miRNAs as a new class of targets in the development of cancer therapies. Several studies have focused on targeting miRNAs as an experimental therapy in vitro or in vivo [85]. Notably, to modulate cancer-associated miRNAs in vivo, two main approaches were established: first, miRNA replacement therapy, which is based on adding the miRNAs missing in cancer cells for restoring their normal functions; second, inhibition of oncogenic miRNAs by using single-stranded chemically modified anti-miR oligonucleotides [85, 88]. The first successful in vivo experiment using anti-miRs in conjunction with locked nucleic acids was successfully applied in African green monkeys with hypercholesterolemia. The experiments resulted in the successful control of triglyceride and cholesterol levels, together with the management of disease manifestations with minimal side effects to herald a new research approach that is equally applicable in cancer [89].

PDAC shares many features with other solid tumors. Numerous studies have reported the significant roles, which miRNAs play in PDAC progression. Furthermore, these studies have also provided important information about cellular features, such as growth, invasive, and metastatic behavior that have been modified or altered in PDAC as a result of miRNAs, thus highlighting, to a large extent, the significance of miRNAs in PDAC progression [90]. High-throughput microarray technologies have been used to extensively profile miRNA signatures in cell lines, normal frozen tissues, formalin-fixed paraffin-embedded tissues (FFPE), blood, and fine needle aspiration biopsy (FNAB) samples, in order to establish a common expression pattern in PDAC [91]. Recently, a meta-analysis reviewed 11 miRNA profiling studies in PDAC and reported 439 miRNAs as deregulated in the 538 PDAC samples that were evaluated [92]. This analysis defines a common pool of

miRNAs	Expression status	Target genes	References
Let-7 family	Downregulated	KRAS, MAPK, c-Myc, STAT3	[94, 104]
miR-181s	Upregulated	TIMP3, TCL1, TGFBI, TRIM2, SIRT1, Bcl2	[91, 105]
miR-26s	Downregulated	MMP2, MMP14, cyclin D1, Mcl-1, Bcl2	[91, 106, 107]
miR-125a	Upregulated	Bcl-w, Bcl2	[108]
miR-192	Downregulated	SERPINE1	[109]
miR-148a,b	Downregulated	DNMT3B, Mtif, CCKBR, BCL2	[90, 91, 110]
miR-200 family	Downregulated	VEGF-A, KRAS, KDR, VEGFR2, ZEB1/2	[100, 111–113]
miR-34a	Downregulated	Notch1/2, Bcl2, SIRIT, CDK4, VEGF	[99, 114–117]
miR-375	Downregulated	PDK1	[90]
miR-124	Downregulated	ITGB1, Rac1, RocK2, EZH1, Bcl2, CDK6	[91, 101, 118]
miR-217	Downregulated	KRAS, SIRIT, c-MYC	[119, 120]
miR-21	Upregulated	PTEN	[121]
miR-132	Upregulated	Rb1, SMAD2	[122, 123]
miR-208	Upregulated	E-cadherin	[106]
miR-196-a	Upregulated	NFKBIA	[124]
miR-100	Upregulated	IGFR1	[90]
miR-155	Upregulated	TP53INP1	[125]
miR-10b	Upregulated	TIP30	[91]

Table 2.
Top frequently deregulated miRNAs in PDAC.

miRNAs that are atypically expressed in PDAC, and the potential renormalization of these miRNAs and/or expression patterns could help create a therapeutic approach in managing this aggressive disease [93].

The commonly deregulated miRNAs are associated with major regulatory genes in several signaling pathways (**Table 2**), which are involved in most aspects of cellular physiology including regulation of cell cycle, differentiation, proliferation, and apoptosis. Notably, altered miRNA expression in PDAC contributes to metastasis and drug resistance [92, 94, 95]. The more frequently deregulated miRNAs in PDAC include miR-21, the expression of which is regulated by KRAS, and correlates with the degree of tumor progression [90]. KRAS is an important molecule in PDAC and is a direct target of miR-96, miR-217, miR-126, and miR-200c. The overexpression of these miRNAs reduces the level of KRAS expression, resulting in decreased cell invasion, migration, and tumor growth [96, 97]. Strikingly, two of these miRNAs, miR-145 and miR-200c, function as a regulatory network in the AKT-PI3K signaling pathway [98]. Conversely, it has been reported that KRAS activation suppresses the expression of the miR-134/145 cluster via the Ras responsive element-binding protein (RREB1) [99]. The miR-200 family is also frequently deregulated in PDAC and plays a significant role in EMT inhibition. One study demonstrated that miR-200 negatively regulates ZEB1 and ZEB2, which are both direct repressors of E-cadherin [100]. In the context of epigenetic modifications, several studies have found TSmiRs in PDAC, including miR-9-1, miR-124s, miR-192, miR-615-5p, and miR-1247, which were hypermethylated [44, 101–103].

6. Conclusions

For the high mortality, poor prognosis, and undefined therapeutic targets in PDAC, the unraveling of the complex molecular layers driving this lethal cancer is a prerequisite for more effective therapeutic strategies and consistent diagnostic markers. The recent research on epigenetic mechanisms has significantly enriched our knowledge about the regulatory characteristics involved in the initiation, progression, and metastasis of PDAC. This book chapter has focused on the most critical epigenetics mechanisms, including DNA methylation, histone modifications, and modulated expression of miRNAs that play a significant role in PDAC tumorigenesis, and could serve as future therapeutic targets. Currently, significant emphasis is still given on detecting somatic genetic alterations in PDAC. However, it seems also promising to investigate the underlying epigenetic mechanisms for completing the full puzzle of altered gene expression in PDAC. The epigenetics field has developed strongly and will continue to advance into a frontier field for PDAC research. Additionally, it is essential to highlight the features of epigenetic mechanisms of gene regulation—their reversibility. This feature provides a ground for specifically targeting the epigenetic changes contributing to PDAC.

Acknowledgements

Alia Abukiwan was funded by the Heidrun-Seibert-Stiftung.

Conflict of Interest

The authors declare no conflict of interest.

Author details

Alia Abukiwan and Martin R. Berger*
Toxicology and Chemotherapy Unit, German Cancer Research Center(DKFZ), Heidelberg, Germany

*Address all correspondence to: m.berger@dkfz.de

References

[1] Ying H et al. Genetics and biology of pancreatic ductal adenocarcinoma. Genes & Development. 2016;**30**(4):355-385

[2] Cowan RW, Maitra A. Genetic progression of pancreatic cancer. Cancer Journal. 2014;**20**(1):80-84

[3] Yuan QY et al. Identification of dysregulated pathways associated with pancreatic cancer by survival analysis. Molecular Medicine Reports. 2015;**11**(1):277-282

[4] Lomberk GA, Urrutia R. The triple-code model for pancreatic cancer: Cross talk among genetics, epigenetics, and nuclear structure. The Surgical Clinics of North America. 2015;**95**(5):935-952

[5] Paradise BD, Barham W, Fernandez-Zapico ME. Targeting epigenetic aberrations in pancreatic cancer, a new path to improve patient outcomes? Cancers (Basel). 2018;**10**(5)

[6] Trager MM, Dhayat SA. Epigenetics of epithelial-to-mesenchymal transition in pancreatic carcinoma. International Journal of Cancer. 2017;**141**(1):24-32

[7] Sharma S, Kelly TK, Jones PA. Epigenetics in cancer. Carcinogenesis. 2010;**31**(1):27-36

[8] Shen H, Laird PW. Interplay between the cancer genome and epigenome. Cell. 2013;**153**(1):38-55

[9] Feinberg AP, Koldobskiy MA, Gondor A. Epigenetic modulators, modifiers and mediators in cancer aetiology and progression. Nature Reviews. Genetics. 2016;**17**(5):284-299

[10] Silverman BR, Shi J. Alterations of epigenetic regulators in pancreatic cancer and their clinical implications. International Journal of Molecular Sciences. 2016;**17**(12)

[11] McCleary-Wheeler AL et al. Insights into the epigenetic mechanisms controlling pancreatic carcinogenesis. Cancer Letters. 2013;**328**(2):212-221

[12] Bird A. DNA methylation patterns and epigenetic memory. Genes & Development. 2002;**16**(1):6-21

[13] Biankin AV et al. Pancreatic cancer genomes reveal aberrations in axon guidance pathway genes. Nature. 2012;**491**(7424):399-405

[14] Sausen M et al. Clinical implications of genomic alterations in the tumour and circulation of pancreatic cancer patients. Nature Communications. 2015;**6**:7686

[15] Kugel S et al. SIRT6 suppresses pancreatic cancer through control of Lin28b. Cell. 2016;**165**(6):1401-1415

[16] Borazanci E et al. Pancreatic cancer: "a riddle wrapped in a mystery inside an enigma". Clinical Cancer Research. 2017;**23**(7):1629-1637

[17] Lahtz C, Pfeifer GP. Epigenetic changes of DNA repair genes in cancer. Journal of Molecular Cell Biology. 2011;**3**(1):51-58

[18] Geisler JP et al. Mismatch repair gene expression defects contribute to microsatellite instability in ovarian carcinoma. Cancer. 2003;**98**(10):2199-2206

[19] Saez GT. DNA injury and repair systems. International Journal of Molecular Sciences. 2018;(7):**19**

[20] Hitchins MP et al. Epigenetic inactivation of a cluster of genes flanking MLH1 in

microsatellite-unstable colorectal cancer. Cancer Research. 2007;**67**(19):9107-9116

[21] Kondo E et al. Not hMSH2 but hMLH1 is frequently silenced by hypermethylation in endometrial cancer but rarely silenced in pancreatic cancer with microsatellite instability. International Journal of Oncology. 2000;**17**(3):535-541

[22] Ye P, Shi Y, Li A. Association between hMLH1 promoter methylation and risk of gastric cancer: A meta-analysis. Frontiers in Physiology. 2018;**9**:368

[23] Shalaby SM et al. Promoter methylation and expression of DNA repair genes MGMT and ERCC1 in tissue and blood of rectal cancer patients. Gene. 2018;**644**:66-73

[24] De Maglio G et al. MGMT promoter methylation status in brain metastases from colorectal cancer and corresponding primary tumors. Future Oncology. 2015;**11**(8):1201-1209

[25] Schmitt AM et al. Prognostic and predictive roles of MGMT protein expression and promoter methylation in sporadic pancreatic neuroendocrine neoplasms. Neuroendocrinology. 2014;**100**(1):35-44

[26] Jin J et al. Aberrant DNA methylation of MGMT and hMLH1 genes in prediction of gastric cancer. Genetics and Molecular Research. 2014;**13**(2):4140-4145

[27] Zuo C et al. O6-methylguanine-DNA methyltransferase gene: Epigenetic silencing and prognostic value in head and neck squamous cell carcinoma. Cancer Epidemiology, Biomarkers & Prevention. 2004;**13**(6):967-975

[28] Rivenbark AG et al. Epigenetic reprogramming of cancer cells via targeted DNA methylation. Epigenetics. 2012;**7**(4):350-360

[29] Lujambio A et al. A microRNA DNA methylation signature for human cancer metastasis. Proceedings of the National Academy of Sciences of the United States of America. 2008;**105**(36):13556-13561

[30] Tan AC et al. Characterizing DNA methylation patterns in pancreatic cancer genome. Molecular Oncology. 2009;**3**(5-6):425-438

[31] Consortium EP. An integrated encyclopedia of DNA elements in the human genome. Nature. 2012;**489**(7414):57-74

[32] Zhang MW et al. DNA methylation in the tumor microenvironment. Journal of Zhejiang University. Science. B. 2017;**18**(5):365-372

[33] Vincent A et al. Genome-wide analysis of promoter methylation associated with gene expression profile in pancreatic adenocarcinoma. Clinical Cancer Research. 2011;**17**(13):4341-4354

[34] Zhu J et al. Gain-of-function p53 mutants co-opt chromatin pathways to drive cancer growth. Nature. 2015;**525**(7568):206-211

[35] Rajamani D, Bhasin MK. Identification of key regulators of pancreatic cancer progression through multidimensional systems-level analysis. Genome Medicine. 2016;**8**(1):38

[36] Huang PH et al. TGFbeta promotes mesenchymal phenotype of pancreatic cancer cells, in part, through epigenetic activation of VAV1. Oncogene. 2017;**36**(16):2202-2214

[37] Galamb O et al. Aberrant DNA methylation of WNT pathway genes in the development and progression

of CIMP-negative colorectal cancer. Epigenetics. 2016;**11**(8):588-602

[38] Zhu W et al. miR-181b modulates multidrug resistance by targeting BCL2 in human cancer cell lines. International Journal of Cancer. 2010;**127**(11):2520-2529

[39] Morita S et al. miR-29 represses the activities of DNA methyltransferases and DNA demethylases. International Journal of Molecular Sciences. 2013;**14**(7):14647-14658

[40] Ramassone A et al. Epigenetics and MicroRNAs in cancer. International Journal of Molecular Sciences. 2018;**19**(2)

[41] Thompson MJ et al. Pancreatic cancer patient survival correlates with DNA methylation of pancreas development genes. PLoS One. 2015;**10**(6):e0128814

[42] Iguchi E et al. Pancreatic cancer, a Mis-interpreter of the epigenetic language. The Yale Journal of Biology and Medicine. 2016;**89**(4):575-590

[43] Gu YM et al. Dickkopf3 overexpression inhibits pancreatic cancer cell growth in vitro. World Journal of Gastroenterology. 2011;**17**(33):3810-3817

[44] Omura N, Goggins M. Epigenetics and epigenetic alterations in pancreatic cancer. International Journal of Clinical and Experimental Pathology. 2009;**2**(4):310-326

[45] Schutte M et al. Abrogation of the Rb/p16 tumor-suppressive pathway in virtually all pancreatic carcinomas. Cancer Research. 1997;**57**(15):3126-3130

[46] Audia JE, Campbell RM. Histone modifications and cancer. Cold Spring Harbor Perspectives in Biology. 2016;**8**(4):a019521

[47] Shanmugam MK et al. Role of novel histone modifications in cancer. Oncotarget. 2018;**9**(13):11414-11426

[48] Kurdistani SK. Histone modifications in cancer biology and prognosis. Progress in Drug Research. 2011;**67**:91-106

[49] Strahl BD, Allis CD. The language of covalent histone modifications. Nature. 2000;**403**(6765):41-45

[50] Zheng M et al. Snail and slug collaborate on EMT and tumor metastasis through miR-101-mediated EZH2 axis in oral tongue squamous cell carcinoma. Oncotarget. 2015;**6**(9):6797-6810

[51] Lin Y, Dong C, Zhou BP. Epigenetic regulation of EMT: The snail story. Current Pharmaceutical Design. 2014;**20**(11):1698-1705

[52] Peinado H et al. Snail mediates E-cadherin repression by the recruitment of the Sin3A/histone deacetylase 1 (HDAC1)/HDAC2 complex. Molecular and Cellular Biology. 2004;**24**(1):306-319

[53] Suganuma T, Workman JL. Crosstalk among histone modifications. Cell. 2008;**135**(4):604-607

[54] Grzenda A, Ordog T, Urrutia R. Polycomb and the emerging epigenetics of pancreatic cancer. Journal of Gastrointestinal Cancer. 2011;**42**(2):100-111

[55] Wang W et al. Polycomb group (PcG) proteins and human cancers: Multifaceted functions and therapeutic implications. Medicinal Research Reviews. 2015;**35**(6):1220-1267

[56] Van der Meulen J, Speleman F, Van Vlierberghe P. The H3K27me3 demethylase UTX in normal development and disease. Epigenetics. 2014;**9**(5):658-668

[57] Wei Y et al. Loss of trimethylation at lysine 27 of histone H3 is a predictor of poor outcome in breast, ovarian, and pancreatic cancers. Molecular Carcinogenesis. 2008;**47**(9):701-706

[58] Yamada N et al. MUC1 expression is regulated by DNA methylation and histone H3 lysine 9 modification in cancer cells. Cancer Research. 2008;**68**(8):2708-2716

[59] Yokoyama S et al. Aberrant methylation of MUC1 and MUC4 promoters are potential prognostic biomarkers for pancreatic ductal adenocarcinomas. Oncotarget. 2016;**7**(27):42553-42565

[60] Grunstein M. Histone acetylation in chromatin structure and transcription. Nature. 1997;**389**(6649):349-352

[61] Marmorstein R, Zhou MM. Writers and readers of histone acetylation: Structure, mechanism, and inhibition. Cold Spring Harbor Perspectives in Biology. 2014;**6**(7):a018762

[62] Demir IE, Ceyhan GO, Friess H. Epigenomic therapies: The potential of targeting SIRT6 for the treatment of pancreatic cancer. Expert Opinion on Therapeutic Targets. 2017;**21**(1):1-3

[63] Campbell MJ, Turner BM. Altered histone modifications in cancer. Advances in Experimental Medicine and Biology. 2013;**754**:81-107

[64] Rivera CM, Ren B. Mapping human epigenomes. Cell. 2013;**155**(1):39-55

[65] Yang H et al. SIRT3-dependent GOT2 acetylation status affects the malate-aspartate NADH shuttle activity and pancreatic tumor growth. The EMBO Journal. 2015;**34**(8):1110-1125

[66] Banerjee T, Chakravarti D. A peek into the complex realm of histone phosphorylation. Molecular and Cellular Biology. 2011;**31**(24):4858-4873

[67] Sawicka A, Seiser C. Histone H3 phosphorylation—a versatile chromatin modification for different occasions. Biochimie. 2012;**94**(11):2193-2201

[68] Prigent C, Dimitrov S. Phosphorylation of serine 10 in histone H3, what for? Journal of Cell Science. 2003;**116**(Pt 18):3677-3685

[69] Choi HS et al. Phosphorylation of histone H3 at serine 10 is indispensable for neoplastic cell transformation. Cancer Research. 2005;**65**(13):5818-5827

[70] Chadee DN et al. Increased Ser-10 phosphorylation of histone H3 in mitogen-stimulated and oncogene-transformed mouse fibroblasts. The Journal of Biological Chemistry. 1999;**274**(35):24914-24920

[71] Aihara H et al. Histone H2A T120 phosphorylation promotes oncogenic transformation via upregulation of Cyclin D1. Molecular Cell. 2016;**64**(1):176-188

[72] Bryant KL et al. KRAS: Feeding pancreatic cancer proliferation. Trends in Biochemical Sciences. 2014;**39**(2):91-100

[73] Espino PS et al. Genomic instability and histone H3 phosphorylation induction by the Ras-mitogen activated protein kinase pathway in pancreatic cancer cells. International Journal of Cancer. 2009;**124**(3):562-567

[74] Winter J et al. Many roads to maturity: microRNA biogenesis pathways and their regulation. Nature Cell Biology. 2009;**11**(3):228-234

[75] Calin GA, Croce CM. MicroRNA signatures in human cancers. Nature Reviews. Cancer. 2006;**6**(11):857-866

[76] Lujambio A, Lowe SW. The microcosmos of cancer. Nature. 2012;**482**(7385):347-355

[77] Wilczynska A, Bushell M. The complexity of miRNA-mediated repression. Cell Death and Differentiation. 2015;**22**(1):22-33

[78] Ha M, Kim VN. Regulation of microRNA biogenesis. Nature Reviews. Molecular Cell Biology. 2014;**15**(8):509-524

[79] Witkos TM, Koscianska E, Krzyzosiak WJ. Practical aspects of microRNA target prediction. Current Molecular Medicine. 2011;**11**(2):93-109

[80] Shin C et al. Expanding the microRNA targeting code: Functional sites with centered pairing. Molecular Cell. 2010;**38**(6):789-802

[81] Chatterjee S, Grosshans H. Active turnover modulates mature microRNA activity in *Caenorhabditis elegans*. Nature. 2009;**461**(7263):546-549

[82] Kunej T et al. Cross talk between microRNA and coding cancer genes. Cancer Journal. 2012;**18**(3):223-231

[83] Esquela-Kerscher A, Slack FJ. Oncomirs—microRNAs with a role in cancer. Nature Reviews. Cancer. 2006;**6**(4):259-269

[84] Zhang B et al. microRNAs as oncogenes and tumor suppressors. Developmental Biology. 2007;**302**(1):1-12

[85] Wu WL et al. Suppressive effects of microRNA-16 on the proliferation, invasion and metastasis of hepatocellular carcinoma cells. International Journal of Molecular Medicine. 2015;**36**(6):1713-1719

[86] Wu W et al. MicroRNA and cancer: Current status and prospective. International Journal of Cancer. 2007;**120**(5):953-960

[87] Pan X, Wang ZX, Wang R. MicroRNA-21: A novel therapeutic target in human cancer. Cancer Biology & Therapy. 2010;**10**(12):1224-1232

[88] Wang Z et al. Targeting miRNAs involved in cancer stem cell and EMT regulation: An emerging concept in overcoming drug resistance. Drug Resistance Updates. 2010;**13**(4-5):109-118

[89] Akbari Moqadam F, Pieters R, den Boer ML. The hunting of targets: Challenge in miRNA research. Leukemia. 2013;**27**(1):16-23

[90] Bloomston M et al. MicroRNA expression patterns to differentiate pancreatic adenocarcinoma from normal pancreas and chronic pancreatitis. JAMA. 2007;**297**(17): 1901-1908

[91] Yonemori K et al. MicroRNA in pancreatic cancer. Journal of Human Genetics. 2016

[92] Hawa Z et al. The miRacle in pancreatic cancer by miRNAs: Tiny angels or devils in disease progression. International Journal of Molecular Sciences. 2016;**17**(6)

[93] Taucher V, Mangge H, Haybaeck J. Non-coding RNAs in pancreatic cancer: Challenges and opportunities for clinical application. Cellular Oncology (Dordrecht). 2016;**39**(4):295-318

[94] Szafranska AE et al. MicroRNA expression alterations are linked to tumorigenesis and non-neoplastic processes in pancreatic ductal adenocarcinoma. Oncogene. 2007;**26**(30):4442-4452

[95] Li Z, Rana TM. Therapeutic targeting of microRNAs: Current status and future challenges. Nature Reviews. Drug Discovery. 2014;**13**(8):622-638

[96] Zhu M et al. microRNA and gene networks in human pancreatic cancer. Oncology Letters. 2013;**6**(4):1133-1139

[97] Kopp F, Wagner E, Roidl A. The proto-oncogene KRAS is targeted by miR-200c. Oncotarget. 2014;**5**(1):185-195

[98] Drakaki A, Iliopoulos D. MicroRNA-gene signaling pathways in pancreatic cancer. Biomedical Journal. 2013;**36**(5):200-208

[99] Jamieson NB et al. MicroRNA molecular profiles associated with diagnosis, clinicopathologic criteria, and overall survival in patients with resectable pancreatic ductal adenocarcinoma. Clinical Cancer Research. 2012;**18**(2):534-545

[100] Park SM et al. The miR-200 family determines the epithelial phenotype of cancer cells by targeting the E-cadherin repressors ZEB1 and ZEB2. Genes & Development. 2008;**22**(7):894-907

[101] Wang P et al. Methylation-mediated silencing of the miR-124 genes facilitates pancreatic cancer progression and metastasis by targeting Rac1. Oncogene. 2014;**33**(4):514-524

[102] Gao W et al. miR-615-5p is epigenetically inactivated and functions as a tumor suppressor in pancreatic ductal adenocarcinoma. Oncogene. 2015;**34**(13):1629-1640

[103] Yi JM et al. Epigenetically altered miR-1247 functions as a tumor suppressor in pancreatic cancer. Oncotarget. 2017;**8**(16):26600-26612

[104] Patel K et al. MicroRNA let-7 downregulates STAT3 phosphorylation in pancreatic cancer cells by increasing SOCS3 expression. Cancer Letters. 2014;**347**(1):54-64

[105] Wald P et al. Prognostic value of microRNA expression levels in pancreatic adenocarcinoma: A review of the literature. Oncotarget. 2017;**8**(42):73345-73361

[106] Kent OA et al. A resource for analysis of microRNA expression and function in pancreatic ductal adenocarcinoma cells. Cancer Biology & Therapy. 2009;**8**(21):2013-2024

[107] Deng M et al. miR-26a suppresses tumor growth and metastasis by targeting FGF9 in gastric cancer. PLoS One. 2013;**8**(8):e72662

[108] Tang L et al. MiR-125a-5p decreases after long non-coding RNA HOTAIR knockdown to promote cancer cell apoptosis by releasing caspase 2. Cell Death & Disease. 2016;**7**:e2137

[109] Botla SK et al. Early epigenetic downregulation of microRNA-192 expression promotes pancreatic cancer progression. Cancer Research. 2016;**76**(14):4149-4159

[110] Zhang R et al. MiR-148a regulates the growth and apoptosis in pancreatic cancer by targeting CCKBR and Bcl-2. Tumour Biology. 2014;**35**(1):837-844

[111] Feng X et al. MiR-200, a new star miRNA in human cancer. Cancer Letters. 2014;**344**(2):166-173

[112] Uhlmann S et al. miR-200bc/429 cluster targets PLCgamma1 and differentially regulates proliferation and EGF-driven invasion than miR-200a/141 in breast cancer. Oncogene. 2010;**29**(30):4297-4306

[113] Chen Y, Zhang L. WITHDRAWN: MiR-200 family and cancer: Function, regulation and signaling. Surgical Oncology. 2014

[114] Luo G et al. Highly lymphatic metastatic pancreatic cancer cells possess stem cell-like properties. International Journal of Oncology. 2013;**42**(3):979-984

[115] Ji Q et al. MicroRNA miR-34 inhibits human pancreatic cancer

tumor-initiating cells. PLoS One. 2009;**4**(8):e6816

[116] Lodygin D et al. Inactivation of miR-34a by aberrant CpG methylation in multiple types of cancer. Cell Cycle. 2008;**7**(16):2591-2600

[117] Nalls D et al. Targeting epigenetic regulation of miR-34a for treatment of pancreatic cancer by inhibition of pancreatic cancer stem cells. PLoS One. 2011;**6**(8):e24099

[118] Hunt S et al. MicroRNA-124 suppresses oral squamous cell carcinoma motility by targeting ITGB1. FEBS Letters. 2011;**585**(1):187-192

[119] Deng S et al. Chronic pancreatitis and pancreatic cancer demonstrate active epithelial-mesenchymal transition profile, regulated by miR-217-SIRT1 pathway. Cancer Letters. 2014;**355**(2):184-191

[120] Zhao WG et al. The miR-217 microRNA functions as a potential tumor suppressor in pancreatic ductal adenocarcinoma by targeting KRAS. Carcinogenesis. 2010;**31**(10):1726-1733

[121] Wei X et al. MicroRNA-21 induces 5-fluorouracil resistance in human pancreatic cancer cells by regulating PTEN and PDCD4. Cancer Medicine. 2016;**5**(4):693-702

[122] Park JK et al. miR-132 and miR-212 are increased in pancreatic cancer and target the retinoblastoma tumor suppressor. Biochemical and Biophysical Research Communications. 2011;**406**(4):518-523

[123] Zhao JL et al. miR-212/132 downregulates SMAD2 expression to suppress the G1/S phase transition of the cell cycle and the epithelial to mesenchymal transition in cervical cancer cells. IUBMB Life. 2015;**67**(5):380-394

[124] Huang F et al. MiR-196a promotes pancreatic cancer progression by targeting nuclear factor kappa-B-inhibitor alpha. PLoS One. 2014;**9**(2):e87897

[125] Gironella M et al. Tumor protein 53-induced nuclear protein 1 expression is repressed by miR-155, and its restoration inhibits pancreatic tumor development. Proceedings of the National Academy of Sciences of the United States of America. 2007;**104**(41):16170-16175

Chapter 6

The Role of DNA Repair and the Epigenetic Markers Left after Repair in Neurologic Functions, Including Memory and Learning

Carol Bernstein and Harris Bernstein

Abstract

In eukaryotic cell nuclei, DNA is wrapped around and firmly associated with histone proteins, forming chromatin. When DNA is damaged, the chromatin structure needs to be loosened to allow repair enzymes to gain access to the damage. This requires modifying the histone proteins. These modifications, called epigenetic alterations, do not alter the base-pair sequence. Repair-associated epigenetic alterations are usually transient, removed when no longer needed for repair. However, some remain after repair. In the human brain, long-lasting novel epigenetic alterations appear to account for the persistence of addictions to such substances as alcohol, nicotine and cocaine. Certain neurodegenerative diseases are caused by inherited mutations in genes necessary for DNA repair. Deficient DNA repair in these diseases is associated with extensive epigenetic alterations that likely have a role in the disease phenotype. Persistent epigenetic alterations due to DNA repair processes, both histone modifications and methylations of DNA, can also have positive consequences. Stimulation of brain activity (e.g. learning and memory formation) is often accompanied by the generation of DNA damage in neuronal DNA, followed by repair associated with persistent epigenetic alterations. In particular, recent research has shown the need for non-homologous end joining and base excision repair in memory formation.

Keywords: DNA repair, epigenetic, histone acetylation, histone methylation, CpG island methylation, addiction, neurodegenerative disease, memory, learning, cognition

1. Introduction

Even in the earliest stages of evolution, damage to the genome was presumably a fundamental problem for life. Thus it is likely that organisms developed processes for repairing genome damages very early. Such repair processes are ordinarily restorative, designed to reestablish the original undamaged genome sequence. During the course of the evolution of lineages leading to mammals, DNA repair processes became more complex, and acquired additional capabilities. One such example is the employment of the DNA double-strand break repair process of non-homologous end joining in the generation of immunological diversity [1].

In chromatin, epigenetic alterations are an integral part of DNA repair processes [2]. Although most epigenetic alterations introduced during DNA repair are transient with restoration of the epigenetic pattern that existed prior to repair, some are long lasting. Epigenetic alterations can enhance or inhibit gene expression without changing the DNA base pair sequence. Examples of epigenetic alterations are hyper- or hypomethylation of cytosines in the DNA sequence, increased or decreased histone H3 and H4 acetylation by histone acetyltransferases or histone deacetylases, and increased or decreased histone methylation by histone methyltransferases or histone demethylases.

In humans, the oxygen demands of the brain are high, constituting about 20% of total body oxygen consumption, while the mass of the brain is only about 2% of body mass [3]. This results in elevated release of reactive oxygen species in the brain that, in turn, cause oxidative DNA damages. Because damages are prevalent, processes that repair DNA damages have a vital role in maintaining the health of brain neurons, and these DNA repair processes can cause epigenetic alterations.

When DNA repair processes are impaired or insufficient, the result can be improper (non-adaptive) epigenetic alterations. Such improper epigenetic alterations in neurons are likely an important underlying cause of certain addictions and neurodegenerative diseases. Several addictive agents cause increased DNA damage in neurons resulting in increased dependence on DNA repair. Addictions are associated with characteristic persistent patterns of epigenetic alterations in the brain. In several neurodegenerative diseases the neurological impairments are caused by inherited mutations in genes that encode proteins employed in DNA repair. These diseases are associated with particular patterns of epigenetic alterations in neurons. It is likely that the neurological impairments suffered by individuals during addiction or neurodegenerative disease are caused, at least in part, by epigenetic alterations resulting from insufficient or faulty DNA repair. That is, insufficient or faulty DNA repair may produce epigenetic alterations that have long-lasting negative consequences at the level of gene expression that manifest as neurological impairment.

Zovkic et al. [4] noted that learning and memory can be broadly defined as lasting alterations of a behavioral output produced in response to a transient environmental input. In order for a brief stimulus to cause a persistent change in behavior, neurons need to undergo some kind of molecular alterations that stabilize a memory into an enduring set of cellular marks. As reviewed by Bird in 2002 [5], in mammals, DNA methylation is adapted for specific cellular memory in development, even over successive cell divisions. This observation of cellular memory indicated that epigenetic mechanisms could provide a molecular basis for neuronal memory formation and maintenance in non-replicating neurons [4]. In addition to DNA methylation/demethylation, it is now known that other mechanisms such as chromatin histone acetylation and histone methylation can also cause persistent epigenetic changes [6].

In the sections below, we review evidence for the following ideas. Neuronal activity causes DNA damages, and repair processes are required to deal with these damages. Such repair processes involve epigenetic alterations, some of which are long lasting. Individuals, addicted to abuse of certain substances that cause DNA damage, have long-lasting epigenetic alterations in brain neurons that appear to be related to the dependency. Also, inherited inability to adequately repair DNA damages can cause epigenetic alterations in neurons associated with neurodegenerative disease. However, long-lasting epigenetic alterations can also be adaptively beneficial. Cognitive functions such as memory and learning in response to external stimuli appear to depend, at least in part, on persistent epigenetic alterations arising during DNA repair processes.

2. Epigenetic alterations required for DNA repair

DNA is condensed in the nucleus of the cell in a highly organized and compact manner, referred to as chromatin (reviewed by Walker and Nestler [7] and Ding et al. [8]). In chromatin, the DNA is packaged with histone proteins to form nucleosomes. DNA repair proteins are recruited and interact with DNA in response to DNA damage. However, the architecture of nucleosomes and the organization of chromatin can present barriers to DNA damage recognition and repair. Epigenetic modifiers play an important role in regulating nucleosome and chromatin structure to facilitate DNA repair. Epigenetic alterations relax certain regions of chromatin to allow access to DNA repair enzymes and also condense certain regions to repress transcription in order to facilitate repair. When repair is complete, epigenetic modifications are largely returned to the state before damage occurred. These roles of epigenetic modifiers in DNA repair have been described as the "access-repair-restore" model [9].

2.1 Histone acetylation

The basic unit of chromatin, the nucleosome, is composed of 147 DNA base pairs wrapped around a histone octamer consisting of two copies of each of the following proteins: H2A, H2B, H3, and H4. The histones also have histone tail extensions, constituting up to 30% by mass of the histones (**Figure 1**). Each histone protein can undergo post translational modifications in which molecules, such as an acetyl group or one (or up to three) methyl group(s), are covalently added to (or removed from)

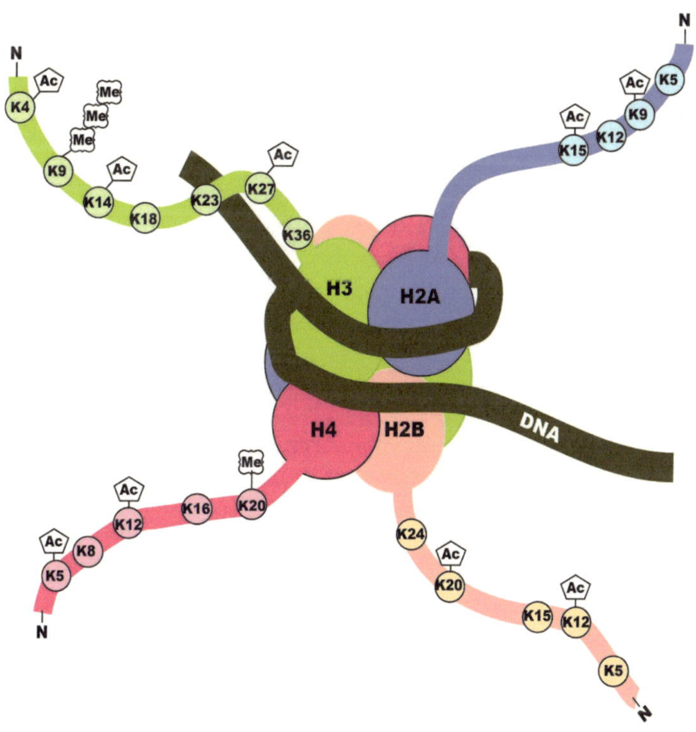

Figure 1.
A nucleosome showing 4 pairs of histones (H2A, H2B, H3, and H4), each pair with the same color. The amino-terminal (N-terminal) tails of one of each pair of histones is shown, labeled with the positions of lysine amino acids (labeled "K" in the single letter code for lysine) that are subject to acetylation or methylation. The number at each lysine indicates its position counting from the amino end of the protein chain. Acetylations (indicated by Ac) and methylations (indicated by Me) are shown in some positions susceptible to these alterations. The DNA, wound around the histone core, is indicated by the dark line.

lysine residues of their amino terminal (N-terminal) tail. The single letter K designates lysine. If an acetyl group is added to a lysine located as the 4th amino acid from the N-terminal tail end of histone 3, this is designated H3K4Ac. These modifications not only alter the structure of the nucleosome but also change the interaction of DNA with the associated histones, thus allowing entry of DNA repair enzymes into chromatin and permitting histones to be moved, if needed, to allow for repair [2]. The epigenetic modifications, if they remain after DNA repair, also can increase or decrease the likelihood of transcription of a given gene near the site of the repaired DNA damage [10].

Acetylation of histone lysines promotes chromatin relaxation to facilitate DNA repair [2]. It is also generally associated with a permissive transcriptional state. By negating the positive charge associated with the lysine residues on histone tails, acetylation promotes an "open" chromatin state.

2.2 Histone methylation

Histone lysine methylation is associated with either activation or repression of gene expression depending on which residues are methylated and whether one, two or three methyl groups are added at that position [11]. For instance enrichment of H3K4Me1 or H3K4Me3 at specific gene regions is correlated positively with increased transcription levels, whereas enrichment of H3K9Me2, H3K9Me3 or H3K27Me3 is negatively correlated with transcription. In response to DNA double-strand breaks, histone methyl transferases are recruited to sites of damage where they catalyze trimethylation of H3K9 and H3K27, thereby repressing transcription in order to facilitate DNA repair [12].

2.3 DNA methylation

An important epigenetic regulator in addition to histone modification is DNA methylation. DNA methylation often occurs with the addition of a methyl group to the DNA sequence cytosine-phosphate-guanine (CpG) at the C5 position (5mC). DNA methylation at gene promoters is generally associated with repression, while methylation within genes has been associated with active transcription [7]. DNA methyl transferase 1 (DNMT1) binds to sites of oxidative damage formed in GC-rich regions of the genome and promotes formation and recruitment of a large epigenetic silencing complex. Localization of these epigenetic modifiers to sites of oxidative damage in promoter CpG islands results in increased DNA methylation.

2.4 Noncoding RNA

Non-coding RNAs provide an additional type of epigenetic regulation. As one example, microRNAs are short sequences of RNA (about 22 bases) that exert a repressive role on gene expression by binding a target sequence on specific mRNAs and blocking translation or inducing degradation. The typical microRNA has about 400 specific target mRNAs. In one report, specific microRNAs collaborated with histone deacetylases and cooperatively regulated several relevant target genes [13].

2.5 Epigenetic alterations allow DNA repair

Figure 2 illustrates some of the actions of epigenetic alterations. Histone acetyltransferases add acetyl groups to histone tails to open chromatin structure to make DNA damages accessible to repair enzymes. If the acetyl groups remain after DNA repair, this allows genes in the area of DNA repair to be switched on. Histone deacetylases remove acetyl groups from histone tails to complete DNA repair and return chromatin to its condensed state existing before DNA repair. Improper actions of histone deacetylases can inappropriately switch genes off.

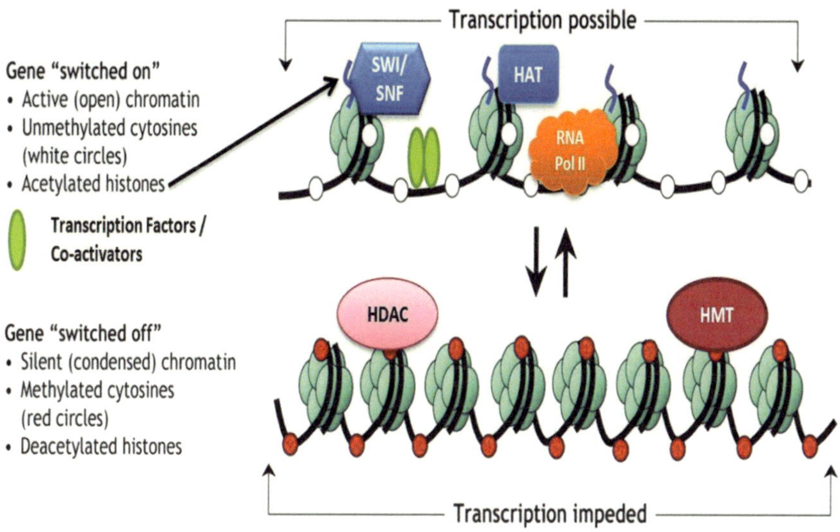

Figure 2.
A gene located in chromatin, with its DNA wrapped around histones. Open chromatin (top image) has been relaxed by acetylation of histone tails. Condensed chromatin (lower image) has been tightened by removal of acetyl groups and addition of methylation of histone tails. Symbols include histone acetyltransferase (HAT), histone deacetylase (HDAC), and histone methyltransferase (HMT). SWI/SNF (not an epigenetic alteration) is a nucleosome-remodeling complex that stimulates gene expression if the epigenetic factors (methylation on cytosines in DNA; acetylations and methylations of lysines in histone tails) allow transcription [14].

In this figure, histone methyltransferase (HMT) is shown as switching a gene off. However, some histone methylations serve to activate genes [11].

DNA gene promoters without methylated cytosines are indicated (in **Figure 2**) as allowing transcription (upper image), and DNA gene promoters with methylated cytosines (in CpG sites) are indicated as impeding transcription. The green vertical ovals represent transcription factors. They are not epigenetic factors, but also regulate gene transcription.

3. Epigenetic remnants (scars) after DNA repair

Dabin et al. [15], in an extensive review, noted that after repair of various types of DNA damages there are a number of types of epigenetic alterations that could potentially remain as scars. These epigenetic alterations include (1) changes in DNA methylation, (2) incorporation into nucleosomes of new histones with a pattern of acetylations or methylations that differ from that in the histones originally present before DNA damage, (3) incorporation into nucleosomes of histone variants such as histone H2AZ, (4) altered acetylation or methylation of histone tails, and even (5) altered histone density at repair sites. Several illustrative reports showing such scars after DNA repair are described below.

3.1 Homologous recombinational repair (HRR) of double-strand breaks leaves epigenetic alterations

Homologous recombinational repair (HRR) modified the DNA methylation pattern of a repaired DNA double-strand break in a green fluorescent protein (GFP) gene inserted into the HeLa cell genome [16]. In different subclones isolated after HRR repair events, the repair created either more highly methylated or less highly methylated cytosines in the GFP gene DNA. HRR also altered local histone H3 methylation, forming H3K9Me2 or H3K9Me3 at repair locations. However, H3K9Me2/3 was selectively retained after HRR only in recombined genes with increased DNA methylation.

During a 2-week period after repair, some transcription-associated demethylation of the repaired DNA was promoted by base excision repair enzymes [16]. Subsequently, the repaired genes displayed stable but diverse methylation profiles. These profiles governed the levels of expression in each clone. These epigenetic alterations (scars) were stable over time and were recovered with the same frequency after 3 years of continuous culture.

3.2 Double-strand break repair by non-homologous end joining leaves epigenetic alterations

DNA repair by non-homologous end joining induces alterations in DNA cytosine methylation and these alterations are a source of permanent epigenetic changes [17]. In a HeLa cell line containing a green fluorescent protein (GFP) based reporter gene, a double-strand break in the gene followed by non-homologous end joining repair created two populations of cells, those with increased DNA methylation in the GFP gene (identified by a dim green color) and those with decreased DNA methylation in the GFP gene (identified by a bright green color). The degree of methylation for each population changed somewhat over the subsequent 4 days, but then remained stable for 24 days. Even though the HeLa cells were undergoing replication, the epigenetic changes produced stable high expressing or low expressing clones.

3.3 Base excision repair is associated with epigenetic alterations

The major forms of oxidative DNA damage are non-bulky lesions such as 8-oxo-2′-deoxyguanosine and thymine glycol that are repaired predominantly by base excision repair. After oxidative DNA damage was increased in HCT116 cells in culture, histone alterations were found in genes with CpG island-containing gene promoters and these histone alterations caused decreased transcription [18]. The histone alterations introduced by increased oxidative damage included reduction in H3K4Me3 and H4K16Ac and an increase in H3K27Me3. DNA methylation was also increased, but primarily in promoters of genes which normally have low basal expression [18].

3.4 Histone replacements during DNA repair

For many types of DNA damage, histones must be removed and replaced during the repair of the damaged DNA [19]. Disruption of nucleosomes in human cells after introduction of double-strand breaks or UV damage occurs with a drop in histone H2B levels and a selective loss of histones H2A and H2B, but not of H3 or H4 at the site of the damage [19]. After DNA repair, new histones (in addition to some pre-existing histones) are deposited at the site of repair. The new histones lack the histone post-translational modifications that existed before the repair. The presence of the differently modified new histones can specifically mark the domain as a site of repair, and remain as a scar [19]. The failure to recycle all of the pre-existing histone marks results in alterations in gene expression [15].

4. Addiction

One of the principal features of addiction is its persistence. The persistent behavioral changes appear to be due to long-lasting changes, resulting from epigenetic alterations affecting gene expression, within particular regions of the brain [20].

4.1 Alcohol

Alcohol can be addictive. About 7% of the US population are alcoholics, with alcohol use disorder [21]. Many negative physiologic consequences of alcoholism are reversible during abstinence. Long-term chronic alcoholics suffer a variety of cognitive deficiencies [22]. Multiyear abstinence resolves many neurocognitive deficits. One exception is lingering deficits in spatial processing [23]. In addition, some frequent long-term consequences are not reversible during abstinence. Alcohol craving (compulsive need to consume alcohol) is usually present long-term among alcoholics [24]. Among 461 individuals who sought help for alcohol problems, follow-up was provided for up to 16 years [25]. By 16 years, 54% of those who tried to remain abstinent without professional help had relapsed, and 39% of those who tried to remain abstinent with help (such as Alcoholics Anonymous) had relapsed.

Long-term, stable consequences of chronic alcohol abuse are thought to be due to stable changes of gene expression resulting from epigenetic alterations within particular regions of the brain [26–28]. For example, in rats exposed to alcohol for up to 5 days, there was an increase in histone 3 lysine 9 acetylation in the pronociceptin promoter in the brain amygdala complex. This acetylation is an activating mark for pronociceptin. The nociceptin/nociceptin opioid receptor system is involved in the reinforcing or conditioning effects of alcohol [29].

4.2 Cigarette smoking

Cigarette smokers (about 21% of the US population in 2013) [30] are usually addicted to nicotine [31]. This is a strong addiction. The proportion of smokers who reported having seriously tried to quit and who managed to quit for 6 months or more was less than 10% [32].

After 7 days of nicotine treatment of mice, the post-translational modifications consisting of acetylation of both histone H3 and histone H4 was increased at the *FosB* promoter in the nucleus accumbens of the brain, causing a 61% increase in FosB expression [33]. This also increases expression of the splice variant *Delta FosB*. In the nucleus accumbens of the brain, Delta FosB functions as a "sustained molecular switch" and "master control protein" in the development of an addiction [34, 35]. Similarly, after 15 days of nicotine treatment of rats, the post-translational modification consisting of threefold increased acetylation of histone H4 occurs at the promoter of the dopamine D1 receptor gene in the prefrontal cortex of the rats. This caused increased dopamine release in the prefrontal cortex reward-related brain region, and such increased dopamine release is recognized as an important factor for addiction [36].

4.3 Cocaine

Cocaine addiction occurs in about 0.5% of the US population. In humans treated for cocaine addiction, the relapse rate after 5 years was 25% [37]. Repeated cocaine administration in mice induces post-translational modifications including hyperacetylation of histone 3 (H3) or histone 4 (H4) at 1696 genes in one brain reward region, the nucleus accumbens, and deacetylation at 206 genes [7, 38]. At least 45 genes, shown in previous studies to be upregulated in the brain nucleus accumbens of mice after chronic cocaine exposure, were found to be associated with post-translational hyperacetylation of histone H3 or histone H4. Many of these individual genes are directly related to aspects of addiction associated with cocaine exposure [38].

4.4 Addictive substances can cause DNA damage

In rodent models, many addictive substances cause DNA damage in the brain. For example, alcohol, through its metabolic product acetaldehyde, induces double-strand breaks in DNA in the mouse brain [39].

Nicotine from cigarette smoke also very likely causes DNA damage in the brain. Nicotine reaches the brain 10–20 seconds after a puff of smoke. The level of nicotine in the brain is 75–80% as high as in the blood or the liver [40]. E-cigarette smoke is composed primarily of nicotine vapors. Nicotine from E-cigarettes, applied to mice (with the dose and duration equivalent in human terms to light E-cigarette smoking for 10 years), caused DNA damages including mutagenic O^6-methyl-deoxyguanosines and γ-hydroxy-1,N_2-propano-deoxyguanosines in the lung, bladder, and heart [41]. These same damages are likely to occur as well in neurons upon exposure to nicotine.

Cocaine [42] and methamphetamine [43, 44] each also cause DNA damage in the brain.

After repair at the sites of DNA damages caused by drugs of addiction, the epigenome may not return entirely to their pre-damage states. Some of the methylations of DNA and/or the acetylations or methylations of histones at the sites of DNA repair may remain and thus become epigenetic scars on chromatin [15]. Such epigenetic scars likely contribute to the persistent epigenetic alterations found in addiction.

5. Neurodegenerative diseases with deficient DNA repair

DNA repair processes in mammalian cells normally involve extensive chromatin remodeling. This remodeling involves epigenetic modifications of chromatin that are usually transient, but may persist. When a protein necessary for proper DNA repair is mutationally defective, epigenetic alterations that deviate from a normal functional pattern can be introduced. In a number of neurodegenerative diseases, such epigenetic alterations appear to significantly underlie the disease phenotype.

We describe below four neurodegenerative diseases, ataxia telangiectasia, Huntington's disease, Aicardi-Goutières syndrome and Cockayne syndrome that have inherited genetic deficiencies due to mutations in genes necessary for DNA repair. We briefly summarize for each disease, the notable neurodegenerative features of the disease, the DNA repair processes that are defective, and the accompanying epigenetic alterations that likely have a role in the etiology of the disease. On the basis of the evidence reviewed, it appears that the proper functioning of the nervous system depends on DNA repair processes that not only restore damaged DNA sequence information, but also promote normal gene expression through the maintenance of an appropriate pattern of epigenetic markers.

5.1 Ataxia telangiectasia (AT)

AT is a multisystem disease characterized by neurodegeneration in the central nervous system. Certain regions of the brain including the cerebellum, are adversely affected in AT resulting in difficulty with movement and coordination. There is also an association with microcephaly. AT is inherited as an autosomal recessive trait, and is caused by mutation of the gene *AT mutated* (*ATM*) that encodes a serine/threonine protein kinase. The wild-type ATM protein has a key role in the DNA damage response. ATM is part of a molecular complex that signals the presence of oxidative DNA damage, including double-strand breaks, and facilitates subsequent repair [45].

ATM protein is employed in chromatin remodeling and in epigenetic alterations that are required for repairing DNA double-strand breaks [45]. ATM mutation causes defects in epigenetic regulation that likely contribute to the rapid postnatal degeneration of the cerebellum that underlies the progressive ataxia observed in AT [45]. AT is associated with histone acetylation alterations, including significant decreases in histone H3 and H4 acetylation [46]. ATM regulates neuron specific epigenetic alterations involving histone deacetylase-4 [45]. In ATM mutant neurons, misallocation of histone deacetylase-4 represses transcription of genes important in neuronal function and synaptic maintenance [45].

5.2 Huntington's disease (HD)

HD typically occurs in midlife. The symptoms include progressive movement disorder, cognitive dysfunction and psychiatric impairment. HD is inherited in an autosomal dominant manner. HD results from an unstable expansion of CAG repeat sequences in exon 1 of the *huntingtin* gene (*HTT*). Several lines of evidence link the HTT protein to repair of DNA damage [47]. HTT is a scaffolding protein that directly participates in oxidative DNA damage repair [48]. The ATM protein recruits HTT to sites of DNA damage. HTT co-localizes with, and acts as a scaffold for, proteins of the DNA damage response pathway in response to oxidative stress. The fibroblasts of HD patients with expanded CAG repeats have deficient oxidative damage repair [48].

Impaired DNA repair in HD also appears to cause deleterious epigenetic alterations that are linked to transcriptional dysregulation. Individuals with HD experience accelerated epigenetic aging of the brain, particularly in the frontal lobe, cingulate gyrus and the parietal lobe. This process is associated with substantial changes in brain DNA methylation levels [49]. Also post-translational modifications of histone proteins are significantly altered in HD patients as well as in HD cellular and animal models [50].

5.3 Aicardi-Goutières syndrome (AGS)

AGS is characterized by early onset, often in early infancy. Features of AGS include neurological dysfunction, psychomotor retardation, seizures, and microcephaly [51]. AGS is an inherited disease and most cases are inherited in an autosomal recessive pattern. AGS arises from mutations in genes encoding proteins TREX 1 (AGS1), RNase H2 (AGS2, 3 and 4) and SAMHD1 (AGS5) [51]. The incorporation of ribonucleotide triphosphates (rNTPs) into DNA is perhaps the most common type of endogenous DNA damage encountered in proliferating cells [52]. Removal of rNTPs incorporated into DNA is referred to as rNTP excision repair. Key players in rNTP excision repair are TREX1 and RNase H2 [52]. RNase H2 is the predominant nuclear enzyme to hydrolyze the RNA strand of RNA/DNA hybrids [53].

TREX1, *RNASEH2* and *SAMHD1* mutations in AGS cells cause common molecular abnormalities including increased levels of RNA:DNA hybrid species and genome-wide DNA hypomethylation, a substantial epigenetic perturbance [51]. AGS2 and AGS4 mutant cells display about a 20% reduction in genomic methylation levels overall, and this reduction is spread along the length of entire chromosomes impacting nearly all compartments including genic, intergenic unique and repeat regions [51].

5.4. Cockayne syndrome (CS)

Due to impaired neurological development, individuals with CS are characteristically mentally retarded and have microcephaly. CS is caused by mutations in the *CSA* and *CSB* genes. CS is inherited as an autosomal recessive trait. Transcription of DNA can be inhibited by DNA damage, and restoration of transcription requires removal of blocking damages by a sub-pathway of nucleotide excision repair that specifically removes transcription-blocking DNA damages. This sub-pathway is referred to as transcription-coupled DNA repair (TCR). In mammals, TCR depends on the CSA and CSB proteins. More than 70% of CS syndrome patients have a mutation in the *CSB* gene. CSA and CSB proteins regulate recruitment of chromatin remodeling and repair factors to stalled RNA polymerase at sites of DNA damage [54, 55].

Among the proteins recruited by CSA and CSB are nucleotide excision repair proteins and histone acetyltransferase, an enzyme that catalyzes chromatin remodeling and epigenetic alteration [54]. CSB can slide histones along DNA and histone chaperone proteins that accept and donate histones can greatly facilitate this process [55]. Nucleosome remodeling by CSB is important for TCR, and inability to efficiently mobilize nucleosomes appears to contribute to the underlying mechanism of CS [55]. The chromatin remodeling activity of CSB appears to create an epigenetic landscape that permits more efficient DNA repair or facilitates transcription resumption after repair is completed [56].

5.5 Perspective on the role of DNA repair in neurodegeneration

The neurodegenerative diseases AT, HD, AGS and CS are due to mutation in genes that encode proteins employed in DNA repair. Inadequate DNA repair can lead directly to cell death and neuron depletion that may be reflected in microcephaly, as is seen in AT, AGS and CS. The defects in DNA repair also cause disruptions in the pattern of epigenetic alteration required for normal neuronal function. These epigenetic alterations likely underlie characteristic features of the disease phenotype. Thus it appears that important functions of the nervous system, including those involved in various aspects of cognition and motor function, depend on the role of intact DNA repair processes in maintaining normal patterns of epigenetic markers.

5.6 Other neurodegenerative diseases deficient in DNA repair

In addition to the four neurodegenerative diseases discussed above, there is also evidence for defective DNA repair in the neurodegenerative diseases amyotrophic lateral sclerosis [57], fragile X syndrome [58], Friedrich's ataxia [59], spinocerebellar ataxia type 1 [60], trichothiodystrophy [61], and xeroderma pigmentosum [62].

Amyotrophic lateral sclerosis is causally linked to mutations in the gene *FUS* [57]. ALS patients with *FUS* mutations have increased neuronal DNA damage. FUS protein functions in the DNA damage response including recruitment to double-strand breaks and homologous recombinational DNA repair. FUS protein also directly interacts with histone deacetylase 1 in response to DNA damage, and this interaction is necessary for efficient DNA repair [57].

Fragile X syndrome is a common form of inherited mental retardation. The fragile X mental retardation protein FMRP is a chromatin-binding protein that functions in the DNA damage response, likely in DNA repair [58]. Fragile X syndrome is caused by loss of expression of the *FMR1* gene, most often due to an expansion of a CGG repeat in the first exon of *FMR1*. The repeat expansion results in abnormal methylation of the promoter region which leads to transcriptional silencing of the *FMR1* gene [63].

Friedreich ataxia, a progressive neurodegenerative disease, is caused by deficient frataxin protein resulting from downregulation of the *FXN* gene. Frataxin is employed in the repair of DNA double-strand breaks [59]. Most individuals with Friedrich ataxia have a homozygous mutation consisting of a GAA trinucleotide repeat expansion within the first intron of the FXN gene. This expansion itself may lead to downregulation of the *FXN* gene. In addition, there is a repressive heterochromatin effect around the *FXN* gene caused by the expanded GAA repeats, consisting of high levels histone methylation of H3K9 and H3K27 [64].

Spinocerebellar ataxia type 1 (SCA1) is an autosomal dominant neurodegenerative disease characterized by progressive motor incoordination. SCA1 results from mutation in the *ATXN1* gene that leads to a pathogenic glutamine-repeat expansion in the protein ataxin-1 (ATXN1). The multifunctional protein TERA/VCP/p97 acts in DNA damage repair. Glutamine-repeat expansion mutant proteins such as mutant ATXN1 impair accumulation and function of TERA/VCP/p67 leading to an increase in unrepaired DNA double-strand breaks [60]. Also mutant *ATXN1* represses gene transcription by decreasing histone acetylation [65].

Trichothiodystrophy (TTD) is an autosomal recessive disorder with a range of clinical neurodevelopmental features and often photosensitivity. All photosensitive TTD individuals have a mutation in the *XPB*, *XPD* or *TTDA* genes that encode subunits of the dual functional repair/transcription factor IIH (TFIIH) [61]. These individuals deficient for TFIIH are defective in nucleotide excision repair, a process that repairs transcription-blocking DNA damages, including UV induced DNA damages, thus explaining their photosensitivity. Induction of DNA damage in cells with *XPB* or *XPD* mutations that cause TTD results in reduced transient DNA strand breaks that are intermediates during DNA repair [66]. Also methylation of histone H3 (H3K9Me3) was reduced in an evaluated model promoter region [66].

Xeroderma pigmentosum (XP) is an autosomal recessive genetic disorder. XP has characteristic neurological manifestations, but the most prominent feature of the condition is sensitivity to sunlight resulting in a high predisposition to UV-induced skin cancer. Seven different complementation groups (genes) *XPA*, *XPB*, *XPC*, *XPD*, *XPE*, *XPF* and *XPG* encode proteins employed in nucleotide excision repair, a process that repairs bulky DNA damages including damages caused by UV-light [62]. XPF and XPG proteins are endonucleases that also trigger chromatin looping and DNA demethylation that promote accurate expression of activated genes [67].

6. Mental activity is associated with DNA damage and repair in the brain

An easy type of DNA damage to measure is the double-strand break. When a double-strand break occurs there is a rapid effect on particular histones near the break. A variant histone, H2AX, is sometimes present in histone cores, and it constitutes about 2–25% of the H2A histones in mammalian chromatin [68]. After a double-strand break, H2AX histones near the break are phosphorylated by the kinases ATM, ATR and DNA-PK [69], allowing formation of H2AX phosphorylated on serine 139 near the break. This histone is then designated γH2AX. γH2AX can be detected as soon as 20 seconds after irradiation of cells (with DNA double-strand break formation), and half maximum accumulation of γH2AX occurs in 1 minute [68]. Chromatin with phosphorylated γH2AX extends to about a million base pairs on each side of a DNA double-strand break [68]. It is easy to detect γH2AX by immunohistochemistry, and these large segments of chromatin with γH2AX are called γH2AX foci.

Learning and new memories occur when mice explore a new, strange environment. This is a low level stimulation. Exploration of a novel environment increased the number of neurons with double-strand breaks in neuronal DNA as measured by γH2AX foci [70]. This occurs in different brain regions but particularly in the dentate gyrus, which is involved in spatial learning and memory. Within 24 hours of break formation, DNA repair occurs with removal of the breaks [70]. When double-strand breaks in this situation were also measured by the comet assay (another simple assay), roughly 30–40% of dentate gyrus nuclei had comet tails indicating double-strand breaks in the nuclear DNA [70].

6.1 Visual stimulation

Another neuronal activity also caused double-strand breaks. Exposure of anesthetized mice to visual stimuli activated the primary visual cortex (V1) of the brain. One eye was exposed to visual stimuli for 15 minutes, while the other was shielded from light. One hour after the visual stimulation began, the number of cells with γH2AX foci in the stimulated contralateral V1 was roughly twice as high as that in the unstimulated ipsilateral V1 [70].

6.2 Optogenetic stimulation

Optogenetic stimulation of a mouse striatum brain region also caused DNA double-strand breaks [70]. Transgenic mice expressing Cre-recombinase in medium spiny neurons of the dorsomedial striatum were used. The Cre-recombinase gene inserted into DNA of the striatum neurons in these mice provides a topoisomerase I like mechanism to carry out site-specific recombination events. Using this system, a viral vector was infused into the striatum, carrying a genetic segment coding for a light sensitive ChR2 protein. The ChR2 gene frequently recombined into the mouse dorsomedial striatum DNA. A glass fiber was then implanted close to the viral injection site. Two weeks later, awake mice were stimulated by light through the glass fiber. This caused neuronal activity in the dorsomedial striatum, resulting in behavioral ipsiversive rotations in mice (mice turning in a circle). The mice were then terminated and the mouse brains examined. The illuminated striata contained many more cells with γH2AX foci than the non-illuminated contralateral striata [70].

6.3 Non-homologous end joining (NHEJ) repair required for long-term memory retention

One form of long-term memory, through associative learning, is contextual fear conditioning [71]. This fear conditioning occurs, for instance, when a rodent is placed in a novel environment (a new context) and is then subjected to an electric shock (e.g. a footshock). This produces robust fear learning, shown by a strong fear response, when the rodent is placed in that context again. Contextual fear conditioning occurs very rapidly (can occur with a single event) and has a lasting effect.

Madabhushi et al. [72] subjected wild-type C57BL/6 mice to a training paradigm for contextual fear conditioning, following which they prepared hippocampal lysates and measured γH2AX levels (as a measure of double-strand breaks in DNA). Elevated γH2AX levels were detectable in hippocampal lysates within 15 minutes after exposure to the fear-conditioning paradigm.

NHEJ, which repairs double-strand breaks in DNA, appears to be needed specifically for consolidation of memory into long-term memory. Contextual fear conditioning in mice increased NHEJ repair activity in the hippocampus brain region measured at 10 and 60 minutes after training [73]. The hippocampus is important in forming memories [74].

When NHEJ repair was active, memories were demonstrated in fear-conditioned mice at 6 and 24 hours after training. Ara-C (cytosine arabinoside) interferes with DNA synthesis. Injecting animals systemically with ara-C 1 hour before exposing them to the conditioning inhibited NHEJ repair [68]. If NHEJ repair was blocked before fear conditioning, memories of fear conditioning were substantially diminished at the 6- and 24-hour time periods tested. Thus it appears that NHEJ repair is required for memory formation. Other cognitive elements were not blocked by ara-C. Mice given ara-C and then subjected to contextual fear conditioning maintained their short-term memory (tested at 30 seconds after training) and exploratory behavior in an open field 24 hours after training. Treatment with ara-C also did not cause general malaise, motor in-coordination, sedation, or anxiety.

7. Long-term memory depends on epigenetic alterations

7.1 Contextual fear memory conditioning causes changes in DNA methylation in brain neurons

Halder et al. [75], in a mouse study, evaluated differently expressed genes and short differentially methylated regions in neurons of the anterior cingulate cortex, a brain region important for associative memory acquisition and maintenance of long-term memory. In the anterior cingulate cortex at 1 hour after contextual fear conditioning, there were 6250 differentially methylated genes with 46,395 differently methylated short regions (700 base pair regions). (Frequently, multiple short differentially methylated regions occurred in a differentially methylated gene.) At 4 weeks after training 1223 differentially methylated genes and 5018 differently methylated short regions persisted. In addition, at 4 weeks after training they found 1700 differentially expressed genes in the anterior cingulate cortex. These findings suggest that long-term memory (4 weeks) is associated with differential methylation of DNA and altered expression of genes.

Halder et al. [75] also evaluated differentially methylated regions and differently expressed genes in the hippocampal CA1 region, a region that is crucial for short-term memory formation during contextual fear conditioning. They found that, in contrast to the anterior cingulate cortex, in the hippocampus there were 1619 differentially methylated regions after 1 hour, but these changes did not persist, and almost none were present after 4 weeks.

Also studying the hippocampus, Duke et al. [76], working with rats, found that at 24 hours after contextual fear conditioning there were more than 5000 differentially methylated regions (500 base pair short regions), but less than 20 differentially methylated regions after context change alone. Hypermethylated differentially methylated regions overlapping differentially expressed genes were associated with decreased gene expression, consistent with the concept that cytosine methylation is often a mechanism for suppressing transcription. Also at 24 hours after contextual fear conditioning, there were more than 2000 differentially methylated regions that were associated with 1048 genes having down-regulated expression and 564 genes having up-regulated expression (usually known to be associated with hypomethylated regions). At 24 hours after training, 9.17% of the genes in the rat genome of hippocampus neurons were differentially methylated. Gene Ontology term analysis was performed, and differentially expressed gene enrichment analysis revealed that many of the genes involved in synaptic functions after fear conditioning were up-regulated.

7.2 The role of base excision repair in memory consolidation

In both the studies of Halder et al. [75] and Duke [76], above, there were on the order of a thousand demethylations of cytosines in neuron genomes during memory consolidation in the brain after contextual fear conditioning. The two likely processes of demethylating cytosine each depend on base excision repair, as shown in **Figure 3**. These processes were reviewed by Bayraktar and Kreutz [77]. There is considerable evidence for the left hand process illustrated in **Figure 3**. In this process there are two or more fast oxidations by one of the ten-eleven translocation methylcytosine dioxygenases (TET1, TET2, TET3), first altering 5-methylcytosine (5mC) to 5-hydroxymethylcytosine (5hmC), and then producing 5-formylcytosine (5fC) followed by

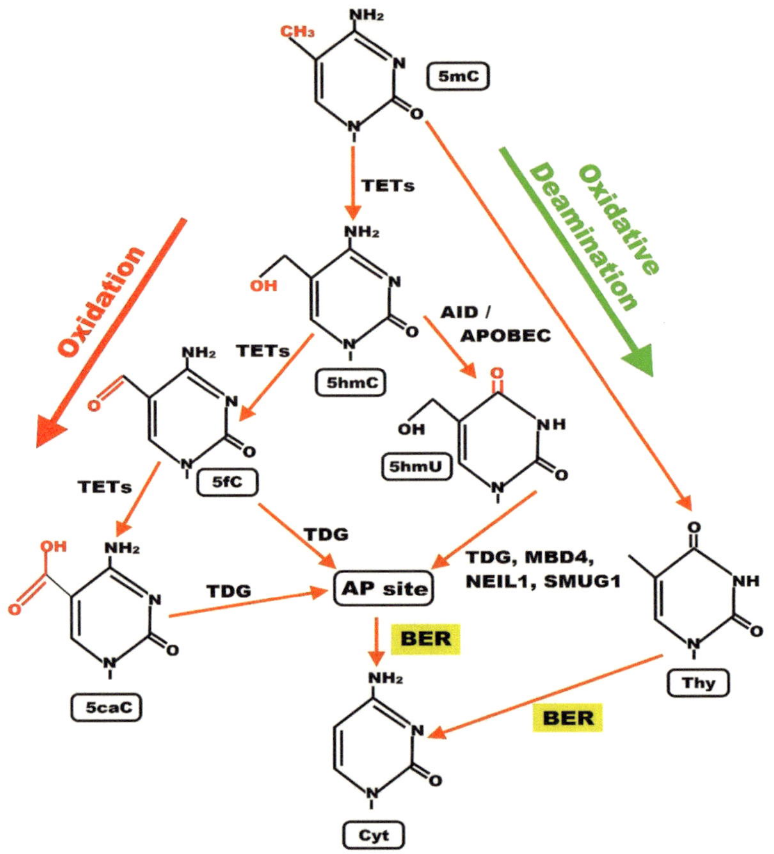

Figure 3.
Demethylation of 5-methylcytosine (5mC) to cytosine (Cyt) in DNA depends on base excision repair (BER) as the final step. In initial steps, the ten-eleven translocation methylcytosine dioxygenase family of enzymes (TET1, TET2, and TET3) each may catalyze the conversion of 5-methylcytosine (5mC) to 5-hydroxymethylcytosine (5hmC) and further steps form 5-formylcytosine (5fC) and 5-carboxylcytosine (5caC). 5fC and 5caC can be excised from DNA by thymine DNA glycosylase (TDG) to form an apyrimidinic site (AP site). AID/APOBEC is a family of cytidine deaminases that can oxidatively deaminate 5mC to 5-hydroxymethyl uracil (5hmU) or 5mC to thymine (Thy). 5hmU can be excised from DNA by TDG, methyl-CpG-binding domain protein 4 (MBD4), endonuclease VIII-like 1 (NEIL1) or single-strand selective monofunctional uracil DNA glycosylase (SMUG1).

5-carboxylcytosine (5caC). Both 5fC and 5caC can be excised by thymine DNA glycosylase (TDG), generating an apyrimidinic (AP) site, which is repaired by base excision repair to place cytosine (cyt) in the DNA opposite guanine. However there is some indication that a cytidine deaminase (AID/APOBEC) enzyme can carry out oxidative deamination of 5mC to 5-hydroxymethyluracil, which is then excised by one of the four enzymes shown, to form an AP site. Alternatively, a cytidine deaminase (AID/APOBEC) may carry out an oxidative deamination of 5mC by to thymine, and the mispair of thymine with guanine is then repaired by base excision repair to generate cytosine paired with guanine in DNA.

Zhang et al. [78] generated homozygous mutant mice deficient in TET1 catalytic activity. These mice were viable and fertile, with no discernible morphological or growth abnormality. The Tet1 deficient mice would be expected to have reduced ability to convert 5mC to cytosine by the TET/base excision repair-dependent pathway. When examined in neural progenitor cells, 478 genes showed elevated promoter DNA methylation levels compared to the wild-type control, while only 32 genes had lower DNA methylation. There was a link between the altered DNA methylation pattern and transcriptional activity. In the neural progenitor cells of TET1 mutant mice 1267 genes were down-regulated with respect to transcription and 498 were up-regulated compared to wild-type. In particular, with TET1 mutant mice, 39 genes were found to be both hyper-methylated and down-regulated in neural progenitor cells isolated from the *dentate gyrus* (part of the brain hippocampus). Four-month-old wild-type and TET1 knockout mice were tested in the Morris water maze. The TET1 deficient mice, with reduced ability to use a pathway dependent on base excision repair, showed impairment in spatial learning and short-term memory.

8. Perspective on the role of DNA repair in cognitive functions

The evidence discussed above in Section 6 clearly indicated that neuronal activity causes DNA double-strand breaks, especially in early response genes after neuronal stimulation. NHEJ repair is required to repair these breaks, and NHEJ repair is required for long-term memory formation. As discussed in Section 7, long-term memory formation depends on large numbers of epigenetic alterations including methylations and demethylations of cytosine in DNA. Although it is known that repair of double-strand breaks by NHEJ repair can leave epigenetic alterations (scars) (including alterations in the pattern of cytosine methylation) after the repair occurs, it is not known whether the NHEJ repair "scars" are a major portion of these epigenetic alterations. About a thousand demethylations occur during long-term memory formation in rats and mice. Base excision repair is central to demethylation of 5mC to cytosine. A deficiency in the TET/base excision repair pathway causes diminished epigenetic demethylations of DNA as well as alterations in memory.

Overall, memory and learning depend on epigenetic alterations. Two forms of DNA repair, NHEJ repair and base excision repair, have essential roles in cognitive functions, and at least base excision repair has a direct role in regulating one major type of epigenetic alteration, the demethylation of 5mC to cytosine in DNA during memory formation.

9. Conclusion

In eukaryotic cell nuclei, DNA is associated with histone proteins in highly organized and compact structures to form chromatin. When the DNA is damaged, repair enzymes need to gain access to the damage, and this requires modification of the compact structure. These modifications, termed epigenetic alterations, include acetylation of histones, methylation of histones and methylation of CpG sequences in DNA. Such epigenetic alterations can allow access of repair enzymes to sites of DNA damage while not disturbing the DNA base-pair sequence.

DNA repair processes are characteristically initiated rapidly and completed in a short period of minutes to hours, but epigenetic alterations introduced by such repair may be retained after repair is completed. A type of epigenetic alteration that can last after repair of a double-strand break is the DNA methylation of CpG islands in gene promoters. Such epigenetic alterations can silence gene expression. Also, several types of oxidative DNA damage are removed by base excision repair. Base excision repair is accompanied by epigenetic alterations of histones that are associated with genes containing CpG islands in their promoters. These epigenetic alterations can cause decreased transcription of the genes.

The persistent behavioral changes that are a prominent feature of addictions appear to be the result of epigenetic alterations that affect gene expression in particular regions of the brain. Specific epigenetic alterations have been found to be associated with addiction to alcohol, nicotine and cocaine. The epigenetic alterations that occur in those particular regions of the brain are considered to be involved with each of the addictions. Nicotine and cocaine, and alcohol through its metabolic product acetaldehyde, cause DNA damage in the brain. Such DNA damage is subject to DNA repair processes that likely cause at least a portion of the long lasting epigenetic alterations found in the brains of addicted individuals.

In humans and other mammals inherited mutations in genes necessary for DNA repair can cause neurodegenerative diseases. Examples of such diseases are ataxia telangiectasia, Huntington's disease, Aicardi-Goutières syndrome and Cockayne syndrome. The deficiencies in DNA repair in these diseases cause disruptions in the pattern of epigenetic alterations required for normal neuronal function. These epigenetic alterations likely underlie key features of the neurodegenerative disease phenotypes.

Learning and new memories occur when mice explore a new, strange environment. Exploration of a novel environment increases the number of neurons with double-strand breaks in neuronal DNA, particularly in the dentate gyrus, which is involved in spatial learning and memory. Another neuronal activity, visual stimulation, was found to cause DNA double-strand breaks. Direct stimulation of the striatum region of the brain also caused DNA double-strand breaks. Memory retention of context associated electric shock events in mice involved induction of double-strand breaks and their repair by the process of non-homologous end joining in the hippocampus, a region of the brain known to be important in forming memories. Inhibition of non-homologous end joining substantially diminished memory retention.

The anterior cingulate cortex is a brain region important for long-term memory formation. Long-term memory (4 weeks in mice) subsequent to a contextual conditioning experience was found to be associated with substantial retention of a differential DNA methylation and gene expression pattern in the anterior cingulate cortex. In addition, differential DNA methylation in the hippocampus appears to be associated with short-term memory formation. Together, long-term and short-term memory formations are associated with on the order of a thousand demethylations of cytosines in neuron genomes during memory consolidation. Demethylation of 5-methylcytosine to cytosine in DNA depends on base excision repair.

In general, the evidence indicates that, in mammals, DNA repair processes can cause epigenetic alterations in chromatin, some of which are long lasting. These epigenetic alterations can have negative consequences on neurological function such as in certain addictions and neurodegenerative diseases. In addition, epigenetic alterations resulting from DNA repair processes, such as non-homologous end joining and base excision repair, appear to have a positive role in facilitating adaptive cognitive capabilities that include memory and learning.

Author details

Carol Bernstein* and Harris Bernstein
Department of Cellular and Molecular Medicine, College of Medicine, University of Arizona, Tucson, Arizona, USA

*Address all correspondence to: bernstein324@yahoo.com

References

[1] Pryor JM, Conlin MP, Carvajal-Garcia J, Luedeman ME, Luthman AJ, Small GW, et al. Ribonucleotide incorporation enables repair of chromosome breaks by nonhomologous end joining. Science. 2018;**361**(6407):1126-1129. DOI: 10.1126/science.aat2477

[2] Dhar S, Gursoy-Yuzugullu O, Parasuram R, Price BD. The tale of a tail: Histone H4 acetylation and the repair of DNA breaks. Philosophical Transactions of the Royal Society of London. Series B, Biological Sciences. 2017;**372**(1731). pii: 20160284). DOI: 10.1098/rstb.2016.0284

[3] Raichle ME, Gusnard DA. Appraising the brain's energy budget. Proceedings of the National Academy of Sciences of the United States of America. 2002;**99**(16):10237-10239. DOI: 10.1073/pnas.172399499

[4] Zovkic JB, Guzman-Karisson MC, Sweatt JD. Epigenetic regulation of memory formation and maintenance. Learning & Memory. 2013;**20**(2):61-74. DOI: 10.1101/lm.026575.112

[5] Bird A. DNA methylation patterns and epigenetic memory. Genes & Development. 2002;**16**(1):6-21. DOI: 10.1101/gad.947102

[6] Budhavarapu VN, Chavez M, Tyler JK. How is epigenetic information maintained through DNA replication? Epigenetics & Chromatin. 2013;**6**(1):32. DOI: 10.1186/1756-8935-6-32

[7] Walker DM, Nestler EJ. Neuroepigenetics and addiction. Handbook of Clinical Neurology. 2018;**148**:747-765. DOI: 10.1016/B978-0-444-64076-5.00048-X

[8] Ding N, Maiuri AR, O'Hagan HM. The emerging role of epigenetic modifiers in repair of DNA damage associated with chronic inflammatory diseases. Mutation Research—Reviews in Mutation Research. Online Sept 28, 2017. In Press. DOI: 10.1016/j.mrrev.2017.09.005

[9] Polo SE, Almouzni G. Chromatin dynamics after DNA damage: The legacy of the access-repair-restore model. DNA Repair (Amst). 2015;**36**:114-121. DOI: 10.1016/j.dnarep.2015.09.014

[10] Eberharter A, Becker PB. Histone acetylation: A switch between repressive and permissive chromatin. Second in review series on chromatin dynamics. EMBO Reports. 2002;**3**(3):224-229. DOI: 10.1093/embo-reports/kvf053

[11] Black JC, Van Rechem C, Whetstine JR. Histone lysine methylation dynamics: Establishment, regulation, and biological impact. Molecular Cell. 2012;**48**(4):491-507. DOI: 10.1016/j.molcel.2012.11.006

[12] Wei S, Li C, Yin Z, Wen J, Meng H, Xue L, et al. Histone methylation in DNA repair and clinical practice: New findings during the past 5-years. Journal of Cancer. 2018;**9**(12):2072-2081. DOI: 10.7150/jca.23427

[13] Swierczynski S, Klieser E, Illig R, Alinger-Scharinger B, Kiesslich T, Neureiter D. Histone deacetylation meets miRNA: Epigenetics and post-transcriptional regulation in cancer and chronic diseases. Expert Opinion on Biological Therapy. 2015;**15**(5):651-664. DOI: 10.1517/14712598.2015.1025047

[14] Wikipedia article "Chromatin remodeling" figure is adapted from Luong, P. Basic Principles of Genetics, Connexions Web site (2009) under a Creative Commons Attribution License (CC-BY 3.0). Further modification of the figure is performed by the image uploader with reference from Davis PK, Brackmann RK. Chromatin

remodeling and cancer. Cancer Biology & Therapy. 2003;**2**:22. Image labeled for non-commercial reuse, licensed under the Creative Commons Attribution 3.0 License

[15] Dabin J, Fortuny A, Polo SE. Epigenome maintenance in response to DNA damage. Molecular Cell. 2016;**62**(5):712-727. DOI: 10.1016/j.molcel.2016.04.006

[16] Russo G, Landi R, Pezone A, Morano A, Zuchegna C, Romano A, et al. DNA damage and repair modify DNA methylation and chromatin domain of the targeted locus: Mechanism of allele methylation polymorphism. Scientific Reports. 2016;**6**:33222. DOI: 10.1038/srep33222

[17] Allen B, Pezone A, Porcellini A, Muller MT, Masternak MM. Non-homologous end joining induced alterations in DNA methylation: A source of permanent epigenetic change. Oncotarget. 2017;**8**(25):40359-40372. DOI: 10.18632/oncotarget.16122

[18] O'Hagan HM, Wang W, Sen S, Destefano Shields C, Lee SS, Zhang YW, et al. Oxidative damage targets complexes containing DNA methyltransferases, SIRT1, and polycomb members to promoter CpG Islands. Cancer Cell. 2011;**20**(5): 606-619. DOI: 10.1016/j.ccr.2011.09.012

[19] Hauer MH, Gasser SM. Chromatin and nucleosome dynamics in DNA damage and repair. Genes & Development. 2017;**31**(22):2204-2221. DOI: 10.1101/gad.307702.117

[20] Nestler EJ, Barrot M, Self DW. DeltaFosB: A sustained molecular switch for addiction. Proceedings of the National Academy of Sciences of the United States of America. 2001;**98**(20):11042-11046. DOI: 10.1073/pnas.191352698

[21] Available from: https://www.niaaa.nih.gov/alcohol-health/overview-alcohol-consumption/alcohol-facts-and-statistics

[22] Oscar-Berman M, Valmas MM, Sawyer KS, Ruiz SM, Luhar RB, Gravitz ZR. Profiles of impaired, spared, and recovered neuropsychologic processes in alcoholism. Handbook of Clinical Neurology. 2014;**125**:183-210. DOI: 10.1016/B978-0-444-62619-6.00012-4

[23] Fein G, Torres J, Price LJ, Di Sclafani V. Cognitive performance in long-term abstinent alcoholic individuals. Alcoholism, Clinical and Experimental Research. 2006;**30**(9):1538-1544. DOI: 10.1111/j.1530-0277.2006.00185.x

[24] Bottlender M, Soyka M. Impact of craving on alcohol relapse during, and 12 months following, outpatient treatment. Alcohol and Alcoholism. 2004;**39**(4):357-361. DOI: 10.1093/alcalc/agh073

[25] Moos RH, Moos BS. Rates and predictors of relapse after natural and treated remission from alcohol use disorders. Addiction. 2006;**101**(2):212-222. DOI: 10.1111/j.1360-0443.2006.01310.x

[26] Krishnan HR, Sakharkar AJ, Teppen TL, Berkel TD, Pandey SC. The epigenetic landscape of alcoholism. International Review of Neurobiology. 2014;**115**:75-116. DOI: 10.1016/B978-0-12-801311-3.00003-2

[27] Jangra A, Sriram CS, Pandey S, Choubey P, Rajput P, Saroha B, et al. Epigenetic modifications, alcoholic brain and potential drug targets. Annals of Neurosciences. 2016;**23**(4):246-260. DOI: 10.1159/000449486

[28] Berkel TD, Pandey SC. Emerging role of epigenetic mechanisms in alcohol

addiction. Alcoholism, Clinical and Experimental Research. 2017;**41**(4): 666-680. DOI: 10.1111/acer.13338

[29] D'Addario C, Caputi FF, Ekström TJ, Di Benedetto M, Maccarrone M, Romualdi P, et al. Ethanol induces epigenetic modulation of prodynorphin and pronociceptin gene expression in the rat amygdala complex. Journal of Molecular Neuroscience. 2013;**49**(2):312-319. DOI: 10.1007/s12031-012-9829-y

[30] Available from: https://www.samhsa.gov/data/sites/default/files/NSDUHresultsPDFWHTML2013/Web/NSDUHresults2013.pdf

[31] Available from: https://www.drugabuse.gov/publications/research-reports/tobacco-nicotine-e-cigarettes/nicotine-addictive

[32] Available from: https://www.ncbi.nlm.nih.gov/pmc/articles/PMC2376894/pdf/0980317.pdf

[33] Levine A, Huang Y, Drisaldi B, Griffin EA Jr, Pollak DD, Xu S, et al. Molecular mechanism for a gateway drug: Epigenetic changes initiated by nicotine prime gene expression by cocaine. Science Translational Medicine. 2011;**3**(107):107-109. DOI: 10.1126/scitranslmed.3003062

[34] Ruffle JK. Molecular neurobiology of addiction: What's all the (Δ) FosB about? The American Journal of Drug and Alcohol Abuse. 2014;**40**(6):428-437. DOI: 10.3109/00952990.2014.933840

[35] Nestler EJ. Epigenetic mechanisms of drug addiction. Neuropharmacology. 2014;**76**(Pt B):259-268. DOI: 10.1016/j.neuropharm.2013.04.004

[36] Gozen O, Balkan B, Yildirim E, Koylu EO, Pogun S. The epigenetic effect of nicotine on dopamine D1 receptor expression in rat prefrontal cortex. Synapse. 2013;**67**(9):545-552. DOI: 10.1002/syn.21659

[37] Simpson DD, Joe GW, Broome KM. A national 5-year follow-up of treatment outcomes for cocaine dependence. Archives of General Psychiatry. 2002;**59**(6):538-544. DOI: 10.1001/archpsyc.59.6.538

[38] Renthal W, Kumar A, Xiao G, Wilkinson M, Covington HE 3rd, Maze I, et al. Genome-wide analysis of chromatin regulation by cocaine reveals a role for sirtuins. Neuron. 2009;**62**(3):335-348. DOI: 10.1016/j.neuron.2009.03.026

[39] Rulten SL, Hodder E, Ripley TL, Stephens DN, Mayne LV. Alcohol induces DNA damage and the Fanconi anemia D2 protein implicating FANCD2 in the DNA damage response pathways in brain. Alcoholism, Clinical and Experimental Research. 2008;**32**(7):1186-1196. DOI: 10.1111/j.1530-0277.2008.00673.x

[40] Hukkanen J, Jacob P 3rd, Benowitz NL.Metabolism and disposition kinetics of nicotine. Pharmacological Reviews 2005;**57**(1):79-115. DOI: 10.1124/pr.57.1.3

[41] Lee HW, Park SH, Weng MW, Wang HT, Huang WC, Lepor H, et al. E-cigarette smoke damages DNA and reduces repair activity in mouse lung, heart, and bladder as well as in human lung and bladder cells. Proceedings of the National Academy of Sciences of the United States of America. 2018;**115**(7):E1560-E1569. DOI: 10.1073/pnas.1718185115

[42] de Souza MF, Gonçales TA, Steinmetz A, Moura DJ, Saffi J, Gomez R, et al. Cocaine induces DNA damage in distinct brain areas of female rats under different hormonal conditions. Clinical and Experimental Pharmacology &

Physiology. 2014;**41**(4):265-269. DOI: 10.1111/1440-1681.12218

[43] Johnson Z, Venters J, Guarraci FA, Zewail-Foote M. Methamphetamine induces DNA damage in specific regions of the female rat brain. Clinical and Experimental Pharmacology & Physiology. 2015;**42**(6):570-575. DOI: 10.1111/1440-1681.12404

[44] Tokunaga I, Ishigami A, Kubo S, Gotohda T, Kitamura O. The peroxidative DNA damage and apoptosis in methamphetamine-treated rat brain. The Journal of Medical Investigation. 2008;**55**(3-4):241-245. DOI: 10.2152/jmi.55.241

[45] Berger ND, Stanley FKT, Moore S, Goodarzi AA. ATM-dependent pathways of chromatin remodeling and oxidative DNA damage responses. Philosophical Transactions of the Royal Society B. 2017;**372**. pll: 20160283. DOI: 10.1098/rstb.2016.0283

[46] Li J, Chen J, Ricupero CL, Hart RP, Schwartz MS, Kusnecov A, et al. Nuclear accumulation of HDAC4 in ATM deficiency promotes neurodegeneration in ataxia telangiectasia. Nature Medicine. 2012;**18**(5):783-790. DOI: 10.1038/nm.2709

[47] Massey TH, Jones L. The central role of DNA damage and repair in CAG repeat diseases. Disease Models & Mechanisms. 2018;**11**(1). pii: dmm031930). DOI: 10.1242/dmm.031930

[48] Maiuri T, Mocle AJ, Hung CL, Xia J, van Roon-Mom WM, Truant R. Huntingtin is a scaffolding protein in the ATM oxidative DNA damage response complex. Human Molecular Genetics. 2017;**26**(2):395-406. DOI: 10.1093/hmg/ddw395

[49] Horvath S, Langfelder P, Kwak S, Aaronson J, Rosinski J, Vogt TF, et al. Huntington's disease accelerates epigenetic aging of human brain and disrupts DNA methylation levels. Aging (Albany NY). 2016;**8**(7):1485-1512. DOI: 10.18632/aging.101005

[50] Glajch KE, Sadri-Vakili G. Epigenetic mechanisms involved in Huntington's disease pathogenesis. Journal of Huntington's Disease. 2015;**4**(1):1-15. DOI: 10.3233/JHD-159001

[51] Lim YW, Sanz LA, Xu X, Hartone SR, Chetin F. Genome-wide DNA hypomethylation and RNA:DNA hybrid accumulation in Aicardi-Goutieres syndrome. eLife. 2015;**4**:08007. DOI: 10.7554/eLife.08007

[52] McKinnon PJ. Genome integrity and disease prevention in the nervous system. Genes & Development. 2017;**31**(12):1180-1194. DOI: 10.1101/gad.301325.117

[53] Reijns MA, Bubeck D, Gibson LC, Graham SC, Baillie GS, Jones EY, et al. The structure of the human RNase H2 complex defines key interaction interfaces relevant to enzyme function and human disease. The Journal of Biological Chemistry. 2011;**286**(12):10530-10539. DOI: 10.1074/jbc.M110.177394

[54] Fousteri M, Vermeulen W, van Zeeland AA, Mullenders LH. Cockayne syndrome A and B proteins differentially regulate recruitment of chromatin remodeling and repair factors to stalled RNA polymerase II in vivo. Molecular Cell. 2006;**23**(4):471-482. DOI: 10.1016/j.molcel.2006.06.029

[55] Cho I, Tsai PF, Lake RJ, Basheer A, Fan HY. ATP-dependent chromatin remodeling by Cockayne syndrome protein B and NAP1-like histone

chaperones is required for efficient transcription-coupled DNA repair. PLoS Genetics. 2013;**9**(4):e1003407. DOI: 10.1371/journal.pgen.1003407

[56] Boetefuer EL, Lake RJ, Fan HY. Mechanistic insights into the regulation of transcription and transcription-coupled DNA repair by Cockayne syndrome protein B. Nucleic Acids Research. 2018;**46**(15):7471-7479. DOI: 10.1093/nar/gky660

[57] Wang WY, Pan L, Su SC, Quinn EJ, Sasaki M, Jimenez JC, et al. Interaction of FUS and HDAC1 regulates DNA damage response and repair in neurons. Nature Neuroscience. 2013;**16**(10):1383-1391. DOI: 10.1038/nn.3514

[58] Alpatov R, Lesch BJ, Nakamoto-Kinoshita M, Blanco A, Chen S, Stützer A, et al. A chromatin-dependent role of the fragile X mental retardation protein FMRP in the DNA damage response. Cell. 2014;**157**(4):869-881. DOI: 10.1016/j.cell.2014.03.040

[59] Khonsari H, Schneider M, Al-Mahdawi S, Chianea YG, Themis M, Parris C, et al. Lentivirus-meditated frataxin gene delivery reverses genome instability in Friedreich ataxia patient and mouse model fibroblasts. Gene Therapy. 2016;**23**(12):846-856. DOI: 10.1038/gt.2016.61

[60] Fujita K, Nakamura Y, Oka T, Ito H, Tamura T, Tagawa K, et al. A functional deficiency of TERA/VCP/p97 contributes to impaired DNA repair in multiple polyglutamine diseases. Nature Communications. 2013;**4**:1816. DOI: 10.1038/ncomms2828

[61] Theil AF, Hoeijmakers JH, Vermeulen W. TTDA: Big impact of a small protein. Experimental Cell Research. 2014;**329**(1):61-68. DOI: 10.1016/j.yexcr.2014.07.008

[62] Koch SC, Simon N, Ebert C, Carell T. Molecular mechanisms of xeroderma pigmentosum (XP) proteins. Quarterly Reviews of Biophysics. 2016;**49**:e5. DOI: 10.1017/S0033583515000268

[63] Serrano M. Epigenetic cerebellar diseases. Handbook of Clinical Neurology. 2018;**155**:227-244. DOI: 10.1016/B978-0-444-64189-2.00015-9

[64] Yandim C, Natisvili T, Festenstein R. Gene regulation and epigenetics in Friedreich's ataxia. Journal of Neurochemistry. 2013;**126**(Suppl 1):21-42. DOI: 10.1111/jnc.12254

[65] Cvetanovic M, Kular RK, Opal P. LANP mediates neuritic pathology in Spinocerebellar ataxia type 1. Neurobiology of Disease. 2012;**48**(3):526-532. DOI: 10.1016/j.nbd.2012.07.024

[66] Singh A, Compe E, Le May N, Egly JM. TFIIH subunit alterations causing xeroderma pigmentosum and trichothiodystrophy specifically disturb several steps during transcription. American Journal of Human Genetics. 2015;**96**(2):194-207. DOI: 10.1016/j.ajhg.2014.12.012

[67] Le May N, Fradin D, Iltis I, Bougnères P, Egly JM. XPG and XPF endonucleases trigger chromatin looping and DNA demethylation for accurate expression of activated genes. Molecular Cell. 2012;**47**(4):622-632. DOI: 10.1016/j.molcel.2012.05.050

[68] Rogakou EP, Pilch DR, Orr AH, Ivanova VS. Bonner WM. DNA double-stranded breaks induce histone H2AX phosphorylation on serine 139. The Journal of Biological Chemistry. 1998;**273**(10):5858-5868

[69] Furuta T, Takemura H, Liao ZY, Aune GJ, Redon C, Sedelnikova OA,

et al. Phosphorylation of histone H2AX and activation of Mre11, Rad50, and Nbs1 in response to replication-dependent DNA double-strand breaks induced by mammalian DNA topoisomerase I cleavage complexes. The Journal of Biological Chemistry. 2003;**278**(22):20303-20312. DOI: 10.1074/jbc.M300198200

[70] Suberbielle E, Sanchez PE, Kravitz AV, Wang X, Ho K, Eilertson K, et al. Physiologic brain activity causes DNA double-strand breaks in neurons, with exacerbation by amyloid-β. Nature Neuroscience. 2013;**16**(5):613-621. DOI: 10.1038/nn.3356

[71] Kim JJ, Jung MW. Neural circuits and mechanisms involved in Pavlovian fear conditioning: A critical review. Neuroscience and Biobehavioral Reviews. 2006;**30**(2):188-202. DOI: 10.1016/j.neubiorev.2005.06.005

[72] Madabhushi R, Gao F, Pfenning AR, Pan L, Yamakawa S, Seo J, et al. Activity-induced DNA breaks govern the expression of neuronal early-response genes. Cell. 2015;**161**(7): 1592-1605. DOI: 10.1016/j.cell.2015.05.032

[73] Colón-Cesario M, Wang J, Ramos X, García HG, Dávila JJ, Laguna J, et al. An inhibitor of DNA recombination blocks memory consolidation, but not reconsolidation, in context fear conditioning. Journal of Neuroscience. 2006;**26**(20):5524-5533. DOI: 10.1523/JNEUROSCI.3050-05.2006

[74] Hansen N. The longevity of hippocampus-dependent memory is orchestrated by the locus coeruleus-noradrenergic system. Neural Plasticity. 2017;**2017**:2727602. DOI: 10.1155/2017/2727602

[75] Halder R, Hennion M, Vidal RO, Shomroni O, Rahman RU, Rajput A, et al. DNA methylation changes in plasticity genes accompany the formation and maintenance of memory. Nature Neuroscience. 2016;**19**(1): 102-110. DOI: 10.1038/nn.4194

[76] Duke CG, Kennedy AJ, Gavin CF, Day JJ, Sweatt JD. Experience-dependent epigenomic reorganization in the hippocampus. Learning & Memory. 2017;**24**(7):278-288. DOI: 10.1101/lm.045112.117

[77] Bayraktar G, Kreutz MR. The role of activity-dependent DNA demethylation in the adult brain and in neurological disorders. Frontiers in Molecular Neuroscience. 2018;**11**:169. DOI: 10.3389/fnmol.2018.00169

[78] Zhang RR, Cui QY, Murai K, Lim YC, Smith ZD, Jin S, et al. Tet1 regulates adult hippocampal neurogenesis and cognition. Cell Stem Cell. 2013;**13**(2):237-245. DOI: 10.1016/j.stem.2013.05.006

Chapter 7

Regulation of Oxidized Base Repair in Human Chromatin by Posttranslational Modification

Shiladitya Sengupta, Chunying Yang, Bradley J. Eckelmann, Muralidhar L. Hegde and Sankar Mitra

Abstract

Base excision repair (BER) is the major pathway for the repair of oxidized bases and apurinic/apyrimidinic (abasic; AP) sites produced by reaction with reactive oxygen/nitrogen species (ROS/RNS). These metabolites are generated spontaneously by endogenous cellular processes and also by environmental agents. Because most of these lesions are promutagenic, linked to diverse disease-associated somatic mutations, as well as heritable single nucleotide polymorphisms (SNPs) in the normal human population, their prompt repair is warranted. Impairment of repair leading to mutation, a hallmark of cancer, underscores the essentiality of BER for maintaining genome integrity in humans and other mammals. In mammals, repair of oxidized bases and other BER substrates is initiated by DNA glycosylases (DGs), which excise the damaged bases and cleave the DNA strands at the resulting AP sites, followed by sequential end processing, gap-filling DNA synthesis, and ligation. *In vitro* BER performed with naked DNA substrates has been extensively studied, which delineates its basic mechanistic steps and subpathways. However, recent interest is directed to unraveling BER in cell chromatin, including its regulation via posttranslational modifications (PTMs), which occurs possibly in concert with nucleosome remodeling. Emerging reports on various PTMs of BER enzymes indicate that the PTMs, while dispensable for the enzymatic activity, regulate overall repair by modulating interactions with other repair proteins and chromatin factors, assembly of BER complexes, as well as turnover of the proteins, and may ultimately dictate the cellular phenotype. Here, we discuss recent advances in the BER field by reviewing the PTMs and how they regulate BER in chromatin.

Keywords: oxidative stress, base oxidation, base excision repair, posttranslational modifications, acetylation, phosphorylation, SUMOylation, methylation, chromatin

1. Introduction

DNA, the genetic repository of all cellular functions, is packaged with histones into chromatin consisting of nucleosome units. One hundred forty-seven base pair (bp) segments in DNA wrap ~1.65 times in a left-handed superhelical turn around a histone octamer consisting of two histone H2A-H2B dimers and a H3-H4 tetramer, which form the nucleosome core; the adjacent nucleosomes are separated by some

50 bp unfolded, linker DNA bound to histone H1 or H5. Organization of DNA into chromatin enables the compaction required to accommodate large eukaryotic genomes inside the cell nucleus. This compaction renders DNA inaccessible to any DNA transaction machinery. Replication and transcription are tightly coordinated with specific interactions of their complexes with DNA [1, 2].

The integrity of DNA is under constant threat, naturally from endogenous sources, as well as by environmental factors in the form of a chemical addition, an alteration in the nitrogen base structure, thereby creating an abnormal nucleotide, or a break in one or both strands of DNA [3–8]. Cellular metabolic processes including mitochondrial respiration and hydrolytic reactions generate reactive molecules, such as reactive oxygen species (ROS), reactive nitrogen species (RNS), and alkylating agents. Some chemical bonds in DNA are susceptible to spontaneous hydrolysis. About 70,000 lesions are generated per cell, per day in humans. Single-strand breaks (SSBs), as well as a plethora of oxidized bases, are formed during oxidative genome damage. In addition, deamination, depurination, depyrimidination, double-strand breaks (DSBs), propano-, etheno-, and malondialdehyde-derived DNA adducts, base propenals, and alkylated bases are also formed endogenously. Environmental factors such as UV rays, ionizing radiation (IR), heat, and chemicals from tobacco smoke and industrial sources pose additional risks to DNA.

2. Oxidative genome damage and oxidized bases

For aerobic organisms, oxygen acts like a double-edged sword; while it is absolutely essential for life, it is also a threat to the life, recognized as the "Oxygen Paradox" [9–11]. ROS, which include the superoxide anion ($O_2^{\bullet-}$), hydrogen peroxide (H_2O_2), singlet oxygen ($^1O_2$), and the hydroxyl radical ($^{\bullet}OH$), along with RNS, for example, peroxynitrite ($ONOO^-$) react with all biological molecules including DNA. The hydroxyl radical having the highest reduction potential is mainly generated from Fenton reaction between reduced redox active metal ions (Fe^{2+}, Cu^+) and H_2O_2 [12], as well as by the IR-induced radiolysis of water [13]. A wide variety of cellular antioxidant defense mechanisms including both redox-buffering enzymatic and nonenzymatic systems have evolved, for example, superoxide dismutases, catalases, glutathione peroxidases, peroxiredoxins, and glutaredoxins; these counteract the detrimental effect of oxidative stress to the biological molecules, and an imbalance in their homeostasis leads to increased damage to the biomolecules [14].

A plethora of oxidized base lesions are generated mostly from guanine (G) in DNA, which has the lowest redox potential among the natural bases. Other lesions including 2-deoxyribose modifications, SSBs, DSBs, and protein-DNA cross-links are also ROS reaction products in DNA [10, 14–17]. Nearly 100 such lesions have been identified; however, because of the lack of sensitivity of the techniques used to identify the lesions and inherent instability of some of them, the total number formed in the genome under a pro-oxidant environment is likely to be much higher [18].

The most commonly formed oxidized base lesion is 7,8-dihydro-8-oxoguanine (8-oxoguanine, 8-oxoG), which was discovered by Kasai and Nishimura in 1983 and coined as 8-hydroxyguanine [19–21]. All the nucleobases are also ionized by IR and by high intensity 266-ns laser photolysis. The DNA bases undergo one-electron oxidation (one electron ionization potential of $G<A<C\sim T$). 8-oxoG is generated at a much higher level (>5-fold) than the combined level of other one-electron base oxidation products. Singlet oxygen ($^1O_2$), the major ROS in UVA-mediated oxidation of DNA, specifically targets G and 2-deoxyribose moiety [22–24]. Other major oxidized base lesions are 5-hydroxy-6-hydrothymine, thymine glycol (TG), cytosine glycol (CG), 5-hydroxycytosine (5-OHC), uracil glycol (UG), 5-hydroxyuracil

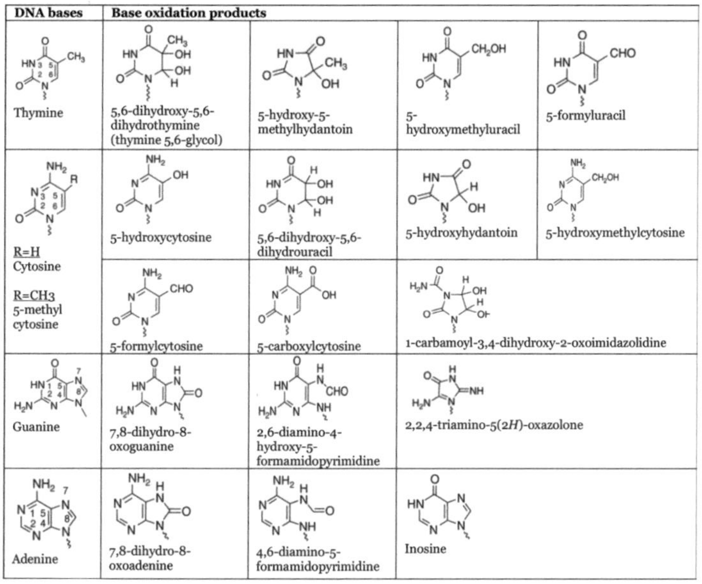

Table 1.
Common oxidized bases detected in DNA.

(5-OHU), 8-hydroxyadenine, and 2-hydroxyadenine [14, 17]. Hypochlorous acid (HOCl), generated by myeloperoxidase in neutrophils during inflammation, chlorinates both DNA and RNA bases [25, 26], and the main products are 5-chlorocytosine, 8-chloroadenine, and 8-chloroguanine. A summary of commonly formed oxidized bases detected in cellular DNA is shown in **Table 1** [16]. Apart from ROS-induced generation of oxidized bases, 5-hydroxymethylcytosine (5hmC), 5-formylcytosine (5fC), and 5-carboxylcytosine (5caC) are formed enzymatically during transcriptional reprogramming involving oxidative demethylation of 5-methyl C (5mC), mostly localized in promoter CpG islands, induced by TET dioxygenases [27, 28]. However, enzymatically generated 5-methyl C oxidation products are produced >2-fold higher than that from direct oxidative damage to DNA [29, 30]. Additionally, tandem base lesions are produced by radicals generated from •OH or one-electron oxidation reactions. Examples include the addition of either 5-(uracilyl)methyl radicals or 6-hydroxy-5,6-dihydrocytosin-5-yl radicals to 5′-adjacent guanine moieties in the DNA of cells exposed to H_2O_2 [31, 32] and formation of a guanine-thymine cross-link upon initial formation of guanine radical cation [33, 34]. One-electron oxidation also leads to DNA-protein cross-links. UVA irradiation of 6-thioguanine-containing DNA forms DNA-protein cross-links in human cells [33, 35].

3. Fate of oxidized bases and accumulation of mutations

ROS-induced oxidized base lesions and AP sites if left unrepaired are replicated by replicative or DNA translesion synthesis (TLS) polymerases [36]. Their misreplication generates mutations, a hallmark of cancer genomes, which account for two-thirds of single base pair substitutions [37–40]. Furthermore, single nucleotide polymorphisms (SNPs), observed in normal human genomes, also likely result from such spontaneous single base pair substitutions. U and 5-OHU, the spontaneous and ROS-induced oxidative deamination product of C, respectively, preferably pair with A during replication, resulting in GC → AT transition mutation; 8-oxoG, the predominant oxidized base lesion mispairs with A, leading to GC → TA transversion mutation [41, 42]. In response to continuous assault by both endogenous and environmental factors, cellular defense mechanisms including diverse DNA repair pathways have evolved in all organisms to correct these base modifications and maintain genomic integrity.

4. Base excision repair of oxidized bases

Base excision repair (BER) is responsible for repairing most oxidized base lesions, AP sites, and DNA SSBs. The basic mechanism of BER first elucidated in *Escherichia coli* is broadly conserved across all organisms, as highlighted in several reviews [43–46]. BER requiring only four or five enzymes in the basic reaction steps is initiated with excision of the damaged base by a monofunctional DNA glycosylase (DG), for example, uracil-DNA glycosylase (UDG) or 3-methyladenine-DNA glycosylase, generating an abasic apurinic/apyrimidinic (AP) site due to hydrolysis of the N-glycosidic bond of the damaged base. The AP endonuclease (APE1 in mammalian cells) cleaves the resulting AP site in the second step and generates 3′ OH and 5′ deoxyribose phosphate (dRP) termini. The DNA polymerase in the third step fills in the single nucleotide gap. In mammalian cells, DNA polymerase β (Pol β) also has intrinsic dRP lyase activity, which cleaves the dRP residue and generates 5′ phosphate; the resulting nick after incorporation of the correct base is sealed by DNA ligase III (Lig III) complexed with XRCC1 in the final step.

The BER initiating DGs for oxidized bases, on the other hand, are bifunctional with intrinsic AP lyase activity. The bifunctional oxidized base-specific DGs further process the AP site via β or βδ lyase reaction. The Nth family of DGs, OGG1, and NTH1, via β eliminations generates 3′ phospho α,β-unsaturated aldehyde (3′ PUA; formally named 3′ phospho 4-hydroxylpentenal) and 5′ phosphate at the strand break. NTH1 prefers oxidized pyrimidines as substrates, and 8-oxoG and ring opened guanine, that is, formamidopyrimidine (Fapy-G), are preferred substrates for OGG1. The Fpg/Nei family DGs NEIL1, NEIL2, NEIL3, discovered by us and others [47–51] catalyze βδ elimination and remove the deoxyribose residue to produce a 3′ phosphate and 5′ phosphate at the strand break. NEILs prefer modified pyrimidine substrates, NEIL1 having preference for ring-opened purines, for example, Fapy-A and Fapy-G. The activity and substrate specificity of NEILs depend on the DNA structure, and NEILs have significant 5-OHU excision activity with single-stranded or bubble, forked DNA. In contrast, OGG1 and NTH1 prefer double-stranded DNA substrates. Usually, the base excision and lyase reactions act in a concerted sequence. However, due to weak lyase activity of OGG1, intact AP sites are the major product after OGG1-catalyzed cleavage of 8-oxoG [52, 53]. All these bifunctional DGs have broad and overlapping substrate range and possess backup activity for many base lesions. This accounts for the fact that only few DGs have been discovered so far for much larger number of oxidized bases and for the nonessentiality of individual DGs.

The 3′ phosphate generated by the NEILs by βδ elimination is a poor substrate for mammalian APE1 and is processed by polynucleotide kinase phosphatase (PNKP) [54–57]. Thus, for oxidized bases, the DGs actually define the subsequent steps. APE1 is responsible for processing the β elimination product of OGG1 and NTH1, whereas PNKP is required for generating 3′-OH termini from 3′ phosphate, a βδ elimination product of NEILs. Furthermore, AP sites and 3′ PUA generated by other DNA glycosylases can also be processed through a NEIL-PNKP-dependent pathway [53, 57]. This alternative repair route provides the functional redundancy in mammalian BER for genome safeguarding against a plethora of endogenous and induced oxidative damages.

BER, in the simplistic model, generates a 1-nucleotide gap after excision of the damaged base and has been termed single nucleotide BER (SN-BER) or short-patch BER (SP-BER). In contrast, long-patch BER (LP-BER) involves repair synthesis of two to eight deoxynucleotides. The 5′ blocking group after oxidation of AP sites cannot be removed by Pol β via its dRP lyase activity. Instead it is removed by 5′-flap endonuclease 1 (FEN-1), which is normally required for removing the 5′ RNA primers from Okazaki fragments during DNA replication. Thus, the subsequent steps of LP-BER are identical to that of DNA replication, utilizing DNA replication machinery, involving DNA polymerases δ/ε (Pol δ/ε) and DNA ligase I (Lig I). These enzymes including FEN-1 are recruited by the sliding clamp PCNA, loaded by replication factor-C (RFC), as in replication [58]. Thus, the choice of LP-BER vs. SN-BER depends on the 5′-terminus at the base cleavage site. With unaltered aldehyde group in deoxyribose, Pol β could carry out SN-BER by excising the 5′-dRP. LP-BER becomes necessary for repairing the oxidized AP sites, which cannot be processed by the 5′ end cleaning lyase activity of Pol β. The nuclear replicative Pol δ/ε lack dRP lyase activity and thus repair synthesis by these enzymes have to follow the LP-BER subpathway. Because Pol β-depleted cells are resistant to oxidative stress, Pol δ/ε can substitute for DNA Pol β and carry out the preferred LP-BER. The BER subpathways are schematically shown in **Figure 1**, adapted from [44].

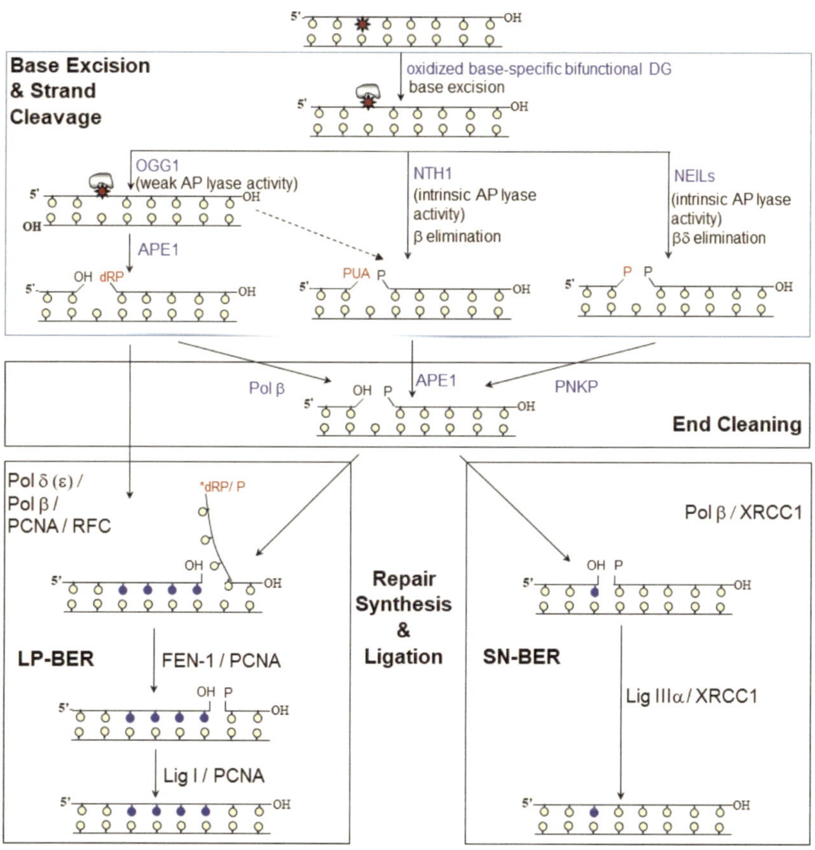

Figure 1.
A schematic representation of oxidized base-specific BER subpathways. The damaged base is represented as ✸. *BER is initiated by the DGs: OGG1, NTH1, NEILs, and converge to common steps for end cleaning, followed by repair synthesis and ligation. See text for details.*

5. Prereplicative BER of oxidized bases

The genomic integrity is particularly vulnerable during replication. Transient single-stranded (ss) DNA serving as a template during DNA replication after unwinding of the duplex genome is particularly vulnerable to ROS, which induces oxidized bases, sugar fragments, as well as strand breaks. Most oxidized bases do not stall replicative DNA polymerases, but they mispair during replication, thereby causing mutations. In contrast, bulky lesions, which stall replicative polymerases, block replisomes so as to allow repair. However, blocked replication may also lead to fork collapse, causing significant alteration in genomic stability. Furthermore, oxidized deoxynucleotides may be incorporated into the progeny strand during replication. If left unrepaired, these mutations could accumulate in progeny cells, a recipe for pathologies linked to genomic instability, including cancer, accelerated aging, and degenerative brain diseases [59, 60]. Repair of oxidative lesions, which are generated at much higher abundance than the bulky adducts in the replicating genome, is thus critical to maintain genomic fidelity. Mammalian cells have developed multiple ways to faithfully repair such base damages via prereplicative repair in the template strand and postreplicative repair in the progeny strand, immediately after replicative synthesis. Both the pathways involve an intricate collaboration of specific repair machinery with the replication proteins, likely via formation of dynamic "preformed" "repair-replication complexes" at the replication fork [61, 62].

Repair of most mutagenic base lesions except 8-oxoG, for example, 5-OHU, TG, 5-OHC, Fapy-A, 8-oxoA, and UG must be carried out prior to replication in order to prevent mutation fixation. How such lesions, which do not block replicative Pol δ, are flagged for prereplicative repair without causing DSBs was unclear. Our recent study showed that the mammalian DG NEIL1 binds to the oxidized lesion sites in ss DNA substrates *in vitro* to facilitate fork regression and participates in prereplicative repair of the damaged base in the reannealed duplex DNA [61, 62]. We compared the function of NEIL1 in stalling the replication fork at the damage sites for the prereplicative repair to the function of a "cow catcher" attached to the front of early steam locomotives that served to push aside animals or debris from the track ahead of the train's traversal, in a simplistic analogy to this exquisitely orchestrated process [63]. The key features of this "cow catcher" model are the ability of NEIL1 to recognize base lesions in ss DNA templates and its nonproductive binding to lesions in ss DNA, which, while preventing lethal DSB formation, causes the stalling of the replication fork. Subsequent fork reversal allows base lesion repair in the reannealed duplex. High expression and activation of NEIL1 in replicating cells, together with its stable physical and functional association with proteins in the DNA replication complex [48, 64–66], are consistent with this surveillance role of NEIL1. The human genome during each cell division may be at higher risk for oxidative damage whose repair would prevent accumulation of mutations in the daughter cells. Thus NEIL1's prereplicative BER function appears to be critical for preventing mutations and maintaining genome fidelity during cell division.

6. Posttranslational modifications of BER proteins

In vitro BER studies, carried out during the last couple of decades, are straightforward, mainly documenting functions of the repair proteins; however, in the complex cellular environment, the pathways are tightly regulated by interactions among the partner proteins in multiprotein complexes, which in turn also dictates the stability of the complexes. The stability and subcellular localization of these proteins are regulated by site-specific posttranslational modifications (PTMs), primarily involving acetylation, methylation, phosphorylation, SUMOylation, ubiquitination, and PARylation. Thus PTMs are at the root of major regulatory processes, by bestowing novel biochemical properties to the modified proteins, including changes in enzymatic activity, subcellular localization, interaction partners, protein stability, and DNA binding. Although purified recombinant BER proteins without any PTMs are proficient in their enzymatic activities, *in cellulo* BER is significantly affected by these PTMs. In this section, we discuss all the major PTMs of BER proteins identified so far.

The hallmark of mammalian DGs and early BER proteins is the presence of nonconserved, intrinsically disordered appendages at the N or C terminus, which are absent in their bacterial orthologs. Some examples are the N-terminal extension in human NTH1 absent in the *E. coli* Nth, C-terminal extension in human NEIL1 which is lacking in *E. coli* Nei, N-terminal extension in human APE1 lacking in *E. coli* Xth [44, 65, 67, 68]. Although the unfolded sequence generally exists at the N or C terminus, this could also exist internally as in Human NEIL2, where it may serve as a linker of the two domains. Analogous to the situation of histones H3 and H4, where mostly all PTMs occur in the disordered N-terminal tail [69, 70], PTMs in many early BER proteins are clustered in their disordered domains. See **Table 2** for the major BER PTMs known so far.

6.1 Acetylation

Acetylation of histones was discovered back in 1963 after the Nobel prize-winning discovery of acetyl CoA [71–74], and acetylation of histones at the ε-amino group of Lys residues in their disordered N-terminal region was shown to suppress their abilities to inhibit transcription [75]. Following these pioneering discoveries that linked histone acetylation to chromatin decondensation and transcriptional activation [76–78], diverse acetylation modifiers were identified and characterized. These include various histone acetyltransferases (HATs) such as E1a-binding protein p300 (p300), CREB-binding protein (CBP), ortholog of yeast transcription regulator Gcn5, TAF(II)250 subunit of transcription factor IID, several members of the MYST family (MOZ, YBF2/SAS3, SAS2, and TIP60) and p300/CBP associated factor (PCAF). Histone deacetylases (HDACs) were subsequently discovered as "erasers," which include distinct members, HDACs1–11 and SIRTs in different transcriptional repressor complexes SIN3, NURD, etc., which regulate acetylation/deacetylation cycle in cells [79–81]. These discoveries set the stage for epigenetic regulation of gene expression. Simultaneously, the concept of "reader" proteins [80, 82] that specifically recognize acetylated Lys residues through their bromodomains was introduced in addition to the "writers" (HATs) and "erasers" (HDACs). Although the first discovered nonhistone protein acetylation dated back in 1997 for the tumor suppressor TP53 [83], the overwhelming numbers of nonhistone protein acetylation, particularly in large macromolecular complexes involved in chromatin remodeling, DNA repair, cell cycle, etc., were appreciated much later, after 2006, from mass spectrometric-based proteomic approaches, and provided the global scenario of "cellular acetylome" [81, 84–86].

6.2 Phosphorylation

Although enzymatic phosphorylation of proteins was discovered in 1954 [87], phosphorylated protein was known much earlier, based on identification of phosphate in vitellin [88], followed by detection of phosphoserine in this protein [89]. During the 1950s, ATP was discovered to be required for phosphorylation when the phosphate group was found to be covalently attached to specific serine/

Functional class	BER protein	PTM and identified site	BER activity	Protein stability	Reference
DNA glycosylases	Uracil DNA glycosylase (UNG)	Phosphorylation; T6, S23, T60, S64, T126	+	–	[127, 128, 213]
		SUMOylation		+	[214]
		Ubiquitination		–	[127, 215, 216]
	Single-strand-selective monofunctional uracil DNA glycosylase 1 (SMUG1)	Ubiquitination		–	[215, 216]
	Methyl CpG-binding domain protein 4, DNA glycosylase (MBD4)	Phosphorylation; S156,S262	+		[217]
	Thymine DNA glycosylase (TDG)	Acetylation; K94, K95, K98	–		[129, 130]
		Phosphorylation; S93, S96, S99	+		[129, 130]
		SUMOylation; K330 K341	– +		[131, 218–221]
		Ubiquitination		–	[222, 223]
	MutY DNA glycosylase homolog (MYH)	Phosphorylation; S524	+		[224, 225]
		Ubiquitination; C-terminal K between aa 475–535		–	[226]
	8-Oxo guanine DNA glycosylase 1 (OGG1)	Acetylation; K338, K341	+		[203]
		Phosphorylation; S326	+		[227, 228]
		Ubiquitination	–	–	[229]
	Nei-like DNA glycosylase 1 (NEIL1)	Acetylation; K296, K297, K298	+	+	[161]
		Phosphorylation; S61, S207, Y263, S269, S306			[230–232]
	Nei-like DNA glycosylase 2 NEIL2	Acetylation; K49, K153	–		[233]
	N-methylpurine DNA glycosylase (MPG)	Acetylation	+		[234]
		Phosphorylation; S172	+		[235]

Functional class	BER protein	PTM and identified site	BER activity	Protein stability	Reference
End processors	Apurinic/ apyrimidinic endonuclease 1 (APE1)	Acetylation; K6, K7, K27, K31, K32, K35	+	+	[135, 136, 236–238]
		Phosphorylation; T233	–		[239, 240]
		Ubiquitination; K6, K7, K24, K25, K27, K31, K32, K35		–	[137, 138, 241]
	Polynucleotide kinase phosphatase (PNKP)	Phosphorylation; S114, S126	+	+	[139–141]
		Ubiquitination; K414, K417, K484		–	[139]
	Flap endonuclease-1 (FEN-1)	Acetylation; K354, K355, K377, K380	–		[242]
		Phosphorylation; S187	–	–	[144, 145]
		Methylation; R192	+	+	[146]
		SUMOylation; K168		–	[143]
DNA polymerases	DNA polymerase β (Pol β)	Acetylation; K72	–		[147]
		Methylation; R137, R83, R152	+		[148, 149]
		Ubiquitination; K41, K61, K81		–	[150, 151]
	DNA polymerases δ (Pol δ)	Phosphorylation; S458 of p68 subunit	–		[243]
DNA ligases	DNA ligase IIIα (Lig IIIα)	Phosphorylation; S123			[244]
		Ubiquitination		–	[150, 245]
Accessory proteins	X-Ray repair cross-complementing 1 (XRCC1)	Phosphorylation; S518, T519, T523, C-terminal linker, T284, S371	+	+	[246–252]
		SUMOylation			[152, 253]
		Ubiquitination; BRCA1 C terminus (BRCT II) motif on the C-terminal end		–	[150, 245, 252]
	Poly(ADP-ribose) polymerase 1 (PARP-1)	Acetylation; K498, K505, K508, K521, K524			[254]
		Phosphorylation; S372, T373	+		[255]
		SUMOylation; K203, K482, and K486			[132, 133]
		Ubiquitination		–	[132, 245, 256]

Table 2.
PTMs of BER proteins.

threonine residues [90, 91]. Subsequently, various kinases that phosphorylate serine/threonine and later tyrosine residues were characterized for their ability to modulate protein functions [91–93]. As with acetylation, phosphorylation induces conformational changes in the protein that stimulates its enzymatic activity and modulates protein-protein interactions [92, 94, 95]. Although the initial studies in protein phosphorylation were focused on cellular communications and signal transduction pathways, eventually the critical role of protein kinases and the relevance of phosphorylation/dephosphorylation events in DNA damage response (DDR) are extensively acknowledged, and mass spectrometry-based global screening approaches enabled identification of diverse phosphorylation targets [96, 97].

6.3 Ubiquitination and SUMOylation

Proteins are also posttranslationally modified via isopeptide bond formation with small proteins, which leads to nonlinear polypeptides [98, 99]. Ubiquitin is the first-discovered and well-characterized member of this growing family of small peptide modifiers, which covalently modify diverse proteins involved in chromatin organization, gene expression, signal transduction, DDR, DNA repair, and protein degradation [100–102]. Ubiquitin signals are generated by an enzymatic cascade involving E1 ubiquitin-activating enzymes, E2 ubiquitin-conjugating enzymes, and E3 ubiquitin ligases. Ubiquitination is a highly dynamic process with deubiquitinases (DUBs) involved in this signaling, and growing evidence indicates the involvement of ubiquitination/deubiquitination in BER, as shown in **Table 2**.

Small ubiquitin-related modifier (SUMO), containing 100 amino acid (aa) residues protein, is ubiquitin-like polypeptide, which is conjugated to substrates in a manner similar to ubiquitination [102, 103]. The SUMO paralogs are synthesized as precursor proteins that are cleaved by a family of SUMO isopeptidases [104]. Mature SUMO is subsequently activated by a heterodimeric E1-activating enzyme Aos1/Uba2 (SAE1/SAE2) forming a thioester bond between its catalytic cysteine and the C-terminal carboxyl group of mature SUMO. Then SUMO is transferred to the catalytic cysteine of the E2-conjugating enzyme Ubc9. In contrast to the ubiquitin system where dozens of E2 enzymes have been identified, Ubc9 is the only known SUMO E2 conjugating enzyme. Finally, an isopeptide bond is formed between SUMO and the substrate by E3 ligases. A consensus SUMO acceptor site has been identified consisting of the sequence ΨKXE, where Ψ is a large hydrophobic amino acid and K is the site of SUMO conjugation [105]. There are at least four SUMO paralogs in humans, SUMO1, SUMO2, SUMO3, and SUMO4, which have more than 1000 protein targets. SUMOylation is highly dynamic and can be reversed by the action of deSUMOylating enzymes (SENPs). SUMOylation regulates protein-protein interactions involving SUMO-interacting motifs (SIMs), and it targets a group of proteins in the same pathway to facilitate association of multiprotein complexes for transcription, nuclear transport, chromatin assembly and modification, chromosome segregation, DNA damage repair, replication, and cell signaling [106, 107].

6.4 PARylation

Poly ADP-ribosylation (PARylation), a crucial PTM that appears rapidly at DNA damage sites, is catalyzed by poly(ADP-ribose) polymerases (PARPs). The human PARP family contains 17 members among which only PARP1, 2, and 3 are involved in DDR [108–111]. PARPs covalently attach the ADP-ribose unit via an ester bond to the carboxyl group of glutamate or aspartate and sometimes also attach to cysteine or lysine of the target proteins [112–114]. PARPs successively transfer ADP-ribose units from NAD^+ to produce PAR chains containing up to 200 ADP-ribose units; however, in many cases, only single mono ADP-ribose moiety is transferred to the target proteins. Strand breaks in DNA activate PARP1, the founding and predominant member of the PARP family; the primary substrate of PARP1 is itself. Many proteins in the DDR pathways as well as the damage processing enzymes interact with PARP1 and/or are PARylated [112, 115]. In cells, PARylation/dePARylation is tightly and dynamically regulated; the PAR polymers are degraded by PAR glycohydrolase (PARG), possessing both exoglycosidic and endoglycosidic activities, and release free ADP-ribose moieties [116–118]. ADP-ribosyl-acceptor hydrolase (ARH) also exhibits PAR-degrading activity, although it has only exoglycosidase activity [119, 120]. Retention of PAR chains in cells triggers apoptotic cell death [121]. Although PARP1 interacts with the SSBR sensor XRCC1, as well as with other BER/SSBR proteins, and enables early recruitment of XRCC1 to the DNA lesions [122–126], there is no convincing evidence for PARylation of BER/SSBR proteins.

6.5 Cross-talks between different PTMs, their regulation, and effect on BER

Proteins employ diverse PTMs sequentially or concurrently to expand their repertoire of functions, thereby impacting global cellular signaling. The best example is the disordered N-terminal tail of histone H3, which has multiple sites for acetylation, methylation, phosphorylation, ubiquitination, and SUMOylation [69, 70]. These PTMS could act synergistically or via reciprocal exclusion to modulate chromatin organization, thus affecting the transcriptome. The same Lys residues (K9, K27) in H3 are targets for both acetylation (marker of active chromatin) and methylation; however, monomethylation of these residues are markers of active chromatin, while di- and trimethylation are associated with repression. Recent evidence on BER enzymes, summarized below, suggests that specific modification at one site can dramatically influence another modification at a different site, which may critically impact BER activity.

Cyclin-dependent kinase (CDK)-mediated phosphorylation of UNG2 (nuclear UDG) in S phase signals its ubiquitination-dependent degradation, and CDK-inhibitor roscovitine prevents such degradation [127, 128]. This suggests that phosphorylation-induced conformational change in UNG2 is a prerequisite for ubiquitination.

In the case of TDG, acetylation inhibits its repair activity by two distinct mechanisms. TDG acetylation at K94, K95, and K98 by p300/CBP suppresses BER by preventing APE1 recruitment to the damage site [129]. Protein kinase C (PKC)-mediated phosphorylation at S93, S96, and S99, close to the acetylation sites, may promote repair by sterically blocking repair-inhibitory acetylation of adjacent lysine residues [130]. On the other hand, SUMOylation at K341 inhibits TDG's interaction with CBP, preventing its acetylation and thereby promoting BER [131].

PARP1, SUMOylated at K203 and K486, is a target for ubiquitination and degradation, which is believed to be the mechanism for its turnover [132]. In contrast, PARP1's SUMOylation at K482 does not degrade the protein, rather stimulates PARylation of chromatin-associated proteins [133]. On the other hand, acetylation of PARP1, which stimulates its transactivation function, is inhibited by K486 SUMOylation. Thus, K486 SUMOylation restrains PARP1's transactivation function [134].

While acetylation of APE1 enhances its stability in chromatin and enzymatic activity [135, 136], CDK5-mediated phosphorylation enhances its ubiquitination and degradation [137, 138]. Thus, it is possible that phosphorylation and acetylation are mutually exclusive, acetylation stabilizing the protein, and phosphorylation guiding to its degradation.

In the case of PNKP, ATM-dependent phosphorylation was shown to prevent ubiquitination and hence its degradation. Thus, in response to oxidative stress, ATM phosphorylates and stabilizes PNKP in order to activate a coordinated DDR pathway [139–141]. Furthermore, PNKP interacts with the deubiquitination enzyme ataxin-3 (ATXN3), which enhances its stability and phosphatase activity [142].

Phosphorylation of FEN-1 by CDK1 at S187 was shown to promote SUMOylation at K168, which enhanced its polyubiquitination-dependent degradation [143]. Phosphorylation inhibits FEN-1's flap endonuclease activity [144, 145], which cross-talks with methylation, a lesser studied PTM of BER proteins. Methylation by arginine methyltransferase 5 at R192 prevents this phosphorylation and thus is proposed to be essential for the repair activities of FEN-1 [146]. Thus, in response to oxidative stress in cycling cells, methylation of FEN-1 could be a critical requirement for LP-BER.

Acetylation of Pol β at K72 inhibits its dRP lyase activity [147], and this could account for acetylation-induced inhibition of enzymatic activity and switch from SN-BER to LP-BER. Methylation of Pol β at R137 has no effect on dRP lyase or DNA polymerase activities but inhibits its interaction with PCNA [148] and could thus be predicted to inhibit LP-BER. In contrast, R83 and R152 methylation enhanced Pol β's DNA binding and increased processivity [149]. Cellular Pol β level appears to be maintained by two ubiquitin E3 ligases, Mule and CHIP. DNA Pol β is monoubiquitinated by Mule, which in turn is recognized and polyubiquitinated by CHIP in undamaged cells. In response to oxidative stress, it is deubiquitinated, thus ensuring its stability and oxidized base damage repair [150, 151].

A recent study shows how PARylation stimulates SUMOylation [152]. In response to DNA strand breaks induced by alkylating agent methylmethanesulfonate (MMS), PARP1 is activated and synthesizes PAR chains; this promotes recruitment of SUMO E3 TOPORS to XRCC1, which facilitates XRCC1 SUMOylation. XRCC1 SUMOylation recruits Pol β at the damaged sites and thus ensures completion of BER.

7. Does chromatin organization affect BER? Understanding BER at the chromatin context

BER, as studied *in vitro* with naked DNA substrates, involves sequential enzymatic steps in which each enzyme utilizes the product of the previous step as the substrate. This observation inspired the prevailing dogma that the sequential steps in BER involves the hand-off process where the product of one step is handed over to the enzyme in the next step [153, 154]. Later steps generate intermediate product lesions that are more toxic than the original lesions. The BER intermediates such as AP sites and SSBs, which are highly mutagenic, interfere with replication and transcription, and hence the entire BER steps must be coordinated once the repair is initiated [155–158]. Cumulating evidence suggests that the BER proteins act in concert beyond simply recognizing and acting upon the product of the previous step, by being present at the site of the original lesion [43, 52, 61, 62, 64, 65, 125, 159, 160]. This is the basis for the emerging paradigm of "preformed BER complexes," named, "BERosomes" in mammalian cells. Being an integral part of complexes, it may be easier for the BER intermediates to be handed over to the next enzyme, which likely undergoes allosteric changes after binding to its substrate. Recent studies in our and collaborators' labs suggest that these "BERosomes" are constitutively chromatin-bound to ensure prompt repair in the event of any threat [62, 135, 161]. Simultaneously, recent interests in the BER field have evolved toward deciphering the role of different chromatin factors and the underlying chromatin remodeling in oxidized base repair.

Several *in vitro* studies showed reduced BER activity with reconstituted core nucleosome particles, where every step during repair of diverse lesions was found to be inhibited by histones [162–170]. Overall BER efficiency is strongly inhibited by the presence of nucleosomes, which interfere with the interaction between the repair proteins and their substrate lesions, thereby compromising physical interaction and catalysis. Because oxidized bases perturb the DNA structure only mildly [170], whether chromatin remodeling occurs during BER was questionable. But, as BER efficiently occurs in cells, the results from these *in vitro* experiments imply that chromatin rearrangement occurs at oxidized DNA damage sites *in cells*, as was shown in the case of repair of DSBs, UV ray-mediated damages, and mismatched base pairs [171–173].

An inverse correlation exists in cells between BER and chromatin compaction. ROS induces assembly of BER complexes preferentially on open chromatin regions [174], as we have also observed that the BER complexes are constitutively present on actively transcribing sequences [175]. Interestingly, BER is involved during active CpG demethylation in promoters, mediated by TET dioxygenase(s) during transcriptional activation [176–180]. The TET proteins oxidize 5mC to 5hmC, 5fC, and 5caC; 5fC and 5caC are the TDG substrates. Thus, this coordination between CpG DNA demethylation, an epigenetic process essential for chromatin decondensation during transcriptional activation, and base damage repair supports our notion that "open-chromatin prefers BER activity across the genomic landscape" and highlights a regulatory link between epigenetics, chromatin remodeling, and BER.

Various ATP-dependent chromatin remodeling (ACR) complexes, which play significant roles in protein/DNA and protein/protein interactions in chromatin and regulate transcription, DNA repair processes such as DSB repair (DSBR), nucleotide excision repair (NER), and cross-link repair, also affect BER. ACR complexes utilize the energy of ATP hydrolysis to restructure nucleosomes on chromatin [181–183], thereby affecting gene expression profile and DNA repair. Four structurally related, but functionally distinct, ACR complex families were identified: SWI/SNF (switching defective/sucrose nonfermenting; most extensively studied), ISWI (imitation switch), CHD (chromodomain, helicase, DNA binding), and INO80 (inositol requiring 80). *In vitro* BER studies with reconstituted nucleosomes showed enhanced repair activity in the presence of purified SWI/SNF or ISW1/ISW2 complexes [184–186]. There are some indirect evidences of ACR during BER in yeast and mammalian cells. Depletion of STH1 (ATPase subunit of RSC, a member of SWI/SNF family) causes genome-wide BER inhibition and thus emphasizes a link between chromatin organization and BER [187]. In a recent study, depletion of ALC1/CHD1L, another member of SWI/SNF, compromises chromatin relaxation, associated with BER inhibition and increased sensitivity to MMS and H_2O_2 in chicken cells [188]. On the contrary, INO80 deficiency in MMS-sensitive yeast cells has no effect on genome-wide BER [189]. K56 acetylation in histone H3 is increased in chromatin of both yeast and mammalian cells following MMS treatment, which generates alkylated base substrates for BER, [190, 191]. H3K56Ac was also found to be enriched at DSBR sites and responsible for SWI/SNF complex recruitment during transcription [192]. Thus, it would be interesting to examine if any specific PTM(s) would target ACR after oxidized base damage and illuminate the phenomenon of ACR during BER. In any event, additional studies are required to test if ACR plays a role in enabling BER in condensed chromatin. It would be also of interest to explore if the BER proteins possess inherent chromatin remodeling activities, similar to the NER proteins, which have SWI/SNF domains [193–195]. Though no known BER proteins have SWI/SNF domains, the XRCC1-Lig IIIα complex could disrupt nucleosomes *in vitro* and enable BER completion [166].

Poly-ADP-ribosylation of histones by PARP1 after genome damage adds negative charge on histones and disrupts histone-DNA interactions, thereby promoting chromatin decondensation and enhancing interaction between the proteins involved in DNA transactions and DNA [111, 196–198]. This could increase DNA accessibility to the BER proteins. Although PARP1's role in regulating transcription is well established, this would link chromatin remodeling to BER.

Nucleosomes pose obstruction to all DNA transactions and are likely disassembled to allow DNA replication, repair, and transcription, followed by their reassembly, which utilizes both parental histones and newly synthesized histones. Such replication-coupled nucleosome assembly in the S phase or replication-independent, transcription-coupled assembly throughout the cell cycle involves histone chaperones functioning at multiple steps of nucleosome formation [172, 199, 200]. Replication-coupled nucleosome assembly is aided by the chromatin assembly factor (CAF-1) and Rtt106 with the help of antisilencing function 1A (ASF1A) protein. Histone cell cycle regulator (HIRA) protein, along with Daxx, mediates replication-independent nucleosome assembly. While exploring chromatin-bound BER complexes, we serendipitously discovered CHAF1A (the largest subunit of CAF-1, along with other subunits CHAF1B and RBBP4), ASF1A, and various H3/H4 variants in the immunoprecipitation complex of NEIL1 or acetylated NEIL1 (201; unpublished). This underscores the importance of the diverse chromatin components in preformed "BERosomes," which could regulate oxidize base repair in chromatin. We showed that ROS-induced oxidized base lesions caused transient dissociation of CHAF1A, ASF1A, and histones from the BER complexes and were restored back after repair completion. The repair activities of NEIL1 and OGG1, as well as complete cellular BER, were found to be inhibited by CAF-1, as well as the CHAF1A monomer [201]. So, we propose a hypothesis of temporal regulation of BER by the histone chaperones, whose dissociation from BER complexes is essential to initiate BER [201]. This has been illustrated in **Figure 2**.

Recently, we discovered acetylation of NEIL1 at the disordered C-terminal K296-K298 by p300, which enhances its activity, and found that acetylated NEIL1 (AcNEIL1) could be detected only in the chromatin fraction and not in the soluble nuclear fraction [161]. Although the nonacetylable NEIL1 3KRmutant (Lys296–298 substituted with Arg) translocates to the nucleus and binds to chromatin, presumably due to retention of positive charges as in the WT enzyme, it forms less stable BER complexes with the histones, histone chaperones, and downstream BER proteins. Thus, as proposed earlier [65], the positive charge cluster in the disordered C-terminal region is required for NEIL1's nonspecific DNA binding, after which acetylation occurs on the chromatin. Hydrophobic interaction of NEIL1 after acetylation-mediated charge neutralization probably stabilizes NEIL1's complexes with nucleosome components and downstream BER proteins. Consequently, cells with acetylable NEIL1 exhibit enhanced BER efficiency and are less sensitive to oxidative stress. It is thus likely that unmodified NEIL1 binds to chromatin nonspecifically, and acetylation specifically at the promoter regions of actively transcribing genes by enhanced p300 activity actually stabilizes NEIL1's (and possibly other DG's) BERosomes on these preferred chromatin regions (**Figure 3**), which warrants further investigation.

In a separate study, while investigating how APE1 repairs AP sites in cells, our collaborator's lab found that acetylated APE1 (AcAPE1), like AcNEIL1, is exclusively and stably chromatin-bound throughout the cell cycle [135]. APE1 undergoes acetylation after binding to AP sites in chromatin, which enhances its enzymatic activity. In the absence of APE1 acetylation, cells accumulated AP sites and exhibited higher sensitivity to DNA damaging agents. We predict that other BER proteins OGG1 and MPG, whose repair activity is enhanced by acetylation, are similarly stabilized in chromatin-bound state.

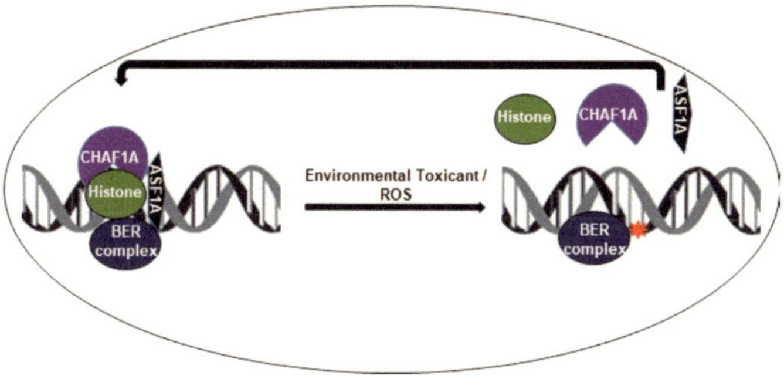

Figure 2.
A schematic showing chromatin-bound BER complexes with histones and histone chaperones. ROS-induced damage causes transient dissociation of histones and histone chaperones to initiate BER, which are restored back after repair completion.

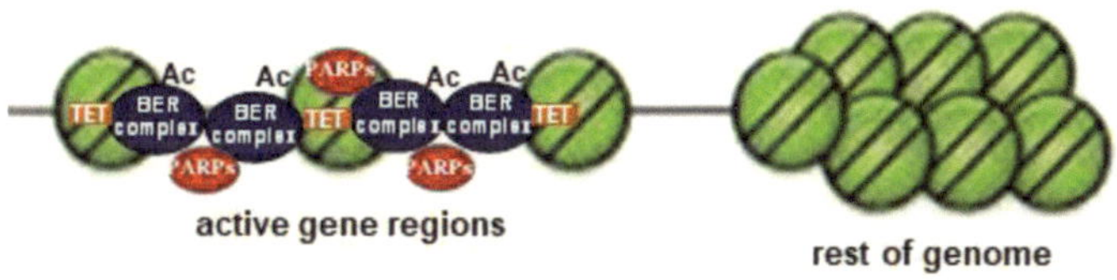

Figure 3.
An illustrative view of "open" chromatin regions, containing bound "BERosomes" with histones, histone chaperones, PARPs, TETs, etc., for preferential repair of these transcriptionally active regions.

8. Future perspectives

The genome-wide impact of various PTMs in the cross-talks among BER proteins, which dictates the overall repair efficiency, thus preserving genomic integrity against genotoxic insults from both endogenous and external oxidative stress, has not been investigated. In this NextGen era, holistic, whole-genome scanning approaches, although a daunting challenge, make it likely to map individual PTMs of BER proteins, the kinetics of their formation and removal, and their correlation with both intrinsic and ROS-induced BER efficiency across the genomic landscape. Because histone PTMs have been well established in chromatin remodeling, it is also important to explore how specific histone PTMs interfere with the BER PTMs.

The Access-Repair-Restore model [182, 202] provides an accepted view of DNA repair in chromatin, where chromatin remodeling is essential for the DNA repair machineries to get access to the damaged DNA. For BER, it is still not clear how chromatin remodeling and the associated histone PTMs initiate BER. The BER complexes constitutively bind to "open" chromatin regions, and chromatin remodeling could assist specific enzyme-substrate binding and enzyme catalysis needed to initiate and propagate BER. Moreover, although chromatin remodeling has been found to enable BER, the enhanced repair activity may be simply due to ROS-induced stimulation of BER genes' expression or their specific PTM (acetylation), as has been shown by us [203–205], along with enhanced substrate binding in "open" chromatin. This may underestimate the contribution of ACR complexes at oxidized base lesion sites to enhance BER. Alternatively, in cells, chromatin remodeling-stimulated BER could be linked to replication and transcription, similar to transcription-coupled NER, which always occurs on "open" chromatin [206]. Indeed, repair of oxidized bases preferentially occurs in the transcribed strand [175], which could be assisted by Cockayne syndrome protein B (CSB), a NER factor, in transcription-coupled but NER-independent fashion [207]. Because BER/SSBR proteins such as PARP1 and APE1 are emerging as potential therapeutic targets [208–212], understanding if and how chromatin remodeling impacts BER activity is crucial to manipulating BER for effective modulation of repair activity in cancer cells. This would provide better efficacy and specificity in cancer therapy.

Acknowledgements

This work was supported by NIH R01 CA158910 (SM), R01 GM105090 (SM), P01 CA092584 (SM), R01 NS088645 (MLH), and HMRI laboratory start-up funds to SM and MLH.

Conflict of interest statement

The authors declare that there are no conflicts of interest associated with this study.

Author details

Shiladitya Sengupta[1,2*], Chunying Yang[1], Bradley J. Eckelmann[1,3], Muralidhar L. Hegde[1,2,4] and Sankar Mitra[1,2]

1 Department of Radiation Oncology, Houston Methodist Research Institute, Houston, Texas, USA

2 Weill Cornell Medical College, Cornell University, New York, New York, USA

3 Texas A&M Health Science Center, College of Medicine, Bryan, Texas, USA

4 Houston Methodist Neurological Institute, Houston, Texas, USA

*Address all correspondence to: sxsengupta@houstonmethodist.org; sengupta.us@gmail.com

References

[1] Talbert PB, Henikoff S. Histone variants on the move: Substrates for chromatin dynamics. Nature Reviews Molecular Cell Biology. 2016;**18**:115

[2] Venkatesh S, Workman JL. Histone exchange, chromatin structure and the regulation of transcription. Nature Reviews Molecular Cell Biology. 2015;**16**:178

[3] Lindahl T, Barnes DE. Repair of endogenous DNA damage. Cold Spring Harbor Symposia on Quantitative Biology. 2000;**65**:127-133

[4] Tubbs A, Nussenzweig A. Endogenous DNA damage as a source of genomic instability in cancer. Cell. 2017;**168**:644-656

[5] De Bont R, van Larebeke N. Endogenous DNA damage in humans: A review of quantitative data. Mutagenesis. 2004;**19**:169-185

[6] Dizdaroglu M. Oxidatively induced DNA damage and its repair in cancer. Mutation Research. Reviews in Mutation Research. 2015;**763**:212-245

[7] Dizdaroglu M, Coskun E, Jaruga P. Measurement of oxidatively induced DNA damage and its repair, by mass spectrometric techniques. Free Radical Research. 2015;**49**:525-548

[8] Lan L, Nakajima S, Oohata Y, Takao M, Okano S, Masutani M, et al. In situ analysis of repair processes for oxidative DNA damage in mammalian cells. Proceedings of the National Academy of Sciences of the United States of America. 2004;**101**:13738-13743

[9] Cadet J, Davies KJA. Oxidative DNA damage & repair: An introduction. Free Radical Biology & Medicine. 2017;**107**:2-12

[10] Cadet J, Douki T, Ravanat JL. Oxidatively generated base damage to cellular DNA. Free Radical Biology & Medicine. 2010;**49**:9-21

[11] Davies KJ. Oxidative stress: The paradox of aerobic life. Biochemical Society Symposium. 1995;**61**:1-31

[12] Winterbourn CC. Reconciling the chemistry and biology of reactive oxygen species. Nature Chemical Biology. 2008;**4**:278-286

[13] Reisz JA, Bansal N, Qian J, Zhao W, Furdui CM. Effects of ionizing radiation on biological molecules—Mechanisms of damage and emerging methods of detection. Antioxidants & Redox Signaling. 2014;**21**:260-292

[14] Storr SJ, Woolston CM, Zhang Y, Martin SG. Redox environment, free radical, and oxidative DNA damage. Antioxidants & Redox Signaling. 2013;**18**:2399-2408

[15] Cadet J, Ravanat JL, TavernaPorro M, Menoni H, Angelov D. Oxidatively generated complex DNA damage: Tandem and clustered lesions. Cancer Letters. 2012;**327**:5-15

[16] Cadet J, Wagner JR. DNA base damage by reactive oxygen species, oxidizing agents, and UV radiation. Cold Spring Harbor Perspectives in Biology. 2013;**5**:a012559

[17] Evans MD, Dizdaroglu M, Cooke MS. Oxidative DNA damage and disease: Induction, repair and significance. Mutation Research. 2004;**567**:1-61

[18] Cadet J, Douki T, Ravanat JL. Measurement of oxidatively generated base damage in cellular DNA. Mutation Research. 2011;**711**:3-12

[19] Kasai H, Nishimura S. Hydroxylation of the C-8 position of deoxyguanosine by reducing agents in

the presence of oxygen. Nucleic Acids Symposium Series. 1983;**12**:165-167

[20] Nishimura S. 8-Hydroxyguanine: From its discovery in 1983 to the present status. Proceedings of the Japan Academy Series B, Physical and Biological Sciences. 2006;**82**: 127-141

[21] Nishimura S. 8-Hydroxyguanine: A base for discovery. DNA Repair (Amst). 2011;**10**:1078-1083

[22] Ravanat JL, Di Mascio P, Martinez GR, Medeiros MH. Singlet oxygen induces oxidation of cellular DNA. The Journal of Biological Chemistry. 2001;**276**:40601-40604

[23] Ravanat JL, Douki T, Cadet J. Direct and indirect effects of UV radiation on DNA and its components. Journal of Photochemistry and Photobiology. B. 2001;**63**:88-102

[24] Ravanat JL, Sauvaigo S, Caillat S, Martinez GR, Medeiros MH, Di Mascio P, et al. Singlet oxygen-mediated damage to cellular DNA determined by the comet assay associated with DNA repair enzymes. Biological Chemistry. 2004;**385**:17-20

[25] Malle E, Furtmuller PG, Sattler W, Obinger C. Myeloperoxidase: A target for new drug development? British Journal of Pharmacology. 2007;**152**:838-854

[26] Masuda M, Suzuki T, Friesen MD, Ravanat JL, Cadet J, Pignatelli B, et al. Chlorination of guanosine and other nucleosides by hypochlorous acid and myeloperoxidase of activated human neutrophils. Catalysis by nicotine and trimethylamine. Journal of Biological Chemitry. 2001;**276**:40486-40496

[27] An J, Rao A, Ko M. TET family dioxygenases and DNA demethylation in stem cells and cancers. Experimental & Molecular Medicine. 2017;**49**:e323

[28] Wu X, Zhang Y. TET-mediated active DNA demethylation: Mechanism, function and beyond. Nature Reviews. 2017;**18**:517-534

[29] Munzel M, Globisch D, Bruckl T, Wagner M, Welzmiller V, Michalakis S, et al. Quantification of the sixth DNA base hydroxymethylcytosine in the brain. Angewandte Chemie (International ed.). 2010;**49**:5375-5377

[30] Pfaffeneder T, Hackner B, Truss M, Munzel M, Muller M, Deiml CA, et al. The discovery of 5-formylcytosine in embryonic stem cell DNA. Angewandte Chemie (International ed.). 2011;**50**: 7008-7012

[31] Hong IS, Carter KN, Sato K, Greenberg MM. Characterization and mechanism of formation of tandem lesions in DNA by a nucleobase peroxyl radical. Journal of the American Chemical Society. 2007;**129**:4089-4098

[32] Jiang Y, Hong H, Cao H, Wang Y. In vivo formation and in vitro replication of a guanine-thymine intrastrand cross-link lesion. Biochemistry. 2007;**46**:12757-12763

[33] Ding S, Kropachev K, Cai Y, Kolbanovskiy M, Durandina SA, Liu Z, et al. Structural, energetic and dynamic properties of guanine(C8)-thymine(N3) cross-links in DNA provide insights on susceptibility to nucleotide excision repair. Nucleic Acids Research. 2012;**40**:2506-2517

[34] Yun BH, Geacintov NE, Shafirovich V. Generation of guanine-thymidine cross-links in DNA by peroxynitrite/ carbon dioxide. Chemical Research in Toxicology. 2011;**24**:1144-1152

[35] Gueranger Q, Kia A, Frith D, Karran P. Crosslinking of DNA repair and replication proteins to DNA in cells treated with 6-thioguanine and UVA. Nucleic Acids Research. 2011;**39**:5057-5066

[36] Prakash S, Johnson RE, Prakash L. Eukaryotic translesion synthesis DNA polymerases: Specificity of structure and function. Annual Review of Biochemistry. 2005;**74**:317-353

[37] Bacolla A, Cooper DN, Vasquez KM. Mechanisms of base substitution mutagenesis in cancer genomes. Genes. 2014;**5**:108-146

[38] Helleday T, Eshtad S, Nik-Zainal S. Mechanisms underlying mutational signatures in human cancers. Nature Reviews. 2014;**15**:585-598

[39] Lawrence MS, Stojanov P, Polak P, Kryukov GV, Cibulskis K, Sivachenko A, et al. Mutational heterogeneity in cancer and the search for new cancer-associated genes. Nature. 2013;**499**:214-218

[40] Tomasetti C, Li L, Vogelstein B. Stem cell divisions, somatic mutations, cancer etiology, and cancer prevention. Science. 2017;**355**:1330-1334

[41] Hsu GW, Ober M, Carell T, Beese LS. Error-prone replication of oxidatively damaged DNA by a high-fidelity DNA polymerase. Nature. 2004;**431**:217-221

[42] Shibutani S, Takeshita M, Grollman AP. Insertion of specific bases during DNA synthesis past the oxidation-damaged base 8-oxodG. Nature. 1991;**349**:431-434

[43] Dutta A, Yang C, Sengupta S, Mitra S, Hegde ML. New paradigms in the repair of oxidative damage in human genome: Mechanisms ensuring repair of mutagenic base lesions during replication and involvement of accessory proteins. Cellular and Molecular Life Sciences. 2015;**72**:1679-1698

[44] Hegde ML, Hazra TK, Mitra S. Early steps in the DNA base excision/single-strand interruption repair pathway in mammalian cells. Cell Research. 2008;**18**:27-47

[45] Mitra S, Hazra TK, Roy R, Ikeda S, Biswas T, Lock J, et al. Complexities of DNA base excision repair in mammalian cells. Molecules and Cells. 1997;**7**:305-312

[46] Mitra S, Izumi T, Boldogh I, Bhakat KK, Hill JW, Hazra TK. Choreography of oxidative damage repair in mammalian genomes. Free Radical Biology & Medicine. 2002;**33**:15-28

[47] Bandaru V, Sunkara S, Wallace SS, Bond JP. A novel human DNA glycosylase that removes oxidative DNA damage and is homologous to *Escherichia coli* endonuclease VIII. DNA Repair (Amst). 2002;**1**:517-529

[48] Hazra TK, Izumi T, Boldogh I, Imhoff B, Kow YW, Jaruga P, et al. Identification and characterization of a human DNA glycosylase for repair of modified bases in oxidatively damaged DNA. Proceedings of the National Academy of Sciences of the United States of America. 2002;**99**:3523-3528

[49] Hazra TK, Kow YW, Hatahet Z, Imhoff B, Boldogh I, Mokkapati SK, et al. Identification and characterization of a novel human DNA glycosylase for repair of cytosine-derived lesions. The Journal of Biological Chemistry. 2002;**277**:30417-30420

[50] Morland I, Rolseth V, Luna L, Rognes T, Bjoras M, Seeberg E. Human DNA glycosylases of the bacterial Fpg/MutM superfamily: An alternative pathway for the repair of 8-oxoguanine and other oxidation products in DNA. Nucleic Acids Research. 2002;**30**:4926-4936

[51] Takao M, Kanno S, Kobayashi K, Zhang QM, Yonei S, van der Horst GT, et al. A back-up glycosylase in Nth1 knock-out mice is a functional Nei (endonuclease VIII) homologue.

The Journal of Biological Chemistry. 2002;**277**:42205-42213

[52] Hill JW, Hazra TK, Izumi T, Mitra S. Stimulation of human 8-oxoguanine-DNA glycosylase by AP-endonuclease: Potential coordination of the initial steps in base excision repair. Nucleic Acids Research. 2001;**29**:430-438

[53] Mokkapati SK, Wiederhold L, Hazra TK, Mitra S. Stimulation of DNA glycosylase activity of OGG1 by NEIL1: Functional collaboration between two human DNA glycosylases. Biochemistry. 2004;**43**:11596-11604

[54] Das A, Wiederhold L, Leppard JB, Kedar P, Prasad R, Wang H, et al. NEIL2-initiated, APE-independent repair of oxidized bases in DNA: Evidence for a repair complex in human cells. DNA Repair (Amst). 2006;**5**:1439-1448

[55] Meijer M, Karimi-Busheri F, Huang TY, Weinfeld M, Young D. Pnk1, a DNA kinase/phosphatase required for normal response to DNA damage by gamma-radiation or camptothecin in Schizosaccharomyces pombe. The Journal of Biological Chemistry. 2002;**277**:4050-4055

[56] Whitehouse CJ, Taylor RM, Thistlethwaite A, Zhang H, Karimi-Busheri F, Lasko DD, et al. XRCC1 stimulates human polynucleotide kinase activity at damaged DNA termini and accelerates DNA single-strand break repair. Cell. 2001;**104**:107-117

[57] Wiederhold L, Leppard JB, Kedar P, Karimi-Busheri F, Rasouli-Nia A, Weinfeld M, et al. AP endonuclease-independent DNA base excision repair in human cells. Molecular Cell. 2004;**15**:209-220

[58] Levin DS, McKenna AE, Motycka TA, Matsumoto Y, Tomkinson AE. Interaction between PCNA and DNA ligase I is critical for joining of Okazaki fragments and long-patch base-excision repair. Current Biology. 2000;**10**:919-922

[59] Maynard S, Fang EF, Scheibye-Knudsen M, Croteau DL, Bohr VA. DNA damage, DNA repair, aging, and neurodegeneration. Cold Spring Harbor Perspectives in Medicine. 2015;**5**:a025130

[60] Roos WP, Thomas AD, Kaina B. DNA damage and the balance between survival and death in cancer biology. Nature Reviews Cancer. 2016;**16**:20-33

[61] Hegde ML, Hegde PM, Bellot LJ, Mandal SM, Hazra TK, Li GM, et al. Prereplicative repair of oxidized bases in the human genome is mediated by NEIL1 DNA glycosylase together with replication proteins. Proceedings of the National Academy of Sciences of the United States of America. 2013;**110**:E3090-E3099

[62] Hegde PM, Dutta A, Sengupta S, Mitra J, Adhikari S, Tomkinson AE, et al. The C-terminal domain (CTD) of human DNA glycosylase NEIL1 is required for forming BERosome repair complex with DNA replication proteins at the replicating genome: Dominant negative function of the CTD. The Journal of Biological Chemistry. 2015;**290**:20919-20933

[63] Rangaswamy S, Pandey A, Mitra S, Hegde ML. Pre-replicative repair of oxidized bases maintains fidelity in mammalian genomes: The cowcatcher role of NEIL1 DNA glycosylase. Genes. 2017;**8**:E175

[64] Hegde ML, Theriot CA, Das A, Hegde PM, Guo Z, Gary RK, et al. Physical and functional interaction between human oxidized base-specific DNA glycosylase NEIL1 and flap endonuclease 1. The Journal of Biological Chemistry. 2008;**283**:27028-27037

[65] Hegde ML, Tsutakawa SE, Hegde PM, Holthauzen LM, Li J, Oezguen N,

et al. The disordered C-terminal domain of human DNA glycosylase NEIL1 contributes to its stability via intramolecular interactions. Journal of Molecular Biology. 2013;**425**:2359-2371

[66] Theriot CA, Hegde ML, Hazra TK, Mitra S. RPA physically interacts with the human DNA glycosylase NEIL1 to regulate excision of oxidative DNA base damage in primer-template structures. DNA Repair. 2010;**9**:643-652

[67] Hegde ML, Hazra TK, Mitra S. Functions of disordered regions in mammalian early base excision repair proteins. Cellular and Molecular Life Sciences. 2010;**67**:3573-3587

[68] Hegde ML, Izumi T, Mitra S. Oxidized base damage and single-strand break repair in mammalian genomes: Role of disordered regions and posttranslational modifications in early enzymes. Progress in Molecular Biology and Translational Science. 2012;**110**:123-153

[69] Zhang C, Liu Y. Retrieving quantitative information of histone PTMs by mass spectrometry. Methods in Enzymology. 2017;**586**:165-191

[70] Zhao Y, Garcia BA. Comprehensive catalog of currently documented histone modifications. Cold Spring Harbor Perspectives in Biology. 2015;7:a025064

[71] Bloch K, Borek E. Biological acetylation of natural amino acids. The Journal of Biological Chemistry. 1946;**164**:483

[72] Lipmann F. Development of the acetylation problem, a personal account. Science. 1954;**120**:855-865

[73] Lipmann F, Kaplan NO, et al. Coenzyme for acetylation, a pantothenic acid derivative. The Journal of Biological Chemistry. 1947;**167**:869

[74] Phillips DM. The presence of acetyl groups of histones. The Biochemical Journal. 1963;**87**:258-263

[75] Allfrey VG, Faulkner R, Mirsky AE. Acetylation and methylation of histones and their possible role in the regulation of RNA synthesis. Proceedings of the National Academy of Sciences of the United States of America. 1964;**51**:786-794

[76] Hebbes TR, Thorne AW, Crane-Robinson C. A direct link between core histone acetylation and transcriptionally active chromatin. The EMBO Journal. 1988;**7**:1395-1402

[77] Turner BM, Birley AJ, Lavender J. Histone H4 isoforms acetylated at specific lysine residues define individual chromosomes and chromatin domains in Drosophila polytene nuclei. Cell. 1992;**69**:375-384

[78] Turner BM, Fellows G. Specific antibodies reveal ordered and cell-cycle-related use of histone-H4 acetylation sites in mammalian cells. European Journal of Biochemistry/FEBS. 1989;**179**:131-139

[79] Marmorstein R, Trievel RC. Histone modifying enzymes: Structures, mechanisms, and specificities. Biochimica et Biophysica Acta. 2009;**1789**:58-68

[80] Marmorstein R, Zhou MM. Writers and readers of histone acetylation: Structure, mechanism, and inhibition. Cold Spring Harbor Perspectives in Biology. 2014;**6**:a018762

[81] Verdin E, Ott M. 50 years of protein acetylation: From gene regulation to epigenetics, metabolism and beyond. Nature Reviews. 2015;**16**:258-264

[82] Dhalluin C, Carlson JE, Zeng L, He C, Aggarwal AK, Zhou MM. Structure and ligand of a histone acetyltransferase bromodomain. Nature. 1999;**399**:491-496

[83] Gu W, Roeder RG. Activation of p53 sequence-specific DNA binding by acetylation of the p53 C-terminal domain. Cell. 1997;**90**:595-606

[84] Choudhary C, Kumar C, Gnad F, Nielsen ML, Rehman M, Walther TC, et al. Lysine acetylation targets protein complexes and co-regulates major cellular functions. Science. 2009;**325**:834-840

[85] Choudhary C, Weinert BT, Nishida Y, Verdin E, Mann M. The growing landscape of lysine acetylation links metabolism and cell signalling. Nature Reviews. 2014;**15**:536-550

[86] Kim SC, Sprung R, Chen Y, Xu Y, Ball H, Pei J, et al. Substrate and functional diversity of lysine acetylation revealed by a proteomics survey. Molecular Cell. 2006;**23**:607-618

[87] Burnett G, Kennedy EP. The enzymatic phosphorylation of proteins. The Journal of Biological Chemistry. 1954;**211**:969-980

[88] Levene PA, Alsberg CL. The cleavage products of vitellin. The Journal of Biological Chemistry. 1906;**2**:127-133

[89] Levene PA, Schormüller A. Serinephosphoric acid obtained on hydrolysis of vitellinic acid. The Journal of Biological Chemistry. 1933;**103**:537-542

[90] Fischer EH, Krebs EG. Conversion of phosphorylase b to phosphorylase a in muscle extracts. The Journal of Biological Chemistry. 1955;**216**:121-132

[91] Lecture KEGN. Protein phosphorylation and cellular regulation I. Bioscience Reports. 1993;**13**:127-142

[92] Barford D, Johnson LN. The allosteric transition of glycogen phosphorylase. Nature. 1989;**340**:609-616

[93] Walsh DA, Perkins JP, Krebs EG. An adenosine 3′,5′-monophosphate-dependant protein kinase from rabbit skeletal muscle. The Journal of Biological Chemistry. 1968;**243**:3763-3765

[94] Pawson T. Specificity in signal transduction: From phosphotyrosine-SH2 domain interactions to complex cellular systems. Cell. 2004;**116**:191-203

[95] Pawson T, Scott JD. Protein phosphorylation in signaling—50 years and counting. Trends in Biochemical Sciences. 2005;**30**:286-290

[96] Bensimon A, Schmidt A, Ziv Y, Elkon R, Wang SY, Chen DJ, et al. ATM-dependent and -independent dynamics of the nuclear phosphoproteome after DNA damage. Science Signaling. 2010;**3**:rs3

[97] Matsuoka S, Ballif BA, Smogorzewska A, McDonald ER 3rd, Hurov KE, Luo J, et al. ATM and ATR substrate analysis reveals extensive protein networks responsive to DNA damage. Science. 2007;**316**: 1160-1166

[98] Psakhye I, Jentsch S. Protein group modification and synergy in the SUMO pathway as exemplified in DNA repair. Cell. 2012;**151**:807-820

[99] Welchman RL, Gordon C, Mayer RJ. Ubiquitin and ubiquitin-like proteins as multifunctional signals. Nature Reviews. 2005;**6**:599-609

[100] Glickman MH, Ciechanover A. The ubiquitin-proteasome proteolytic pathway: Destruction for the sake of construction. Physiological Reviews. 2002;**82**:373-428

[101] Hershko A, Ciechanover A. The ubiquitin system for protein degradation. Annual Review of Biochemistry. 1992;**61**:761-807

[102] Pickart CM. Ubiquitin enters the new millennium. Molecular Cell. 2001;**8**:499-504

[103] Kim KI, Baek SH, Chung CH. Versatile protein tag, SUMO: Its enzymology and biological function. Journal of Cellular Physiology. 2002;**191**:257-268

[104] Mukhopadhyay D, Dasso M. Modification in reverse: The SUMO proteases. Trends in Biochemical Sciences. 2007;**32**:286-295

[105] Rodriguez MS, Dargemont C, Hay RT. SUMO-1 conjugation in vivo requires both a consensus modification motif and nuclear targeting. The Journal of Biological Chemistry. 2001;**276**:12654-12659

[106] Geiss-Friedlander R, Melchior F. Concepts in sumoylation: A decade on. Nature Reviews. 2007;**8**:947-956

[107] Kerscher O. SUMO junction-what's your function? New insights through SUMO-interacting motifs. EMBO Reports. 2007;**8**:550-555

[108] Gibson BA, Kraus WL. New insights into the molecular and cellular functions of poly(ADP-ribose) and PARPs. Nature Reviews. 2012;**13**:411-424

[109] Juarez-Salinas H, Levi V, Jacobson EL, Jacobson MK. Poly(ADP-ribose) has a branched structure in vivo. The Journal of Biological Chemistry. 1982;**257**:607-609

[110] Hottiger MO. Nuclear ADP-ribosylation and its role in chromatin plasticity, cell differentiation, and epigenetics. Annual Review of Biochemistry. 2015;**84**:227-263

[111] Rouleau M, Patel A, Hendzel MJ, Kaufmann SH, Poirier GG. PARP inhibition: PARP1 and beyond. Nature Reviews. Cancer. 2010;**10**:293-301

[112] D'Amours D, Desnoyers S, D'Silva I, Poirier GG. Poly(ADP-ribosyl)ation reactions in the regulation of nuclear functions. The Biochemical Journal. 1999;**342**(Pt 2):249-268

[113] Tallis M, Morra R, Barkauskaite E, Ahel I. Poly(ADP-ribosyl)ation in regulation of chromatin structure and the DNA damage response. Chromosoma. 2014;**123**:79-90

[114] Vyas S, Chang P. New PARP targets for cancer therapy. Nature Reviews Cancer. 2014;**14**:502-509

[115] Daniels CM, Ong SE, Leung AK. The promise of proteomics for the study of ADP-ribosylation. Molecular Cell. 2015;**58**:911-924

[116] Dunstan MS, Barkauskaite E, Lafite P, Knezevic CE, Brassington A, Ahel M, et al. Structure and mechanism of a canonical poly(ADP-ribose) glycohydrolase. Nature Communications. 2012;**3**:878

[117] Kim IK, Kiefer JR, Ho CM, Stegeman RA, Classen S, Tainer JA, et al. Structure of mammalian poly(ADP-ribose) glycohydrolase reveals a flexible tyrosine clasp as a substrate-binding element. Nature Structural & Molecular Biology. 2012;**19**:653-656

[118] Ueda K, Oka J, Naruniya S, Miyakawa N, Hayaishi O. Poly ADP-ribose glycohydrolase from rat liver nuclei, a novel enzyme degrading the polymer. Biochemical and Biophysical Research Communications. 1972;**46**:516-523

[119] Mueller-Dieckmann C, Kernstock S, Lisurek M, von Kries JP, Haag F, Weiss MS, et al. The structure of human ADP-ribosylhydrolase 3 (ARH3) provides insights into the reversibility of protein ADP-ribosylation. Proceedings of the National Academy of Sciences of the United States of America. 2006;**103**:15026-15031

[120] Niere M, Mashimo M, Agledal L, Dolle C, Kasamatsu A, Kato J, et al. ADP-ribosylhydrolase 3 (ARH3), not poly(ADP-ribose) glycohydrolase (PARG) isoforms, is responsible for degradation of mitochondrial matrix-associated poly(ADP-ribose). The Journal of Biological Chemistry. 2012;**287**:16088-16102

[121] Wang Y, Kim NS, Haince JF, Kang HC, David KK, Andrabi SA, et al. Poly(ADP-ribose) (PAR) binding to apoptosis-inducing factor is critical for PAR polymerase-1-dependent cell death (parthanatos). Science Signaling. 2011;**4**:ra20

[122] Caldecott KW. Single-strand break repair and genetic disease. Nature Reviews. 2008;**9**:619-631

[123] Dantzer F, de La Rubia G, Menissier-De Murcia J, Hostomsky Z, de Murcia G, Schreiber V. Base excision repair is impaired in mammalian cells lacking poly(ADP-ribose) polymerase-1. Biochemistry. 2000;**39**:7559-7569

[124] Harris JL, Jakob B, Taucher-Scholz G, Dianov GL, Becherel OJ, Lavin MF. Aprataxin, poly-ADP ribose polymerase 1 (PARP-1) and apurinic endonuclease 1 (APE1) function together to protect the genome against oxidative damage. Human Molecular Genetics. 2009;**18**:4102-4117

[125] Hegde ML, Hegde PM, Arijit D, Boldogh I, Mitra S. Human DNA glycosylase NEIL1's interactions with downstream repair proteins is critical for efficient repair of oxidized DNA base damage and enhanced cell survival. Biomolecules. 2012;**2**:564-578

[126] Liu L, Kong M, Gassman NR, Freudenthal BD, Prasad R, Zhen S, et al. PARP1 changes from three-dimensional DNA damage searching to one-dimensional diffusion after auto-PARylation or in the presence of APE1. Nucleic Acids Research. 2017;**45**:12834-12847

[127] Fischer JA, Muller-Weeks S, Caradonna S. Proteolytic degradation of the nuclear isoform of uracil-DNA glycosylase occurs during the S phase of the cell cycle. DNA Repair (Amst). 2004;**3**:505-513

[128] Hagen L, Kavli B, Sousa MM, Torseth K, Liabakk NB, Sundheim O, et al. Cell cycle-specific UNG2 phosphorylations regulate protein turnover, activity and association with RPA. The EMBO Journal. 2008;**27**:51-61

[129] Tini M, Benecke A, Um SJ, Torchia J, Evans RM, Chambon P. Association of CBP/p300 acetylase and thymine DNA glycosylase links DNA repair and transcription. Molecular Cell. 2002;**9**:265-277

[130] Mohan RD, Litchfield DW, Torchia J, Tini M. Opposing regulatory roles of phosphorylation and acetylation in DNA mispair processing by thymine DNA glycosylase. Nucleic Acids Research. 2010;**38**:1135-1148

[131] Mohan RD, Rao A, Gagliardi J, Tini M. SUMO-1-dependent allosteric regulation of thymine DNA glycosylase alters subnuclear localization and CBP/p300 recruitment. Molecular and Cellular Biology. 2007;**27**:229-243

[132] Martin N, Schwamborn K, Schreiber V, Werner A, Guillier C, Zhang XD, et al. PARP-1 transcriptional activity is regulated by sumoylation upon heat shock. The EMBO Journal. 2009;**28**:3534-3548

[133] Ryu H, Al-Ani G, Deckert K, Kirkpatrick D, Gygi SP, Dasso M, et al. PIASy mediates SUMO-2/3 conjugation of poly(ADP-ribose) polymerase 1 (PARP1) on mitotic chromosomes. The Journal of Biological Chemistry. 2010;**285**:14415-14423

[134] Messner S, Schuermann D, Altmeyer M, Kassner I, Schmidt D, Schar P, et al. Sumoylation of poly(ADP-ribose) polymerase 1 inhibits its acetylation and restrains transcriptional coactivator function. FASEB Journal: Official Publication of the Federation of American Societies for Experimental Biology. 2009;**23**:3978-3989

[135] Roychoudhury S, Nath S, Song H, Hegde ML, Bellot LJ, Mantha AK, et al. Human apurinic/apyrimidinic endonuclease (APE1) is acetylated at DNA damage sites in chromatin, and acetylation modulates its DNA repair activity. Molecular and Cellular Biology. 2017;**37**:16

[136] Sengupta S, Mantha AK, Song H, Roychoudhury S, Nath S, Ray S, et al. Elevated level of acetylation of APE1 in tumor cells modulates DNA damage repair. Oncotarget. 2016;**7**:75197-75209

[137] Busso CS, Iwakuma T, Izumi T. Ubiquitination of mammalian AP endonuclease (APE1) regulated by the p53-MDM2 signaling pathway. Oncogene. 2009;**28**:1616-1625

[138] Meisenberg C, Tait PS, Dianova II, Wright K, Edelmann MJ, Ternette N, et al. Ubiquitin ligase UBR3 regulates cellular levels of the essential DNA repair protein APE1 and is required for genome stability. Nucleic Acids Research. 2012;**40**:701-711

[139] Parsons JL, Khoronenkova SV, Dianova II, Ternette N, Kessler BM, Datta PK, et al. Phosphorylation of PNKP by ATM prevents its proteasomal degradation and enhances resistance to oxidative stress. Nucleic Acids Research. 2012;**40**:11404-11415

[140] Segal-Raz H, Mass G, Baranes-Bachar K, Lerenthal Y, Wang SY, Chung YM, et al. ATM-mediated phosphorylation of polynucleotide kinase/phosphatase is required for effective DNA double-strand break repair. EMBO Reports. 2011;**12**:713-719

[141] Zolner AE, Abdou I, Ye R, Mani RS, Fanta M, Yu Y, et al. Phosphorylation of polynucleotide kinase/phosphatase by DNA-dependent protein kinase and ataxia-telangiectasia mutated regulates its association with sites of DNA damage. Nucleic Acids Research. 2011;**39**:9224-9237

[142] Chatterjee A, Saha S, Chakraborty A, Silva-Fernandes A, Mandal SM, Neves-Carvalho A, et al. The role of the mammalian DNA end-processing enzyme polynucleotide kinase 3′-phosphatase in spinocerebellar ataxia type 3 pathogenesis. PLoS Genetics. 2015;**11**:e1004749

[143] Guo Z, Kanjanapangka J, Liu N, Liu S, Liu C, Wu Z, et al. Sequential posttranslational modifications program FEN1 degradation during cell-cycle progression. Molecular Cell. 2012;**47**:444-456

[144] Guo Z, Qian L, Liu R, Dai H, Zhou M, Zheng L, et al. Nucleolar localization and dynamic roles of flap endonuclease 1 in ribosomal DNA replication and damage repair. Molecular and Cellular Biology. 2008;**28**:4310-4319

[145] Henneke G, Koundrioukoff S, Hubscher U. Phosphorylation of human Fen1 by cyclin-dependent kinase modulates its role in replication fork regulation. Oncogene. 2003;**22**:4301-4313

[146] Guo Z, Zheng L, Xu H, Dai H, Zhou M, Pascua MR, et al. Methylation of FEN1 suppresses nearby phosphorylation and facilitates PCNA binding. Nature Chemical Biology. 2010;**6**:766-773

[147] Hasan S, El-Andaloussi N, Hardeland U, Hassa PO, Burki C, Imhof R, et al. Acetylation regulates the DNA end-trimming activity of

DNA polymerase beta. Molecular Cell. 2002;**10**:1213-1222

[148] El-Andaloussi N, Valovka T, Toueille M, Hassa PO, Gehrig P, Covic M, et al. Methylation of DNA polymerase beta by protein arginine methyltransferase 1 regulates its binding to proliferating cell nuclear antigen. FASEB Journal: Official Publication of the Federation of American Societies for Experimental Biology. 2007;**21**:26-34

[149] El-Andaloussi N, Valovka T, Toueille M, Steinacher R, Focke F, Gehrig P, et al. Arginine methylation regulates DNA polymerase beta. Molecular Cell. 2006;**22**:51-62

[150] Parsons JL, Tait PS, Finch D, Dianova II, Allinson SL, Dianov GL. CHIP-mediated degradation and DNA damage-dependent stabilization regulate base excision repair proteins. Molecular Cell. 2008;**29**:477-487

[151] Parsons JL, Tait PS, Finch D, Dianova II, Edelmann MJ, Khoronenkova SV, et al. Ubiquitin ligase ARF-BP1/Mule modulates base excision repair. The EMBO Journal. 2009;**28**:3207-3215

[152] Hu LY, Chang CC, Huang YS, Chou WC, Lin YM, Ho CC, et al. SUMOylation of XRCC1 activated by poly (ADP-ribosyl)ation regulates DNA repair. Human Molecular Genetics. 2018;**27**:2306-2317

[153] Prasad R, Shock DD, Beard WA, Wilson SH. Substrate channeling in mammalian base excision repair pathways: Passing the baton. The Journal of Biological Chemistry. 2010;**285**:40479-40488

[154] Wilson SH, Kunkel TA. Passing the baton in base excision repair. Nature Structural Biology. 2000;**7**:176-178

[155] Clauson CL, Oestreich KJ, Austin JW, Doetsch PW. Abasic sites and strand breaks in DNA cause transcriptional mutagenesis in *Escherichia coli*. Proceedings of the National Academy of Sciences of the United States of America. 2010;**107**:3657-3662

[156] Fu D, Calvo JA, Samson LD. Balancing repair and tolerance of DNA damage caused by alkylating agents. Nature Reviews Cancer. 2012;**12**:104-120

[157] Goodman MF. Error-prone repair DNA polymerases in prokaryotes and eukaryotes. Annual Review of Biochemistry. 2002;**71**:17-50

[158] Tornaletti S, Maeda LS, Hanawalt PC. Transcription arrest at an abasic site in the transcribed strand of template DNA. Chemical Research in Toxicology. 2006;**19**:1215-1220

[159] Della-Maria J, Hegde ML, McNeill DR, Matsumoto Y, Tsai MS, Ellenberger T, et al. The interaction between polynucleotide kinase phosphatase and the DNA repair protein XRCC1 is critical for repair of DNA alkylation damage and stable association at DNA damage sites. The Journal of Biological Chemistry. 2012;**287**:39233-39244

[160] Waters TR, Gallinari P, Jiricny J, Swann PF. Human thymine DNA glycosylase binds to apurinic sites in DNA but is displaced by human apurinic endonuclease 1. The Journal of Biological Chemistry. 1999;**274**:67-74

[161] Sengupta S, Yang C, Hegde ML, Hegde PM, Mitra J, Pandey A, et al. Acetylation of oxidized base repair-initiating NEIL1 DNA glycosylase required for chromatin-bound repair complex formation in the human genome increases cellular resistance to oxidative stress. DNA Repair (Amst). 2018;**66-67**:1-10

[162] Cole HA, Tabor-Godwin JM, Hayes JJ. Uracil DNA glycosylase activity on nucleosomal DNA depends on rotational orientation of targets.

The Journal of Biological Chemistry. 2010;**285**:2876-2885

[163] Hinz JM. Impact of abasic site orientation within nucleosomes on human APE1 endonuclease activity. Mutation Research. 2014;**766-767**:19-24

[164] Hinz JM, Mao P, McNeill DR, Wilson DM 3rd. Reduced nuclease activity of apurinic/apyrimidinic endonuclease (APE1) variants on nucleosomes: Identification of access residues. The Journal of Biological Chemistry. 2015;**290**:21067-21075

[165] Hinz JM, Rodriguez Y, Smerdon MJ. Rotational dynamics of DNA on the nucleosome surface markedly impact accessibility to a DNA repair enzyme. Proceedings of the National Academy of Sciences of the United States of America. 2010;**107**:4646-4651

[166] Odell ID, Barbour JE, Murphy DL, Della-Maria JA, Sweasy JB, Tomkinson AE, et al. Nucleosome disruption by DNA ligase III-XRCC1 promotes efficient base excision repair. Molecular and Cellular Biology. 2011;**31**:4623-4632

[167] Odell ID, Newick K, Heintz NH, Wallace SS, Pederson DS. Non-specific DNA binding interferes with the efficient excision of oxidative lesions from chromatin by the human DNA glycosylase, NEIL1. DNA Repair (Amst). 2010;**9**:134-143

[168] Odell ID, Wallace SS, Pederson DS. Rules of engagement for base excision repair in chromatin. Journal of Cellular Physiology. 2013;**228**:258-266

[169] Prasad A, Wallace SS, Pederson DS. Initiation of base excision repair of oxidative lesions in nucleosomes by the human, bifunctional DNA glycosylase NTH1. Molecular and Cellular Biology. 2007;**27**:8442-8453

[170] Rodriguez Y, Smerdon MJ. The structural location of DNA lesions in nucleosome core particles determines accessibility by base excision repair enzymes. The Journal of Biological Chemistry. 2013;**288**:13863-13875

[171] House NC, Koch MR, Freudenreich CH. Chromatin modifications and DNA repair: Beyond double-strand breaks. Frontiers in Genetics. 2014;**5**:296

[172] Ransom M, Dennehey BK, Tyler JK. Chaperoning histones during DNA replication and repair. Cell. 2010;**140**:183-195

[173] Rodriges Blanko E, Kadyrova LY, Kadyrov FA. DNA mismatch repair interacts with CAF-1- and ASF1A-H3-H4-dependent histone (H3-H4)2 tetramer deposition. The Journal of Biological Chemistry. 2016;**291**:9203-9217

[174] Amouroux R, Campalans A, Epe B, Radicella JP. Oxidative stress triggers the preferential assembly of base excision repair complexes on open chromatin regions. Nucleic Acids Research. 2010;**38**:2878-2890

[175] Banerjee D, Mandal SM, Das A, Hegde ML, Das S, Bhakat KK, et al. Preferential repair of oxidized base damage in the transcribed genes of mammalian cells. The Journal of Biological Chemistry. 2011;**286**:6006-6016

[176] He YF, Li BZ, Li Z, Liu P, Wang Y, Tang Q, et al. Tet-mediated formation of 5-carboxylcytosine and its excision by TDG in mammalian DNA. Science. 2011;**333**:1303-1307

[177] Ito S, Shen L, Dai Q, Wu SC, Collins LB, Swenberg JA, et al. Tet proteins can convert 5-methylcytosine to 5-formylcytosine and 5-carboxylcytosine. Science. 2011;**333**:1300-1303

[178] Kohli RM, Zhang Y. TET enzymes, TDG and the dynamics of DNA demethylation. Nature. 2013;**502**:472-479

[179] Maiti A, Drohat AC. Thymine DNA glycosylase can rapidly excise 5-formylcytosine and 5-carboxylcytosine: Potential implications for active demethylation of CpG sites. The Journal of Biological Chemistry. 2011;**286**:35334-35338

[180] Weber AR, Krawczyk C, Robertson AB, Kusnierczyk A, Vagbo CB, Schuermann D, et al. Biochemical reconstitution of TET1-TDG-BER-dependent active DNA demethylation reveals a highly coordinated mechanism. Nature Communications. 2016;**7**:10806

[181] Clapier CR, Cairns BR. The biology of chromatin remodeling complexes. Annual Review of Biochemistry. 2009;**78**:273-304

[182] Hinz JM, Czaja W. Facilitation of base excision repair by chromatin remodeling. DNA Repair (Amst). 2015;**36**:91-97

[183] Narlikar GJ, Sundaramoorthy R, Owen-Hughes T. Mechanisms and functions of ATP-dependent chromatin-remodeling enzymes. Cell. 2013;**154**:490-503

[184] Menoni H, Gasparutto D, Hamiche A, Cadet J, Dimitrov S, Bouvet P, et al. ATP-dependent chromatin remodeling is required for base excision repair in conventional but not in variant H2A.Bbd nucleosomes. Molecular and Cellular Biology. 2007;**27**:5949-5956

[185] Menoni H, Shukla MS, Gerson V, Dimitrov S, Angelov D. Base excision repair of 8-oxoG in dinucleosomes. Nucleic Acids Research. 2012;**40**:692-700

[186] Nakanishi S, Prasad R, Wilson SH, Smerdon M. Different structural states in oligonucleosomes are required for early versus late steps of base excision repair. Nucleic Acids Research. 2007;**35**:4313-4321

[187] Czaja W, Mao P, Smerdon MJ. Chromatin remodelling complex RSC promotes base excision repair in chromatin of *Saccharomyces cerevisiae*. DNA Repair (Amst). 2014;**16**:35-43

[188] Tsuda M, Cho K, Ooka M, Shimizu N, Watanabe R, Yasui A, et al. ALC1/CHD1L, a chromatin-remodeling enzyme, is required for efficient base excision repair. PLoS One. 2017;**12**:e0188320

[189] Czaja W, Bespalov VA, Hinz JM, Smerdon MJ. Proficient repair in chromatin remodeling defective ino80 mutants of *Saccharomyces cerevisiae* highlights replication defects as the main contributor to DNA damage sensitivity. DNA Repair (Amst). 2010;**9**:976-984

[190] Haldar D, Kamakaka RT. *Schizosaccharomyces pombe* Hst4 functions in DNA damage response by regulating histone H3 K56 acetylation. Eukaryotic Cell. 2008;**7**:800-813

[191] Vempati RK, Jayani RS, Notani D, Sengupta A, Galande S, Haldar D. p300-mediated acetylation of histone H3 lysine 56 functions in DNA damage response in mammals. The Journal of Biological Chemistry. 2010;**285**:28553-28564

[192] Xu F, Zhang K, Grunstein M. Acetylation in histone H3 globular domain regulates gene expression in yeast. Cell. 2005;**121**:375-385

[193] Citterio E, Rademakers S, van der Horst GT, van Gool AJ, Hoeijmakers JH, Vermeulen W. Biochemical and biological characterization of

wild-type and ATPase-deficient Cockayne syndrome B repair protein. The Journal of Biological Chemistry. 1998;**273**:11844-11851

[194] Citterio E, Van Den Boom V, Schnitzler G, Kanaar R, Bonte E, Kingston RE, et al. ATP-dependent chromatin remodeling by the Cockayne syndrome B DNA repair-transcription-coupling factor. Molecular and Cellular Biology. 2000;**20**:7643-7653

[195] Yu S, Owen-Hughes T, Friedberg EC, Waters R, Reed SH. The yeast Rad7/Rad16/Abf1 complex generates superhelical torsion in DNA that is required for nucleotide excision repair. DNA Repair (Amst). 2004;**3**:277-287

[196] Kim MY, Mauro S, Gevry N, Lis JT, Kraus WL. NAD+-dependent modulation of chromatin structure and transcription by nucleosome binding properties of PARP-1. Cell. 2004;**119**:803-814

[197] Kim MY, Zhang T, Kraus WL. Poly(ADP-ribosyl)ation by PARP-1: 'PAR-laying' NAD+ into a nuclear signal. Genes & Development. 2005;**19**:1951-1967

[198] Rouleau M, Aubin RA, Poirier GG. Poly(ADP-ribosyl)ated chromatin domains: Access granted. Journal of Cell Science. 2004;**117**:815-825

[199] Groth A, Rocha W, Verreault A, Almouzni G. Chromatin challenges during DNA replication and repair. Cell. 2007;**128**:721-733

[200] Burgess RJ, Zhang Z. Histone chaperones in nucleosome assembly and human disease. Nature Structural & Molecular Biology. 2013;**20**:14-22

[201] Yang C, Sengupta S, Hegde PM, Mitra J, Jiang S, Holey B, et al. Regulation of oxidized base damage repair by chromatin assembly factor 1 subunit A. Nucleic Acids Research. 2017;**45**:739-748

[202] Polo SE, Almouzni G. Chromatin dynamics after DNA damage: The legacy of the access-repair-restore model. DNA Repair (Amst). 2015;**36**:114-121

[203] Bhakat KK, Mokkapati SK, Boldogh I, Hazra TK, Mitra S. Acetylation of human 8-oxoguanine-DNA glycosylase by p300 and its role in 8-oxoguanine repair in vivo. Molecular and Cellular Biology. 2006;**26**:1654-1665

[204] Das A, Hazra TK, Boldogh I, Mitra S, Bhakat KK. Induction of the human oxidized base-specific DNA glycosylase NEIL1 by reactive oxygen species. The Journal of Biological Chemistry. 2005;**280**:35272-35280

[205] Sengupta S, Mantha AK, Mitra S, Bhakat KK. Human AP endonuclease (APE1/Ref-1) and its acetylation regulate YB-1-p300 recruitment and RNA polymerase II loading in the drug-induced activation of multidrug resistance gene MDR1. Oncogene. 2011;**30**:482-493

[206] Hanawalt PC, Spivak G. Transcription-coupled DNA repair: Two decades of progress and surprises. Nature Reviews. 2008;**9**:958-970

[207] Menoni H, Wienholz F, Theil AF, Janssens RC, Lans H, Campalans A, et al. The transcription-coupled DNA repair-initiating protein CSB promotes XRCC1 recruitment to oxidative DNA damage. Nucleic Acids Research. 2018;**46**:7747-7756

[208] Abbotts R, Madhusudan S. Human AP endonuclease 1 (APE1): From mechanistic insights to druggable target in cancer. Cancer Treatment Reviews. 2010;**36**:425-435

[209] Al-Safi RI, Odde S, Shabaik Y, Neamati N. Small-molecule inhibitors

of APE1 DNA repair function: An overview. Current Molecular Pharmacology. 2012;**5**:14-35

[210] Thakur S, Sarkar B, Cholia RP, Gautam N, Dhiman M, Mantha AK. APE1/Ref-1 as an emerging therapeutic target for various human diseases: Phytochemical modulation of its functions. Experimental & Molecular Medicine. 2014;**46**:e106

[211] Ferrarotto R, Cardnell R, Su S, Diao L, Eterovic AK, Prieto V, et al. Poly ADP-ribose polymerase-1 as a potential therapeutic target in Merkel cell carcinoma. Head & Neck. 2018;**40**:1676-1684

[212] Drean A, Lord CJ, Ashworth A. PARP inhibitor combination therapy. Critical Reviews in Oncology/Hematology. 2016;**108**:73-85

[213] Lu X, Bocangel D, Nannenga B, Yamaguchi H, Appella E, Donehower LA. The p53-induced oncogenic phosphatase PPM1D interacts with uracil DNA glycosylase and suppresses base excision repair. Molecular Cell. 2004;**15**:621-634

[214] Ma KW, Au SW, Waye MM. Over-expression of SUMO-1 induces the up-regulation of heterogeneous nuclear ribonucleoprotein A2/B1 isoform B1 (hnRNP A2/B1 isoform B1) and uracil DNA glycosylase (UDG) in hepG2 cells. Cell Biochemistry and Function. 2009;**27**:228-237

[215] Schrofelbauer B, Hakata Y, Landau NR. HIV-1 Vpr function is mediated by interaction with the damage-specific DNA-binding protein DDB1. Proceedings of the National Academy of Sciences of the United States of America. 2007;**104**:4130-4135

[216] Schrofelbauer B, Yu Q, Zeitlin SG, Landau NR. Human immunodeficiency virus type 1 Vpr induces the degradation of the UNG and SMUG uracil-DNA glycosylases. Journal of Virology. 2005;**79**:10978-10987

[217] Kim MS, Kondo T, Takada I, Youn MY, Yamamoto Y, Takahashi S, et al. DNA demethylation in hormone-induced transcriptional derepression. Nature. 2009;**461**:1007-1012

[218] Coey CT, Drohat AC. Defining the impact of sumoylation on substrate binding and catalysis by thymine DNA glycosylase. Nucleic Acids Research. 2018;**46**:5159-5170

[219] Coey CT, Fitzgerald ME, Maiti A, Reiter KH, Guzzo CM, Matunis MJ, et al. E2-mediated small ubiquitin-like modifier (SUMO) modification of thymine DNA glycosylase is efficient but not selective for the enzyme-product complex. The Journal of Biological Chemistry. 2014;**289**:15810-15819

[220] Smet-Nocca C, Wieruszeski JM, Leger H, Eilebrecht S, Benecke A. SUMO-1 regulates the conformational dynamics of thymine-DNA glycosylase regulatory domain and competes with its DNA binding activity. BMC Biochemistry. 2011;**12**:4

[221] Steinacher R, Schar P. Functionality of human thymine DNA glycosylase requires SUMO-regulated changes in protein conformation. Current Biology. 2005;**15**:616-623

[222] Shibata E, Dar A, Dutta A. CRL4Cdt2 E3 ubiquitin ligase and proliferating cell nuclear antigen (PCNA) cooperate to degrade thymine DNA glycosylase in S phase. The Journal of Biological Chemistry. 2014;**289**:23056-23064

[223] Slenn TJ, Morris B, Havens CG, Freeman RM Jr, Takahashi TS, Walter JC. Thymine DNA glycosylase is a CRL4Cdt2 substrate. The Journal of Biological Chemistry. 2014;**289**:23043-23055

[224] Kundu S, Brinkmeyer MK, Eigenheer RA, David SS. Ser 524 is a phosphorylation site in MUTYH and Ser 524 mutations alter 8-oxoguanine (OG): A mismatch recognition. DNA Repair (Amst). 2010;**9**:1026-1037

[225] Parker AR, O'Meally RN, Sahin F, Su GH, Racke FK, Nelson WG, et al. Defective human MutY phosphorylation exists in colorectal cancer cell lines with wild-type MutY alleles. The Journal of Biological Chemistry. 2003;**278**:47937-47945

[226] Dorn J, Ferrari E, Imhof R, Ziegler N, Hubscher U. Regulation of human MutYH DNA glycosylase by the E3 ubiquitin ligase mule. The Journal of Biological Chemistry. 2014;**289**:7049-7058

[227] Dantzer F, Luna L, Bjoras M, Seeberg E. Human OGG1 undergoes serine phosphorylation and associates with the nuclear matrix and mitotic chromatin in vivo. Nucleic Acids Research. 2002;**30**:2349-2357

[228] Hu J, Imam SZ, Hashiguchi K, de Souza-Pinto NC, Bohr VA. Phosphorylation of human oxoguanine DNA glycosylase (alpha-OGG1) modulates its function. Nucleic Acids Research. 2005;**33**:3271-3282

[229] Fantini D, Moritz E, Auvre F, Amouroux R, Campalans A, Epe B, et al. Rapid inactivation and proteasome-mediated degradation of OGG1 contribute to the synergistic effect of hyperthermia on genotoxic treatments. DNA Repair (Amst). 2013;**12**:227-237

[230] Bian Y, Song C, Cheng K, Dong M, Wang F, Huang J, et al. An enzyme assisted RP-RPLC approach for in-depth analysis of human liver phosphoproteome. Journal of Proteomics. 2014;**96**:253-262

[231] Prakash A, Cao VB, Doublie S. Phosphorylation sites identified in the NEIL1 DNA glycosylase are potential targets for the JNK1 kinase. PLoS One. 2016;**11**:e0157860

[232] Sui S, Wang J, Yang B, Song L, Zhang J, Chen M, et al. Phosphoproteome analysis of the human Chang liver cells using SCX and a complementary mass spectrometric strategy. Proteomics. 2008;**8**:2024-2034

[233] Bhakat KK, Hazra TK, Mitra S. Acetylation of the human DNA glycosylase NEIL2 and inhibition of its activity. Nucleic Acids Research. 2004;**32**:3033-3039

[234] Likhite VS, Cass EI, Anderson SD, Yates JR, Nardulli AM. Interaction of estrogen receptor alpha with 3-methyladenine DNA glycosylase modulates transcription and DNA repair. The Journal of Biological Chemistry. 2004;**279**:16875-16882

[235] Agnihotri S, Burrell K, Buczkowicz P, Remke M, Golbourn B, Chornenkyy Y, et al. ATM regulates 3-methylpurine-DNA glycosylase and promotes therapeutic resistance to alkylating agents. Cancer Discovery. 2014;**4**:1198-1213

[236] Bhakat KK, Izumi T, Yang SH, Hazra TK, Mitra S. Role of acetylated human AP-endonuclease (APE1/Ref-1) in regulation of the parathyroid hormone gene. The EMBO Journal. 2003;**22**:6299-6309

[237] Fantini D, Vascotto C, Marasco D, D'Ambrosio C, Romanello M, Vitagliano L, et al. Critical lysine residues within the overlooked N-terminal domain of human APE1 regulate its biological functions. Nucleic Acids Research. 2010;**38**:8239-8256

[238] Lirussi L, Antoniali G, Vascotto C, D'Ambrosio C, Poletto M, Romanello M, et al. Nucleolar accumulation of APE1 depends on charged lysine residues that undergo acetylation upon genotoxic

stress and modulate its BER activity in cells. Molecular Biology of the Cell. 2012;**23**:4079-4096

[239] Yacoub A, Kelley MR, Deutsch WA. The DNA repair activity of human redox/repair protein APE/Ref-1 is inactivated by phosphorylation. Cancer Research. 1997;**57**:5457-5459

[240] Huang E, Qu D, Zhang Y, Venderova K, Haque ME, Rousseaux MW, et al. The role of Cdk5-mediated apurinic/apyrimidinic endonuclease 1 phosphorylation in neuronal death. Nature Cell Biology. 2010;**12**:563-571

[241] Busso CS, Wedgeworth CM, Izumi T. Ubiquitination of human AP-endonuclease 1 (APE1) enhanced by T233E substitution and by CDK5. Nucleic Acids Research. 2011;**39**:8017-8028

[242] Hasan S, Stucki M, Hassa PO, Imhof R, Gehrig P, Hunziker P, et al. Regulation of human flap endonuclease-1 activity by acetylation through the transcriptional coactivator p300. Molecular Cell. 2001;**7**:1221-1231

[243] Rahmeh AA, Zhou Y, Xie B, Li H, Lee EY, Lee MY. Phosphorylation of the p68 subunit of Pol delta acts as a molecular switch to regulate its interaction with PCNA. Biochemistry. 2012;**51**:416-424

[244] Dong Z, Tomkinson AE. ATM mediates oxidative stress-induced dephosphorylation of DNA ligase IIIalpha. Nucleic Acids Research. 2006;**34**:5721-5279

[245] Kang HC, Lee YI, Shin JH, Andrabi SA, Chi Z, Gagne JP, et al. Iduna is a poly(ADP-ribose) (PAR)-dependent E3 ubiquitin ligase that regulates DNA damage. Proceedings of the National Academy of Sciences of the United States of America. 2011;**108**:14103-14108

[246] Chou WC, Wang HC, Wong FH, Ding SL, Wu PE, Shieh SY, et al. Chk2-dependent phosphorylation of XRCC1 in the DNA damage response promotes base excision repair. The EMBO Journal. 2008;**27**:3140-3150

[247] Levy N, Martz A, Bresson A, Spenlehauer C, de Murcia G, Menissier-de Murcia J. XRCC1 is phosphorylated by DNA-dependent protein kinase in response to DNA damage. Nucleic Acids Research. 2006;**34**:32-41

[248] Loizou JI, El-Khamisy SF, Zlatanou A, Moore DJ, Chan DW, Qin J, et al. The protein kinase CK2 facilitates repair of chromosomal DNA single-strand breaks. Cell. 2004;**117**:17-28

[249] Luo H, Chan DW, Yang T, Rodriguez M, Chen BP, Leng M, et al. A new XRCC1-containing complex and its role in cellular survival of methyl methanesulfonate treatment. Molecular and Cellular Biology. 2004;**24**:8356-8365

[250] Parsons JL, Dianova II, Finch D, Tait PS, Strom CE, Helleday T, et al. XRCC1 phosphorylation by CK2 is required for its stability and efficient DNA repair. DNA Repair (Amst). 2010;**9**:835-841

[251] Strom CE, Mortusewicz O, Finch D, Parsons JL, Lagerqvist A, Johansson F, et al. CK2 phosphorylation of XRCC1 facilitates dissociation from DNA and single-strand break formation during base excision repair. DNA Repair (Amst). 2011;**10**:961-969

[252] Wei L, Nakajima S, Hsieh CL, Kanno S, Masutani M, Levine AS, et al. Damage response of XRCC1 at sites of DNA single strand breaks is regulated by phosphorylation and ubiquitylation after degradation of poly(ADP-ribose). Journal of Cell Science. 2013;**126**:4414-4423

[253] Gocke CB, Yu H, Kang J. Systematic identification and

analysis of mammalian small ubiquitin-like modifier substrates. The Journal of Biological Chemistry. 2005;**280**:5004-5012

[254] Hassa PO, Haenni SS, Buerki C, Meier NI, Lane WS, Owen H, et al. Acetylation of poly(ADP-ribose) polymerase-1 by p300/CREB-binding protein regulates coactivation of NF-kappaB-dependent transcription. The Journal of Biological Chemistry. 2005;**280**:40450-40464

[255] Kauppinen TM, Chan WY, Suh SW, Wiggins AK, Huang EJ, Swanson RA. Direct phosphorylation and regulation of poly(ADP-ribose) polymerase-1 by extracellular signal-regulated kinases 1/2. Proceedings of the National Academy of Sciences of the United States of America. 2006;**103**:7136-7141

[256] Kashima L, Idogawa M, Mita H, Shitashige M, Yamada T, Ogi K, et al. CHFR protein regulates mitotic checkpoint by targeting PARP-1 protein for ubiquitination and degradation. The Journal of Biological Chemistry. 2012;**287**:12975-12984

Section 4

DNA Repair and Cellular Processes

Chapter 8

The Role of DNA Repair in Cellular Aging Process

Francisco Alejandro Lagunas-Rangel and Rosa María Bermúdez-Cruz

Abstract

Aging is defined as the time-dependent decline of functional properties. One common denominator of aging is mitochondrial dysfunction and accumulation of genetic damage throughout life. In fact, the imperfect maintenance of nuclear and mitochondrial DNA likely represents a critical contributor of aging. Each day, the integrity and stability of DNA are challenged by exogenous physical, chemical, or biological agents, as well as by endogenous processes, including DNA replication mistakes, spontaneous hydrolytic reactions, and reactive oxygen species. In this way, DNA repair systems have evolved a complex network that is collectively able of dealing with most of the damages inflicted. However, their efficiency may decrease with age and, therefore, influence the rate of aging. Thus, the purpose of this work is to summarize the recent knowledge in cellular aging process and its link with DNA repair systems, with a particular emphasis on the molecular mechanisms associated.

Keywords: DNA damage, DNA repair, BER, NER, MMR, HR, NHEJ

1. Introduction

Aging is a complex biological process that results in a progressive loss of physiological integrity. Overall, aging is a consequence of accumulation of cellular damage and is characterized by nine hallmarks: genomic instability, telomere attrition, epigenetic alterations, cellular senescence, mitochondrial dysfunction, loss of proteostasis, deregulated nutrient sensing, stem cell exhaustion, and altered intercellular communication (**Figure 1**) [1]. Although aging may involve damage to various cellular constituents, there is evidence suggesting that DNA constitutes the key target in this process [2]; consequently, genomic instability is the main factor of aging [3–5]. Genome instability has been implicated as a cause of aging since unrepaired DNA damage, DNA mutations, and epimutations accumulate in an age-related manner [3]. In the same way, the notion that multi-system premature aging syndromes are mainly caused by defects in genome maintenance or affect genome function highlights the role of genome integrity in aging [6]. Meanwhile, normal aging is accompanied by telomere shortening with cell division due to the "end-replication problem" and telomere end processing. Currently, there is a wide body of evidence associating reduction in the length of telomeres with failure of cell division and senescence of normal cells, and oxidative stress and inflammation can contribute to the rate of attrition of telomere length [7]. Age-related changes involve alterations in DNA methylation patterns and posttranslational modification of histones such as increased histone H4K16 acetylation [8], H4K20 trimethylation [9], or H3K4 trimethylation [10], as well as decreased H3K9 methylation [11] or H3K27 trimethylation [12]. At the same time, with aging there is also a global heterochromatin loss and redistribution [13], thus affecting the expression of several genes, mainly those involved in DNA repair, cellular proliferation, differentiation, and cell-cycle regulation, and therefore triggering the emergence of other hallmarks of aging [14, 15]. Cellular senescence is a process that has become an important contributor in aging since it imposes a permanent proliferative arrest of cells in response to various stressors such as DNA damage and telomere loss [16]. Furthermore, as cells and organisms age, mitochondria suffer a decline in their integrity and function, tending to diminish the efficacy of the respiratory chain and thus reducing ATP generation, increasing electron leakage and ROS production that can damage DNA, proteins, and lipids, among other important biomolecules [17]. Proteostasis involves mechanisms for correct folding proteins and mechanisms for the degradation of proteins, which act in a coordinated fashion to prevent the accumulation of damaged components and assuring the continuous renewal of intracellular proteins. There is evidence that aging is associated with perturbed proteostasis, thus favoring the development of several diseases [18]. Recent data have shown that anabolic signaling accelerates aging; in agreement with this, caloric-restricted diet decreases nutrient signaling and as a result, a long life span is promoted since DNA repair systems are improved; on the other hand, protein homeostasis decreases ROS production and delays cellular senescence [19]. Decline in the regenerative potential of tissues is one of the most obvious characteristics of aging, where stem cell exhaustion is also important and explained by a decreased cell-cycle activity. Interestingly, this correlates with the accumulation of DNA damage, telomere shortening, and overexpression of cell-cycle inhibitory proteins such as p16INK4a, increasing the relevancy of DNA repair systems [20]. Finally, aging also involves changes at the level of intercellular communication, where neurohormonal signaling tends to be deregulated together with composition of the peri- and extracellular environment

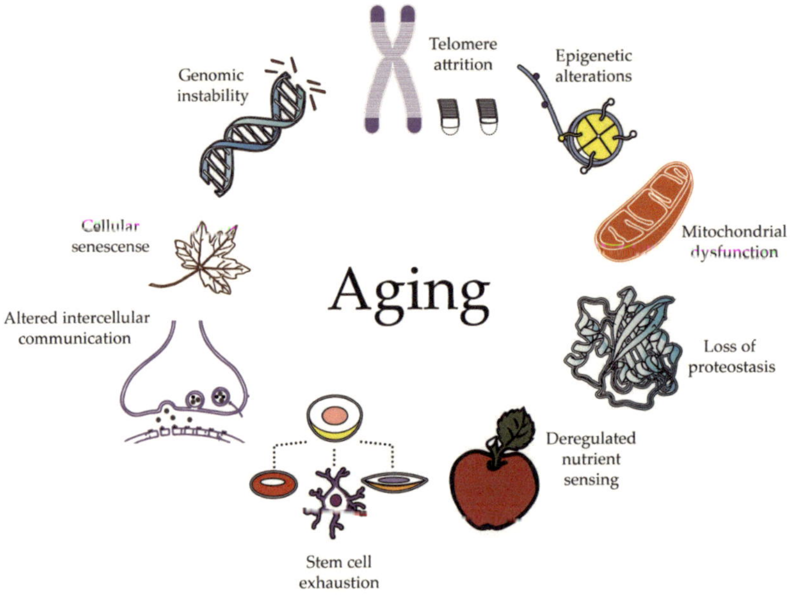

Figure 1.
The hallmarks of aging. The figure illustrates nine hallmarks previously described [1] and where age-related changes in DNA repair systems have important roles to promote the development of this phenotype.

and immune system, specially increasing inflammatory reactions and declining immunosurveillance against pathogens and premalignant cells [21]. In this way, our work focuses on describing the molecular bases that associate DNA damage and the cell aging process, with a special emphasis in DNA repair systems.

2. Age-related changes in DNA repair

Each day, the integrity and stability of DNA are challenged by exogenous physical, chemical, or biological agents, as well as by endogenous processes, including DNA replication mistakes, spontaneous hydrolytic reactions, and reactive oxygen species (ROS). Thus, depending on the source of damage, DNA can be affected in different ways, including nucleotide alterations, bulky adducts, single-strand breaks (SSB), and double-strand breaks (DSB). To combat threats posed by DNA damage, cells have evolved complex and finely regulated mechanisms collectively referred to as DNA damage response (DDR) which detects DNA lesions, signals their presence, and promotes their repair [22–24]. However, according with the genome maintenance hypothesis of aging, DNA repair can itself be subject to age-related changes and deterioration, allowing accumulation of damages (**Figure 2**). The wide diversity of DNA-lesion types requires multiple, largely distinct DNA repair mechanisms that differ in their components, whereas some lesions are subject to direct protein-mediated reversal, most are repaired by a sequence of catalytic events mediated by multiple proteins [22]. Thus, cells with defects in key proteins involved in DDR have been shown an accelerated aging phenotype caused by the accumulation of mutations and epimutations that eventually cause malfunction of the cells, senescence, or apoptosis [25].

2.1 Response to DNA single-strand breaks (SSBs)

2.1.1 Base excision repair (BER)

BER pathway corrects DNA damage from oxidation, deamination, alkylation, and other small DNA alterations that do not distort the overall structure of double helix. In general, BER is initiated by a DNA glycosylase that recognizes and

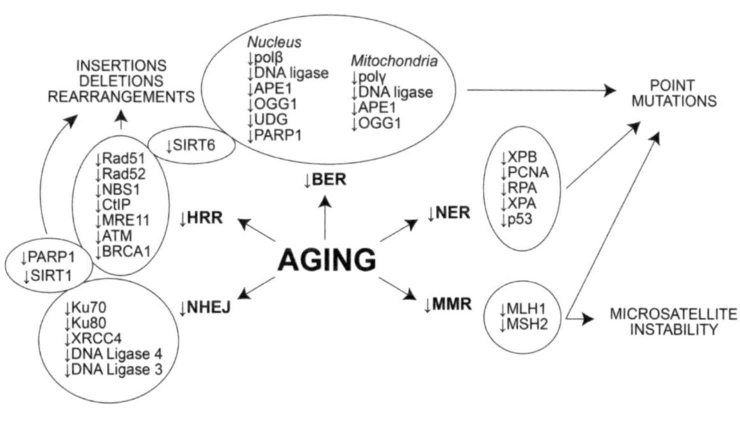

Figure 2.
Age-related changes in DNA repair and their consequences. Aging involves deterioration of DNA repair systems allowing the damages to accumulate and eventually cause a malfunction of the cells. In general, all age-related changes in DNA repair pathways promote genomic instability in different ways. Decline in efficiency and fidelity of BER and NER leads to point mutations, whereas inefficient MMR leads to microsatellite instability and point mutations. Meanwhile, deficiencies in NHEJ and HRR result in deletions and genomic rearrangements.

removes the damaged base, leaving an abasic (apurinic/apyrimidinic; AP) site that is subsequently processed by an AP endonuclease (APE), an exonuclease, a DNA polymerase, a ligase, and many other ancillary factors in a short-patch repair or long-patch repair [26]. Notably, several pieces of evidence indicate that the efficacy of BER may negatively change with age, and it has a significant impact in longevity together with homologous recombination repair (HRR) [27]. Age-related changes in the BER mechanism have been studied mainly in neuronal extracts where it constitutes the main repair pathway. In this way, an overall deficiency in several factors has been observed [28], where DNA polymerase β (pol β) together with DNA ligase [29] and APE1 activities [30, 31] seem to be the most limiting factors. Interestingly, an age-dependent attenuation in the transcriptional activation of pol β and APE1 was observed in response to DNA damage [32] together with APE1 accumulation in the nucleus and mitochondria [33]. Aging has also been shown to have a significant effect on cleavage efficacy of tetrahydrofuran:A, U:G mispair, U:A base pair, thymine glycol:A, and 8-oxo-7,8-dihydroguanine:C [34]. Thus, senescent human fibroblasts as well as leukocytes from old donors showed higher basal level of AP sites than young donors. However, after a challenge with the oxidizing agent H_2O_2 or the alkylating agent methyl methanesulfonate (MMS), the number of AP sites increased quickly in young cells, whereas in senescent and older cells, they were observed to grow slowly with a concomitant loss of viability, suggesting a decrease in DNA glycosylase activity, mainly in OGG1 8-oxoguanine and 3-methyladenine DNA glycosylases [35], although other reports have also mentioned a decrease in the UDG uracil-DNA glycosylase [28]. Because polyADP-ribosylation (PARylation) levels are linked to downstream mechanisms in DNA repair together with other cellular deficiencies as cell-cycle arrest, cell survival, cell death, and/or cell transformation, a decline in PARP1 activity is important since it has been linked with the age in humans and rats [36]. Further, a decrease in the interaction between the endonuclease VIII-like NEIL1 and PARP1 was observed in old mice when compared to young mice [37], which also could be associated with the decrease in PARP1 activity. Meanwhile, a significant decrease in the expression of SIRT6 has been reported to have a relevant role in BER because it regulates repair activity through a PARP1-dependent pathway [38]. Since sirtuins can function as metabolic sensors, they could also be related with a significative increase in pol β [39] and APE activities [30] under caloric restricted diets. Consequently, BER pathway showed to be deficient when repairing age-downregulated genes in comparison with genes that are not affected by age [40].

On the other hand, the mitochondrial free radical theory of aging states that free radicals generated in mitochondria are strongly related with the intrinsic aging process, mainly due to the accumulation of oxidative damage and derived mutations in mitochondrial DNA (mtDNA) mainly in D-loop region. mtDNA is more susceptible to oxidative damage than the nuclear genome, presumably because of the physical proximity of the source of ROS and lack of histones [41]. BER is the predominant and best understood DNA repair pathway in mitochondria involving at least four components, a DNA glycosylase, an AP endonuclease (or other mechanism for processing abasic sites), DNA polymerase γ (pol γ), and DNA ligase [42]. Recently, pol β was also detected in mitochondrial protein extracts, where it is required to provide enhanced mtDNA BER activity [43]. In a similar way to nuclear BER, in rat brain mitochondria, there is a marked age-dependent decline in mitochondrial BER activity, as indicated by a pol β, pol γ, ligase, APE1 endonuclease, and OGG1 glycosylase activities [44]. Interestingly, activity of mitochondrial OGG1 AE8-oxoguanine DNA glycosylase increases in mouse liver mitochondria according with the age [45]. However, a significant fraction of the OGG1 remains in the outer membrane and intermembrane space in an immature form, presumably because its import into the mitochondrial matrix is impaired as a consequence of aging. In addition, a nearly identical phenomenon was observed with the mitochondrial uracil-DNA glycosylase [46].

2.1.2 Nucleotide excision repair (NER)

NER is the primary pathway for repairing a wide range bulky DNA lesions, including UV-induced photoproducts (cyclopyrimidine dimers [CPDs], 6–4 photoproducts [6-4PPs]), adducts formed by mutagens in the environment such as benzo[a]pyrene or some aromatic amines, some oxidative endogenous lesions such as cyclopurines, and adducts formed by cancer chemotherapeutic drugs such as cisplatin. NER can be initiated by two subpathways: global genome NER (GG-NER) where the participation of XPC-RAD23B is involved and the transcription-coupled NER (TC-NER) where RNA polymerase interacts with CSA, CSB, and XAB2. Both converge to complete the excision process requiring the core NER factors RPA, XPA, TFIIH, XPD, XPB, XPG, and ERCC1–XPF, among other auxiliary proteins [47]. NER activity decreases with aging possibly because there is a transcriptional downregulation of NER genes together with an altered protein function or processing and a decrease in energy production [48]. In this manner, it was previously observed that aged human skin [49] and fibroblasts [50] showed decreased levels of XPB, PCNA, RPA, XPA, and p53, and more importantly the UVB-induced pyrimidine dimers were removed in a slower manner than in younger counterparts [50]. Interestingly, the effect of age on the repair of UV-induced DNA damage varies for transcribed and nontranscribed DNA, decreasing considerably in unexpressed DNA [51, 52] but improving in both cases under calorie restricted diets [52]. Furthermore, UV-induced damage and repair in telomeres showed to be slower and less frequent than in other regions of the genome such as active genes [53]. Additionally, ERCC1 and XPF, which are considered as the rate-limiting members in NER, also showed an age-dependent decline in their relative expression levels [54]. Because XPC, XPB, and XPF appear to be dependent on the activation status of the IGF-1R, decreased levels of IGF-1R observed with aging also contributed with the decline of NER pathway [55]. Meanwhile, in an assay based in plasmid reactivation after UV damage, cells from older donors introduced an increased number of mutations in the transfected plasmid, which suggests that not only the repair is less efficient with age but also more mistakes are made [51].

2.1.3 Mismatch repair (MMR)

The mismatched nucleotides in the DNA can result from polymerase misincorporation errors, recombination between imperfectly matched sequences, chemical or physical damage to nucleotides, and deamination of 5-methylcytosine (5mC) mostly during replication. MMR pathway consists of four major heterodimeric complexes, MutL homolog (MutL)α, MutLβ, MutS homolog (MutS)α, and MutSβ. MutLα involves MLH1 and PMS2, whereas MutLβ consist of MLH1 and PMS1. Meanwhile, MutSα consists of MSH2 and MSH6, and MutSβ is constituted by MSH2 and MSH3. Thus, MutSα complex recognizes single mispaired bases, whereas MutSβ detects mispaired runs of 3–6 bases. MutSα or MutSβ recruits MutLα or MutLβ and forms a tetrameric complex that serves as a base for the recruitment of excision and repair machinery [56]. MMR removes mispaired bases preventing mutations [57], and defects in this pathway are strongly associated with a substantial destabilization of microsatellites, which are tandemly repeated sequences (from 1 to 6 bp), highly polymorphic, interspersed in the genome, and susceptible to slippage during replication [58]. Previously, a decline in MMR function and efficiency correlation with age was observed [59, 60], especially in microsatellite sequences [61] where age-related methylation of the MLH1 [62, 63] and MSH2 [64] promoters could be associated to microsatellite instability (MSI). Interestingly, MLH1 shores showed a decrease in methylation with increasing age [65]. Shores are regions of the genome around CpG islands with lower GC content and with the ability to control gene expression.

2.2 Response to DNA double-strand breaks (DSBs)

2.2.1 Homologous recombination repair (HRR)

With aging there is an increase in DNA double-strand breaks [66]. However, it is unknown whether this increase is a consequence of accumulation of unrepaired DSBs or progressively delayed repair events, possibly as a reflection of an inherently limited capacity to process DSBs [67]. To repair this kind of DNA damage, HRR, considered a highly reliable pathway, allows the cell to access and copy information from the intact DNA sequence into the sister chromatid. Notably, HRR is restricted to late S to G2 phases when chromosomes are aligned [68]. RAD51 and other members of the RAD52 epistasis group as RAD50, MRE11, and XRS2 are needed for HRR. The efficiency of HRR is enhanced by mediator proteins that promote the loading of RAD51 onto ssDNA, RAD52 among them [69]. HR-mediated repair efficiency declines precipitously during cellular aging together with a decline of RAD51, RAD51C, RAD52, NBS1, CTIP, and MRE11 levels [66, 70]. Furthermore, in human and mice oocytes, a decrease in expression of BRCA1 and ATM [71] and an impaired recruitment of RAD51 to DNA damage sites during aging [72] were observed, which could force cells to utilize the error-prone NHEJ pathway. At the same time, in older mice a lower activity of the ATM kinase that results in less p53 phosphorylation was reported, thus affecting apoptosis, cell-cycle arrest, and senescence [73]. In addition to the above, the decrease in the levels of PARP1 [36] and SIRT6 [38] not only affects BER pathway but also has a relevant role in HRR since supplementation of recombinant SIRT6 was able to partly restore HR activity [70]. This could be related to a higher binding of DBC1 to PARP1 inhibiting its enzymatic activity as well as the change in NAD+ levels [74]. Decreased NAD+ levels observed with age also reduce activity of other sirtuins as SIRT1 and SIRT7 together with PARP1, reducing NHEJ and HRR pathways [75]. Although HRR is essential, its activity must be carefully controlled in order to maintain genomic integrity [76]. Previously, it has been demonstrated that frequency of recombinant cells is highly variable among tissues, from very low levels in the brain and stomach to very frequent in the pancreas and spleen. Additionally, de novo recombination events indeed accumulate in mice colonic somatic stem cells with age [77].

2.2.2 Nonhomologous end joined (NHEJ)

In human cells, NHEJ is the major pathway for the repair of DSBs, where two ends of DNA with little or no sequence homology are brought together and repaired. NHEJ can act throughout most of the cell cycle but predominantly in G1 phase [68]. NHEJ is divided into two subpathways: the classical NHEJ pathway (c NHEJ), in which DNA-PKcs, Ku70/Ku80 heterodimers, Artemis, XRCC4, XLF, and DNA Ligase 4 are involved, and the alternative NHEJ pathway (alt-NHEJ), comprised of the repair factors PARP1 and DNA ligase 3 [78]. Both NHEJ pathways are associated with changes in DNA sequence, where c-NHEJ causes deletions and insertions, whereas alt-NHEJ propitiates the loss of genetic information between microhomologies on chromosomes [79]. NHEJ becomes inefficient and more error-prone during cellular senescence, thus favoring genomic instability and higher incidence of cancer in the elderly [80, 81]. Furthermore, NHEJ-mediated VDJ recombination in B lymphocytes is impaired, reducing class switch recombination efficiency and contributing to reduced humoral repertoire and impaired immunity with aging [82]. Frequency of microhomology-mediated end joining (MMEJ) increases as a compensatory mechanism; however, at the same time, it favors that more mistakes are generated [81]. Ku 70 and 80 proteins decreased their expression at least twofold in two lines of senescent human fibroblast; at the same time, their localization was changed concentrating them in the nucleus when compared with young cells where they are present in both the nucleus and cytoplasm [83]. Cytoplasmic Ku proteins could serve as a reserve (pool) that is recruited to the nucleus upon DNA damage; therefore in senescent cells these proteins are unavailable to repair new lesions [25]. Additionally, binding activity of the Ku 70/80 heterodimers to broken DNA ends also declines with aging [66]. Notably, mice and cells deleted for either Ku70 or Ku80 exhibited not solely NHEJ disruption but also altered BER [84]. On the other hand, decreased expression of XRCC4, DNA ligase 4, and DNA ligase 3 has been observed, and this implicates that during the aging process, NHEJ becomes more inefficient and inaccurate, leaving more damage sites repaired with a loss of additional genetic information [72]. Interestingly, aging increases DNA-PK activity phosphorylating HSP90α and decreasing its chaperone function in AMPK, which is critical for mitochondrial biogenesis and energy metabolism [85]. Consistently, DNA ligase 4 and Ku80 gene promoters were frequently observed as hypermethylated in elderly people, which could be associated with the silencing expression of both genes [86]. However, as mentioned for other DNA repair mechanisms, caloric restriction diet improves NHEJ activity possibly through SIRT1 and FOXO activity [87].

3. Conclusions

Aging is a consequence of damage accumulation in different cellular constituents and where DNA damage is one of the most important. Every day there are thousands of insults that affect DNA, either due to endogenous factors (such as metabolism) or exogenous factor like contact with radiation sources or exposure to toxic substances; but only a minimal amount (less than 0.02%) accumulates as permanent damage, while the rest is totally repaired. However, if only one gene is not repaired and its function is important as that of a proto-oncogene, a tumor suppressor, or any DNA repair genes, this could lead to accumulation of mutations, and then DNA damage checkpoints can halt the cell cycle and induce cellular senescence or apoptosis, or well erroneous repair or replicative bypass of lesions can result in mutations and chromosomal aberrations leading the cells to transform into cancer cells.

Notably, DNA repair systems are able of dealing with most of the damages inflicted to DNA; however, their efficiency decrease with age, permitting that point mutations, insertions, deletions, and rearrangements, among others, occur more frequently and accumulate over time. This is due in part to the fact that critical proteins involved in DNA repair significantly decrease their expression in an age-related manner. In **Figure 2**, the main age-related changes reported over the different mechanisms of DNA repair together with their consequences that globally cause genomic instability and favor cellular senescence and cancer are summarized.

Overall, this area needs to be more exploited in order to improve our quality of life and prevent or delay the harmful effects of aging. Thus, the more knowledge we acquire about the natural cell aging process and its interrelation with the mechanisms of DNA repair, the closer we will be to develop drugs, therapies, or even vaccines that could help us to prolong our life.

Acknowledgements

FALR is recipient of a doctoral scholarship (application number 2018-000012-01NACF-07226) from the National Council of Science and Technology, CONACyT.

Conflict of interest

The authors declare no conflict of interest.

Author details

Francisco Alejandro Lagunas-Rangel and Rosa María Bermúdez-Cruz*
Department of Genetics and Molecular Biology, Center for Research and Advanced Studies of the National Polytechnic Institute (CINVESTAV), Mexico

*Address all correspondence to: roberm@cinvestav.mx

References

[1] López-Otín C, Blasco MA, Partridge L, Serrano M, Kroemer G. The hallmarks of aging. Cell. 2013 Jun;**153**(6, 6):1194-1217

[2] Lenart P, Krejci L. DNA, the central molecule of aging. Mutation Research: Fundamental and Molecular Mechanisms of Mutagenesis. 2016 Apr;**786**:1-7

[3] Vijg J, Suh Y. Genome instability and aging. Annual Review of Physiology. 2013 Feb;**75**(1):645-668

[4] Vijg J, Dong X, Milholland B, Zhang L. Genome instability: A conserved mechanism of ageing? Essays in Biochemistry. 2017 Jul;**61**(3):305-315

[5] Lombard DB, Chua KF, Mostoslavsky R, Franco S, Gostissa M, Alt FW. DNA repair, genome stability, and aging. Cell. 2005 Feb;**120**(4):497-512

[6] Vermeij WP, Hoeijmakers JH, Pothof J. Aging: Not all DNA damage is equal. Current Opinion in Genetics and Development. 2014 Jun;**26**:124-130

[7] Prasad KN, Wu M, Bondy SC. Telomere shortening during aging: Attenuation by antioxidants and anti-inflammatory agents. Mechanisms of Ageing and Development. 2017 Jun;**164**(April):61-66

[8] Dang W, Steffen KK, Perry R, Dorsey JA, Johnson FB, Shilatifard A, et al. Histone H4 lysine 16 acetylation regulates cellular lifespan. Nature. 2009 Jun;**459**(7248):802-807

[9] Nelson DM, Jaber-Hijazi F, Cole JJ, Robertson NA, Pawlikowski JS, Norris KT, et al. Mapping H4K20me3 onto the chromatin landscape of senescent cells indicates a function in control of cell senescence and tumor suppression through preservation of genetic and epigenetic stability. Genome Biology. 2016 Dec;**17**(1):158

[10] Cruz C, Della Rosa M, Krueger C, Gao Q, Horkai D, King M, et al. Tri-methylation of histone H3 lysine 4 facilitates gene expression in ageing cells. eLife. 2018 Oct;7:1-24

[11] Djeghloul D, Kuranda K, Kuzniak I, Barbieri D, Naguibneva I, Choisy C, et al. Age-associated decrease of the histone methyltransferase SUV39H1 in HSC perturbs heterochromatin and B lymphoid differentiation. Stem Cell Reports. 2016 Jun;**6**(6):970-984

[12] Ma Z, Wang H, Cai Y, Wang H, Niu K, Wu X, et al. Epigenetic drift of H3K27me3 in aging links glycolysis to healthy longevity in Drosophila. eLife. 2018 May;**7**:1-33

[13] Tsurumi A, Li W. Global heterochromatin loss. Epigenetics. 2012 Jul;**7**(7):680-688

[14] Booth LN, Brunet A. The aging epigenome. Molecular Cell. 2016 Jun;**62**(5):728-744

[15] Zane L, Sharma V, Misteli T. Common features of chromatin in aging and cancer: Cause or coincidence? Trends in Cell Biology. 2014 Nov;**24**(11):686-694

[16] Childs BG, Durik M, Baker DJ, van Deursen JM. Cellular senescence in aging and age-related disease: From mechanisms to therapy. Nature Medicine. 2015 Dec;**21**(12): 1424-1435

[17] Chistiakov DA, Sobenin IA, Revin VV, Orekhov AN, Bobryshev YV. Mitochondrial aging and age-related dysfunction of mitochondria. BioMed Research International. 2014;**2014**:1-7

[18] Klaips CL, Jayaraj GG, Hartl FU. Pathways of cellular proteostasis in aging and disease. The Journal of Cell Biology. 2018 Jan;**217**(1):51-63

[19] López-Otín C, Galluzzi L, Freije JMP, Madeo F, Kroemer G. Metabolic control of longevity. Cell. 2016 Aug;**166**(4):802-821

[20] Kosan C, Heidel F, Godmann M, Bierhoff H. Epigenetic erosion in adult stem cells: Drivers and passengers of aging. Cell. 2018 Nov;**7**(12):237

[21] Rebelo-Marques A, De Sousa Lages A, Andrade R, Ribeiro CF, Mota-Pinto A, Carrilho F, et al. Aging hallmarks: The benefits of physical exercise. Front Endocrinol (Lausanne). 2018 May;**9**(May):1-15

[22] Jackson SP, Bartek J. The DNA-damage response in human biology and disease. Nature. 2009 Oct;**461**(7267):1071-1078

[23] Ciccia A, Elledge SJ. The DNA damage response: Making it safe to play with knives. Molecular Cell. 2010 Oct;**40**(2):179-204

[24] Harper JW, Elledge SJ. The DNA damage response: Ten years after. Molecular Cell. 2007 Dec;**28**(5):739-745

[25] Gorbunova V, Seluanov A, Mao Z, Hine C. Changes in DNA repair during aging. Nucleic Acids Research. 2007 Nov;**35**(22):7466-7474

[26] Krokan HE, Bjoras M. Base excision repair. Cold Spring Harbor Perspectives in Biology. 2013 Apr;**5**(4):a012583-a012583

[27] Debrabant B, Soerensen M, Flachsbart F, Dato S, Mengel-From J, Stevnsner T, et al. Human longevity and variation in DNA damage response and repair: Study of the contribution of sub-processes using competitive gene-set analysis. European Journal of Human Genetics. 2014 Sep;**22**(9):1131-1136

[28] Swain U, Rao KS. Age-dependent decline of DNA base excision repair activity in rat cortical neurons. Mechanisms of Ageing and Development. 2012 Apr;**133**(4):186-194

[29] Krishna TH, Mahipal S, Sudhakar A, Sugimoto H, Kalluri R, Rao KS. Reduced DNA gap repair in aging rat neuronal extracts and its restoration by DNA polymerase beta and DNA-ligase. Journal of Neurochemistry. 2005 Feb;**92**(4):818-823

[30] Kisby GE, Kohama SG, Olivas A, Churchwell M, Doerge D, Spangler E, et al. Effect of caloric restriction on base-excision repair (BER) in the aging rat brain. Experimental Gerontology. 2010 Mar;**45**(3):208-216

[31] Li M, Yang X, Lu X, Dai N, Zhang S, Cheng Y, et al. APE1 deficiency promotes cellular senescence and premature aging features. Nucleic Acids Research. 2018 Jun;**46**(11):5664-5677

[32] Cabelof DC, Raffoul JJ, Ge Y, Van Remmen H, Matherly LH, Heydari AR. Age-related loss of the DNA repair response following exposure to oxidative stress. The Journals of Gerontology. Series A, Biological Sciences and Medical Sciences. 2006 May;**61**(5):427-434

[33] Szczesny B, Mitra S. Effect of aging on intracellular distribution of abasic (AP) endonuclease 1 in the mouse liver. Mechanisms of Ageing and Development. 2005 Oct;**126**(10):1071-1078

[34] Pons B, Belmont A-S, Masson-Genteuil G, Chapuis V, Oddos T, Sauvaigo S. Age-associated modifications of base excision repair activities in human skin fibroblast extracts. Mechanisms of Ageing and Development. 2010 Nov;**131**(11-12):661-665

[35] Atamna H, Cheung I, Ames BN. A method for detecting abasic sites in living cells: Age-dependent changes in base excision repair. Proceedings of the

National Academy of Sciences. 2000 Jan;**97**(2):686-691

[36] Grube K, Bürkle A. Poly(ADP-ribose) polymerase activity in mononuclear leukocytes of 13 mammalian species correlates with species-specific life span. Proceedings of the National Academy of Sciences of the United States of America. 1992 Dec;**89**(24):11759-11763

[37] Noren Hooten N, Fitzpatrick M, Kompaniez K, Jacob KD, Moore BR, Nagle J, et al. Coordination of DNA repair by NEIL1 and PARP-1: A possible link to aging. Aging (Albany NY). 2012 Oct;**4**(10):674-685

[38] Xu Z, Zhang L, Zhang W, Meng D, Zhang H, Jiang Y, et al. SIRT6 rescues the age related decline in base excision repair in a PARP1-dependent manner. Cell Cycle. 2015 Jan;**14**(2):269-276

[39] Cabelof D. Caloric restriction promotes genomic stability by induction of base excision repair and reversal of its age-related decline. DNA Repair (Amst). 2003 Mar;**2**(3):295-307

[40] Lu T, Pan Y, Kao S-Y, Li C, Kohane I, Chan J, et al. Gene regulation and DNA damage in the ageing human brain. Nature. 2004 Jun;**429**(6994):883-891

[41] Yakes FM, Van Houten B. Mitochondrial DNA damage is more extensive and persists longer than nuclear DNA damage in human cells following oxidative stress. Proceedings of the National Academy of Sciences. 1997 Jan;**94**(2):514-519

[42] Prakash A, Doublié S. Base excision repair in the mitochondria. Journal of Cellular Biochemistry. 2015 Aug;**116**(8):1490-1499

[43] Sykora P, Kanno S, Akbari M, Kulikowicz T, Baptiste BA, Leandro GS, et al. DNA polymerase beta participates in mitochondrial DNA repair. Molecular and Cellular Biology. 2017 Aug;**37**(16):1-20

[44] Chen D, Cao G, Hastings T, Feng Y, Pei W, O'Horo C, et al. Age-dependent decline of DNA repair activity for oxidative lesions in rat brain mitochondria. Journal of Neurochemistry. 2002 Jun;**81**(6, 6): 1273-1284

[45] de Souza-Pinto N, Hogue B, Bohr V. DNA repair and aging in mouse liver: 8-oxodG glycosylase activity increase in mitochondrial but not in nuclear extracts. Free Radical Biology and Medicine. 2001 Apr;**30**(8):916-923

[46] Szczesny B, Hazra TK, Papaconstantinou J, Mitra S, Boldogh I. Age-dependent deficiency in import of mitochondrial DNA glycosylases required for repair of oxidatively damaged bases. Proceedings of the National Academy of Sciences. 2003 Sep;**100**(19):10670-10675

[47] Schärer OD. Nucleotide excision repair in eukaryotes. Cold Spring Harbor Perspectives in Biology. 2013 Oct;**5**(10):a012609

[48] Meyer JN, Boyd WA, Azzam GA, Haugen AC, Freedman JH, Van Houten B. Decline of nucleotide excision repair capacity in aging *Caenorhabditis elegans*. Genome Biology. 2007;**8**(5):R70

[49] Yamada M, Udono MU, Hori M, Hirose R, Sato S, Mori T, et al. Aged human skin removes UVB-induced pyrimidine dimers from the epidermis more slowly than younger adult skin in vivo. Archives of Dermatological Research. 2006 Jan;**297**(7):294-302

[50] Goukassian D, Gad F, Yaar M, Eller MS, Nehal US, Gilchrest BA. Mechanisms and implications of the age-associated decrease in DNA repair capacity. The FASEB Journal. 2000 Jul;**14**(10):1325-1334

[51] Moriwaki S-I, Ray S, Tarone RE, Kraemer KH, Grossman L. The effect of donor age on the processing of UV-damaged DNA by cultured human cells: Reduced DNA repair capacity and increased DNA mutability. Mutation Research/DNA Repair. 1996 Oct;**364**(2):117-123

[52] Guo ZM, Heydari A, Richardson A. Nucleotide excision repair of actively transcribed versus nontranscribed DNA in rat hepatocytes: Effect of age and dietary restriction. Experimental Cell Research. 1998;**245**(1):228-238

[53] Kruk PA, Rampino NJ, Bohr VA. DNA damage and repair in telomeres: Relation to aging. Proceedings of the National Academy of Sciences. 1995 Jan;**92**(1):258-262

[54] Deng XD, Gao Q, Zhang W, Zhang B, Ma Y, Zhang LX, et al. The age-related expression decline of ERCC1 and XPF for forensic age estimation: A preliminary study. Journal of Forensic and Legal Medicine. 2017 Jul;**49**:15-19

[55] Loesch MM, Collier AE, Southern DH, Ward RE, Tholpady SS, Lewis DA, et al. Insulin-like growth factor-1 receptor regulates repair of ultraviolet B-induced DNA damage in human keratinocytes in vivo. Molecular Oncology. 2016 Oct;**10**(8):1245-1254

[56] Liu D, Keijzers G, Rasmussen LJ. DNA mismatch repair and its many roles in eukaryotic cells. Mutation Research/Reviews in Mutation. 2017 Jul;**773**:174-187

[57] Li GM. Mechanisms and functions of DNA mismatch repair. Cell Research. 2008 Jan;**18**(1):85-98

[58] Coolbaugh-Murphy MI, Xu J, Ramagli LS, Brown BW, Siciliano MJ. Microsatellite instability (MSI) increases with age in normal somatic cells. Mechanisms of Ageing and Development. 2005 Oct;**126**(10):1051-1059

[59] Annett K, Duggan O, Freeburn R, Hyland P, Pawelec G, Barnett Y. An investigation of DNA mismatch repair capacity under normal culture conditions and under conditions of supra-physiological challenge in human CD4+T cell clones from donors of different ages. Experimental Gerontology. 2005 Dec;**40**(12):976-981

[60] Yehuda AB, Globerson A, Krichevsky S, Bar On H, Kidron M, Friedlander Y, et al. Ageing and the mismatch repair system. Mechanisms of Ageing and Development. 2001 Jan;**121**(1-3):173-179

[61] Neri S, Gardini A, Facchini A, Olivieri F, Franceschi C, Ravaglia G, et al. Mismatch repair system and aging: Microsatellite instability in peripheral blood cells from differently aged participants. The Journals of Gerontology. Series A, Biological Sciences and Medical Sciences. 2005 Mar;**60**(3):285-292

[62] Nakagawa H, Nuovo GJ, Zervos EE, Martin EW, Salovaara R, Aaltonen LA, et al. Age-related hypermethylation of the 5′ region of MLH1 in normal colonic mucosa is associated with microsatellite-unstable colorectal cancer development. Cancer Research. 2001 Oct;**61**(19):6991-6995

[63] Kenyon J, Fu P, Lingas K, Thomas E, Saurastri A, Santos Guasch G, et al. Humans accumulate microsatellite instability with acquired loss of MLH1 protein in hematopoietic stem and progenitor cells as a function of age. Blood. 2012 Oct;**120**(16):3229-3236

[64] Conde-Pérezprina JC, Luna-López A, López-Diazguerrero NE, Damián-Matsumura P, Zentella A, Königsberg M. Msh2 promoter region hypermethylation as a marker of aging-related deterioration in old retired female breeder mice. Biogerontology. 2008 Oct;**9**(5):325-334

[65] Savio AJ, Lemire M, Mrkonjic M, Gallinger S, Zanke BW, Hudson TJ, et al. MLH1 region polymorphisms show a significant association with CpG Island shore methylation in a large cohort of healthy individuals. PLoS One. 2012 Dec;**7**(12):e51531

[66] Frasca D, Barattini P, Tirindelli D, Guidi L, Bartoloni C, Errani A, et al. Effect of age on DNA binding of the ku protein in irradiated human peripheral blood mononuclear cells (PBMC). Experimental Gerontology. 1999 Aug;**34**(5):645-658

[67] White RR, Vijg J. Do DNA double-strand breaks drive aging? Molecular Cell. 2016 Sep;**63**(5):729-738

[68] Zhao X, Wei C, Li J, Xing P, Li J, Zheng S, et al. Cell cycle-dependent control of homologous recombination. Acta Biochimica et Biophysica Sinica (Shanghai). 2017 Aug;**49**(8):655-668

[69] Sung P, Klein H. Mechanism of homologous recombination: Mediators and helicases take on regulatory functions. Nature Reviews. Molecular Cell Biology. 2006 Oct;**7**(10):739-750

[70] Mao Z, Tian X, Van Meter M, Ke Z, Gorbunova V, Seluanov A. Sirtuin 6 (SIRT6) rescues the decline of homologous recombination repair during replicative senescence. Proceedings of the National Academy of Sciences. 2012 Jul;**109**(29):11800-11805

[71] Titus S, Li F, Stobezki R, Akula K, Unsal E, Jeong K, et al. Impairment of BRCA1-related DNA double-strand break repair leads to ovarian aging in mice and humans. Science Translational Medicine. 2013 Feb;**5**(172):172ra21, 172ra21

[72] Li Z, Zhang W, Chen Y, Guo W, Zhang J, Tang H, et al. Impaired DNA double-strand break repair contributes to the age-associated rise of genomic instability in humans. Cell Death and Differentiation. 2016 Nov;**23**(11):1765-1777

[73] Feng Z, Hu W, Teresky AK, Hernando E, Cordon-Cardo C, Levine AJ. Declining p53 function in the aging process: A possible mechanism for the increased tumor incidence in older populations. Proceedings of the National Academy of Sciences. 2007 Oct;**104**(42):16633-16638

[74] Li J, Bonkowski MS, Moniot S, Zhang D, Hubbard BP, Ling AJY, et al. A conserved NAD + binding pocket that regulates protein-protein interactions during aging. Science. 2017 Mar;**355**(6331):1312-1317

[75] Mendelsohn AR, Larrick JW. The NAD+/PARP1/SIRT1 axis in aging. Rejuvenation Research. 2017 Jun;**20**(3):244-247

[76] Guirouilh-Barbat J, Lambert S, Bertrand P, Lopez BS. Is homologous recombination really an error-free process? Frontiers in Genetics. 2014 Jun;**5**(Jun):1-15

[77] Sukup-Jackson MR, Kiraly O, Kay JE, Na L, Rowland EA, Winther KE, et al. Rosa26-GFP direct repeat (RaDR-GFP) mice reveal tissue- and age-dependence of homologous recombination in mammals in vivo. PLoS Genetics. 2014 Jun;**10**(6):e1004299

[78] Rulten SL, Grundy GJ. Non-homologous end joining: Common interaction sites and exchange of multiple factors in the DNA repair process. BioEssays. 2017 Mar;**39**(3):1600209

[79] Rodgers K, McVey M. Error-prone repair of DNA double-strand breaks. Journal of Cellular Physiology. 2016 Jan;**231**(1):15-24

[80] Seluanov A, Mittelman D, Pereira-Smith OM, Wilson JH, Gorbunova V. DNA end joining becomes less efficient

and more error-prone during cellular senescence. Proceedings of the National Academy of Sciences. 2004 May;**101**(20):7624-7629

[81] Vaidya A, Mao Z, Tian X, Spencer B, Seluanov A, Gorbunova V. Knock-in reporter mice demonstrate that DNA repair by non-homologous end joining declines with age. PLoS Genetics. 2014 Jul;**10**(7):e1004511

[82] Puthiyaveetil AG, Caudell DL. Non homologous end joining-mediated DNA break repair is impaired in B lymphocytes of aging mice. Molecular Immunology. 2013 Jan;**53**(1-2):79-87

[83] Seluanov A, Danek J, Hause N, Gorbunova V. Changes in the level and distribution of Ku proteins during cellular senescence. DNA Repair (Amst). 2007 Dec;**6**(12):1740-1748

[84] Choi YJ, Li H, Son MY, Wang X, Fornsaglio JL, Sobol RW, et al. Deletion of individual Ku subunits in mice causes an NHEJ-independent phenotype potentially by altering apurinic/apyrimidinic site repair. PLoS One. 2014 Jan;**9**(1):e86358

[85] Park S, Gavrilova O, Brown AL, Soto JE, Bremner S, Kim J, et al. DNA-PK promotes the mitochondrial, metabolic, and physical decline that occurs during aging. Cell Metabolism. 2017 May;**25**(5):1135-1146.e7

[86] Martín-Guerrero I, de Prado E, Lopez-Lopez E, Ardanaz M, Vitoria JC, Parada LA, et al. Methylation of the nonhomologous end joining repair pathway genes does not explain the increase of translocations with aging. Age (Omaha). 2014 Dec;**36**(6):9730

[87] Lee JE, Heo JI, Park SH, Kim JH, Kho YJ, Kang HJ, et al. Calorie restriction (CR) reduces age-dependent decline of non-homologous end joining (NHEJ) activity in rat tissues. Experimental Gerontology. 2011 Nov;**46**(11):891-896

Chapter 9

Hepatocarcinoma Angiogenesis and DNA Damage Repair Response: An Update

Xi-Dai Long, Zhou-Ximao Long, Xiao-Ying Huang, Jin-Guang Yao, Qiang Xia and Yan Deng

Abstract

Hepatocarcinoma is one of the most common lethal human malignant tumors, mainly because of active angiogenesis. This kind of high angiogenesis often accounts for early metastasis, rapid recurrence, and poor survival. Growing evidence has proved that hepatocarcinoma angiogenesis is closely associated with multiple risk factors, such as DNA damages resulting from hepatitis B and C virus infection, aflatoxin B1 exposure, ethanol intake, and obesity. Genetic alterations and genomic instability, probably resulting from low DNA damage repair response (DRR) and the following unrepaired DNA lesions, are also increasingly recognized as important risk factors of hepatocarcinoma angiogenesis. Dysregulation of DRRs and signaling to cell cycle checkpoints involving in DRR pathways may accelerate the accumulation of DNA damages and trigger the dysregulation of angiogenesis-related genes and the progression of hepatocarcinoma. In this review, we discussed DNA damages/DRRs and angiogenesis during hepatocarcinogenesis and their interactive regulations. Hopefully, the review will also remind the medical researchers and clinic doctors of further understanding and validating the values of DNA damages/DRRs in hepatocarcinoma angiogenesis.

Keywords: hepatocarcinoma, angiogenesis, DNA damage, DNA damage repair response

1. Introduction

Hepatocellular carcinoma, also termed as hepatocarcinoma, is one of the most common malignant tumors, with more than 500,000 new cases per year [1]. Until recently, it has been frequent to consider hepatocarcinoma as a tumor with low incidence in the western world but with high incidence in the eastern countries [1]. However, increasing data exhibit that the incidence of this tumor has increased in both western and eastern countries. Etiologically, several risk factors, including hepatitis B virus (HBV), hepatitis C virus (HCV), aflatoxin B1 (AFB1), and alcohol, have been identified for increasing disease incidence worldwide [2]. Although molecular mechanisms of hepatocarcinoma caused by these risk factors have not still been clear, chronic and permanent liver damage and damage response may play a vital role. Macrocosmically, liver damage consists of a series of pathological changes, such as chronic hepatitis, liver cirrhosis, nodular hyperplasia, and

IntechOpen

dysplasia [3]. Microcosmically, chronic DNA damage, including the formation of DNA adducts, DNA strand break and bulk, gene mutations, and genomic instability, is the most important type [4].

Because of early blood metastasis and high death rate of this malignancy, it has become the third most common cause of cancer-associated deaths worldwide. This death risk could be explained by high angiogenesis capacities of hepatocarcinoma [1, 2]. Increasing evidence has exhibited that hepatocarcinoma patients with high microvessel density (MVD) in tumor tissues would feature a poor prognosis, and angiogenesis has been regarded as an important marker predicting the risk of invasiveness and metastasis [5]. This chapter summarizes the latest findings in hepatocarcinoma angiogenesis, DNA damage, and damage repair response (DRR). We also try to shed light on the effects of DNA damage and dysregulation of DRR on tumor angiogenesis.

2. Angiogenesis and regulation in hepatocarcinoma

2.1 Angiogenesis process in hepatocarcinoma

Several previous reviews have summarized the angiogenesis in hepatocarcinoma [5–7]. In brief, angiogenesis is a kind of crucial biological function and survival potential for normal organism development, growth, and adaptation to new environment. The dynamic balance between increasing and decreasing potential of angiogenesis is essential in the different physiological and pathological conditions, such as injury cure, damage repair, inflammatory procession, tumor progression, blindness, and ischemia. Hepatocarcinoma angiogenesis was extensively studied via cell models, experimental animal models, and human tumor samples [5–7]. Accumulating data have proved that local hypoxia in tumor tissues and the change in genome resulting from genetic or environmental risk factors will lead to the secretion and synthetics of angiogenetic regulative factors and triggering angiogenesis [8–10]. In hepatocarcinoma tissues, the process of angiogenesis consists of the following several stages: sprouting, extracellular matrix component (ECMs) reconstruction, endothelial cell (EC) migration and proliferation, lumen formation, and stabilization of newborn vessels (**Figure 1**) [11].

The establishment of conditions allowing ECs proliferation and migration, which often results from local hypoxia, first facilitates endothelial sprouting and budding. During this stage, hypoxia induces the secretion and synthetics of angiogenetic factors, such as nitric oxide (NO), vascular endothelial growth factor (VEGF), CD31, angiopoietin-1, and so on [11]. The NO-induced vasodilation and VEGF-caused high permeability result in the extravasation of plasma components (including fibrinogen and fibrin). Together with ECMs, these plasma components lay down and form provisional scaffolds for migrating ECs. The basement membranes and ECMs (mainly consisting of collagen I and IV and laminin) are next degraded, and subsequently, ECs migrate into local sites and proliferate. Increasing proliferation of ECs in the local hypoxia tissues leads to the formation of nascent vessels with lumen. After that, nascent vessels are recruited and structurally stabilized under the conditions of physical forces and a series of molecules such as platelet-derived growth factor β (PDFG-β), angiopoietin-1, angiopoietin-2, VEGF, and transforming growth factor β1 (TGF-β1) [7, 11, 12].

Vessels in hepatocarcinoma differ from other liver diseases or normal vessels [5, 11, 13]. First, tumor vessels typically appear as irregular diameter and abnormal branching patterns [5]. Second, pericytes of vessels are often incompletely covered or lost; furthermore, their basement membranes are also incomplete [11]. Third, tumor vessels sometimes form irregular channels and the walls of these channels are

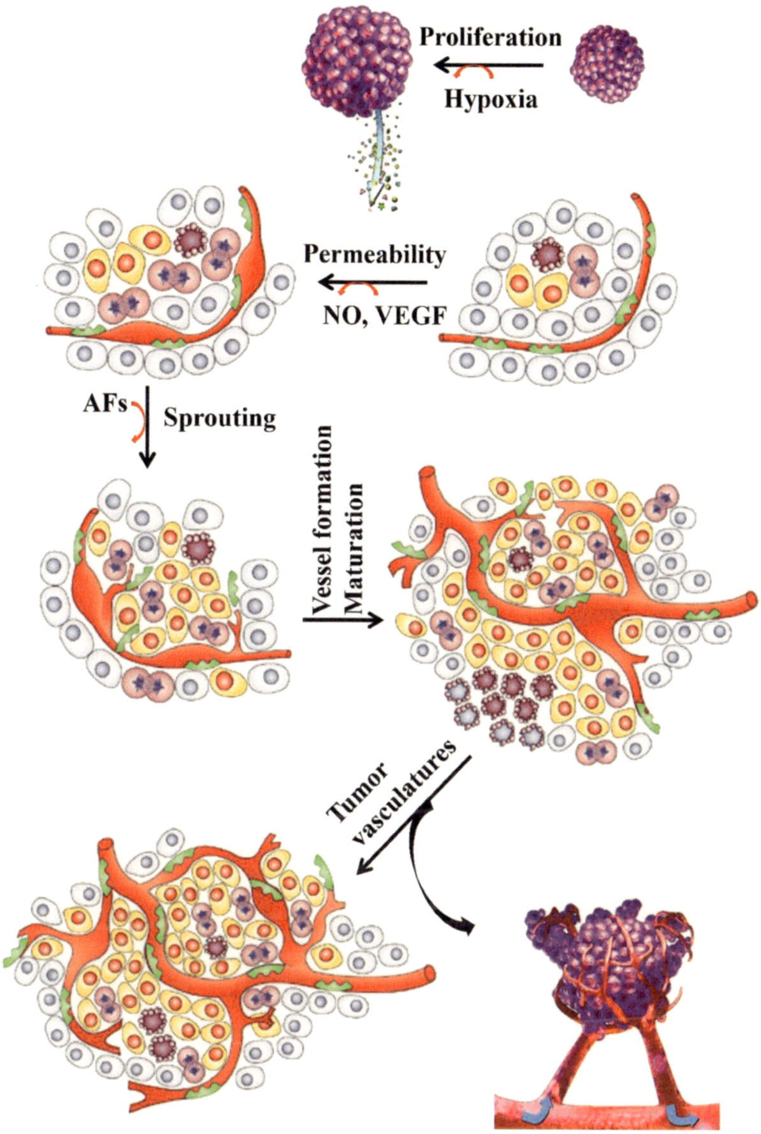

Figure 1.
Angiogenesis procession in hepatocarcinoma. The procession of angiogenesis consists of: (1) sprouting and budding; (2) ECM remodeling; (3) EC proliferation and migration; (4) lumen formation and three-D organization; and (5) stabilization of nascent vessels.

comprised of cancer cells. Moreover, the endothelial cells may be replaced by cancer cells partially or completely. Finally, angiogenesis in hepatocarcinoma not only appears abnormal architecture but also accompanies abnormal molecular expression and regulation [6, 14]. These characteristics result in abnormal structures and function for hepatocarcinoma; however, they can provide some important cues for early diagnosis and therapeutic strategies for cases with hepatocarcinoma.

2.2 Angiogenesis regulation in hepatocarcinoma

A series of angiogenic and antiangiogenic factors (**Tables 1** and **2**) regulate the angiogenesis process in hepatocarcinoma [5]. During the process of hepatocarcinoma angiogenesis, hypoxia and VEGF family play a vital role. Hypoxia in local

No.	Active factors	Effects	Process involved in hepatocarcinoma
AF01	NO	Stimulating vasodilation	Increasing vessel permeably
AF02	VEGF family members	(1) Increasing vascular permeability (2) inducing EC proliferation (3) Progressing leukocyte adhesion (4) Regulating neovascular lumen diameter	(1) Sprouting and budding (2) Vessel growth 3-D organization
AF03	VEGF-R	Integrate angiogenic and survival signals	Vessel growth
AF04	NRP-1	Integrate angiogenic and survival signals	Vessel growth
	Angiopoietins	Inducing EC proliferation	Vessel growth
	IL-4	Inducing EC proliferation	Vessel growth
	IL-8	Inducing EC proliferation	Vessel growth
	Hepatocyte growth factor	Inducing EC proliferation	Vessel growth
	Tissue factor	Inducing EC proliferation	Vessel growth
	Fibronectin	Progressing ECM remodeling	
AF05	Integrins avb3	(1) ECM receptors, intercellular communication (2) Mobilized during EC migration (3) Regulating neovascular lumen diameter	ECM remodeling and EC migration Newborn vessel stabilization
AF06	Integrins avb5	(1) ECM receptors, intercellular communication (2) Mobilized during EC migration (3) Regulating neovascular lumen diameter	ECM remodeling and EC migration Newborn vessel stabilization
AF07	Integrins a6b1	(1) ECM receptors, intercellular communication (2) Mobilized during EC migration (3) Regulating neovascular lumen diameter	ECM remodeling and EC migration Newborn vessel stabilization
AF08	uPA	(1) Remodeling ECM (2) Releasing and activating growth factors	ECM remodeling and EC migration Newborn vessel stabilization
AF09	Plasminogen activators	(1) Remodeling ECM (2) Releasing and activating growth factors	ECM remodeling and EC migration Newborn vessel stabilization
AF10	MMPs	(1) Remodeling ECM (2) Releasing and activating growth factors	ECM remodeling and EC migration Newborn vessel stabilization
AF11	Heparinases	(1) Remodeling ECM (2) Releasing and activating growth factors	ECM remodeling and EC migration Newborn vessel stabilization
AF12	chymases	(1) Remodeling ECM (2) Releasing and activating growth factors	ECM remodeling and EC migration Newborn vessel stabilization
AF13	Tryptases	(1) Remodeling ECM (2) Releasing and activating growth factors	ECM remodeling and EC migration Newborn vessel stabilization
AF14	Cathepsins	(1) Remodeling ECM (2) Releasing and activating growth factors	ECM remodeling and EC migration Newborn vessel stabilization

No.	Active factors	Effects	Process involved in hepatocarcinoma
AF15	PlGF	Inducing EC proliferation	Vessel growth
AF16	aFGF	Inducing EC proliferation	Vessel growth
AF17	bFGF	Inducing EC proliferation	Vessel growth
	FGF-R1	Receptor for aFGF	Vessel growth
	FGF-R2	Receptor for bFGF	Vessel growth
AF18	HGF	Inducing EC proliferation	Vessel growth
	c-Met	Receptor for HGF	Vessel growth
AF19	TGF-a	Inducing EC proliferation	Vessel growth
AF20	TGF-b	Inducing EC proliferation	Vessel growth
	EGF-R	Receptor for TGF-a and TGF-b	Vessel growth
AF21	MCP-1 and other chemokines	Pleiotropic role in angiogenesis	Newborn vessel stabilization
AF22	MEF2C	Regulating neovascular lumen diameter	Newborn vessel stabilization
AF23	Ephrin's	Determining branching and arterial/ venous specification	Newborn vessel stabilization
AF24	PDGF-B and receptors	Recruiting pericytes	Newborn vessel stabilization
AF25	Ang-1	(1) Stabilizing intercellular contacts (2) Inhibiting permeability	Newborn vessel stabilization
AF26	Ang-2	Ang-1 antagonist (destabilizes vessels; causes EC death)	Vessel regression
AF27	Tie-2	Receptor for Ang-1 and Ang-2	Newborn vessel stabilization
AF28	TGF- 1	(1) Promoting vessel maturation (2) stimulating ECM generation (3) Inducing differentiation of mesenchymal cells to pericytes	ECM remodeling and EC migration
AF29	Endoglin	(1) Promoting vessel maturation (2) stimulating ECM generation (3) Inducing differentiation of mesenchymal cells to pericytes	ECM remodeling and EC migration
AF30	Cyr61	(1) Stimulating directed migration of EC through an AVB integrin-dependent pathway (2) Acting as ECM modifiers (3) Promoting EC survival	ECM remodeling and EC migration
AF31	Fisp12	(1) Stimulating directed migration of EC through an AVB integrin-dependent pathway (2) Acting as ECM modifiers (3) Promoting EC survival	ECM remodeling and EC migration

Abbreviations: *VEGF, vascular endothelial growth factor; ECM, extracellular matrix component; EC, endothelial cell; PEDF, Pigment epithelium-derived factor; platelet and endothelial cell adhesion molecule 1; TIMPs, Tissue inhibitor of metalloproteases; IFN, interferon; MMPs, matrix metalloproteinases; Ang, angiopoietin; IL, interleukin; PIGF, placenta growth factor; HGF, hepatocyte growth factor; TGF, transforming growth factor; EGF, epidermal growth factor.*

Table 1.
Angiogenesis active regulative factors in hepatocarcinoma.

No.	Active factors	Effects	Process involved in hepatocarcinoma
IF01	Arrestin	Suppressing VEGF-regulating vessel growth	Vessel growth
IF02	Canstatin	(1) Interruption of stable cell-ECM connections (2) Inducing EC apoptosis	Vessel regression
IF03	Interleukin 12	Suppressing EC cell proliferation	Vessel growth
IF04	PEDF	Suppressing EC cell proliferation	Vessel growth
IF05	VE-cadherin	(1) Adhering junction molecules (2) Intercellular adhesion (3) Providing vessel tightness	Newborn vessel stabilization
IF06	PECAM-1	(1) Adhering junction molecules (2) Intercellular adhesion (3) Providing vessel tightness	Newborn vessel stabilization
IF07	Plakoglobin	(1) Adhering junction molecules (2) Intercellular adhesion (3) Providing vessel tightness	Newborn vessel stabilization
IF08	b-Catenin	(1) Adhering junction molecules (2) Intercellular adhesion (3) Providing vessel tightness	Newborn vessel stabilization
IF09	Claudins	(1) Tightening junction molecules (2) Intercellular adhesion (3) Providing vessel tightness	Newborn vessel stabilization
IF10	Occludin	(1) Tightening junction molecules (2) Intercellular adhesion (3) Providing vessel tightness	Newborn vessel stabilization
IF11	JAM-1	(1) Tightening junction molecules (2) Intercellular adhesion (3) Providing vessel tightness	Newborn vessel stabilization
IF12	JAM-2	(1) Tightening junction molecules (2) Intercellular adhesion (3) Providing vessel tightness	Newborn vessel stabilization
IF13	JAM-3	(1) Tightening junction molecules (2) Intercellular adhesion (3) Providing vessel tightness	Newborn vessel stabilization
IF14	Connexins	(1) Gap junction molecules (2) Facilitating intercellular communication	Newborn vessel stabilization
IF15	Integrins avb3	Suppressing VEGF- and Flk-1-mediated EC survival	Vessel growth
IF16	Integrins avb5	Suppressing VEGF- and Flk-1-mediated EC survival	Vessel growth
IF17	PAI-1	(1) Inhibiting ECM degradation by MMPs (2) Inhibiting EC proliferation	ECM remodeling and EC migration
IF18	TIMPs	(1) Inhibiting ECM degradation by MMPs (2) Inhibiting EC proliferation	ECM remodeling and EC migration
IF19	Angiostatin and related plasminogen fragments	Suppressing tumor angiogenesis	Vessel growth
IF20	Endostatin	Suppressing EC cell proliferation	Vessel growth

No.	Active factors	Effects	Process involved in hepatocarcinoma
IF21	Antithrombin III	Suppressing EC cell proliferation	Vessel growth
IF22	IFN-a	Suppressing EC cell proliferation	Vessel growth
IF23	IFN-b	Suppressing EC cell proliferation	Vessel growth
IF24	LIF	Suppressing EC cell proliferation	Vessel growth
IF25	PF4	Suppressing EC cell proliferation	Vessel growth
IF26	TSP-1	Inhibiting lumen formation	Vessel regression
IF27	Ang-1 (excess)	Making vessels too tight and inhibiting sprouting	Newborn vessel stabilization
IF28	Ang-2	Facilitating sprouting in the presence of VEGF	Vessel regression
IF29	sTie-2	Inhibitor for Ang-1 and Ang-2	Vessel regression
IF30	sFlt-1	Inhibitor for VEGF family	(1) Sprouting and budding (2) Vessel growth 3-D organization
IF31	Thrombospondin-1	Suppressing EC cell proliferation	Vessel growth
IF32	Thrombospondin-2	Suppressing EC cell proliferation	Vessel growth
IF33	Tumstatin	Suppressing EC cell proliferation	Vessel growth
IF34	Vasostatin	Suppressing EC cell proliferation	Vessel growth

Abbreviations: *VEGF, vascular endothelial growth factor; ECM, extracellular matrix component; EC, endothelial cell; PEDF, Pigment epithelium-derived factor; platelet and endothelial cell adhesion molecule 1; TIMPs, Tissue inhibitor of metalloproteases; IFN, interferon; MMPs, matrix metalloproteinases; Ang, angiopoietin.*

Table 2.
Angiogenesis inhibitive regulative factors in hepatocarcinoma.

tumor tissues, an important pathophysiological phenomenon caused by rapid growth of tumor, leads to the expression of hypoxia-inducible factor (HIF)-1α, which is a key inducible factor for angiogenesis in hypoxia tissues [7, 14]. On the one hand, HIF-1α can induce the expression of hypoxia-response-related genes like NO, VEGF, transforming growth factor (TGF) α and β, adrenomedullin (ADM), LDL-receptor-related protein 1 (LRP1), and leptin; on the other hand, local hypoxia status in tumor tissues also downregulates the expression of antiangiogenic factors such as thrombospondin-1 (TS1) and -2 (TS2) [15–17]. Additionally, growing literature has shown that lots of factors, including genetic or acquired alterations in the oncogenes (i.e., Ras, c-Jun, and Myc) and tumor suppressor genes (i.e., TP53), Hepatitis B Virus X (HBx) protein, chromobox 4, and DNA damage induced by chronic inflammation and AFB1 exposure, can increase the expression proangiogenic factors [18–23]. For example, HBx protein has a potential for increasing HIF-1α expression via promoting transcriptional and translational activity and therefore accelerating angiogenesis during carcinogenesis process of hepatocarcinoma [24]. Recent studies have reported that chromobox 4 (a known transcriptional regulator and also a SUMO E3 enzyme) can promote angiogenesis via stabilizing HIF-1 in hepatocarcinoma [18, 19]. VEGF (including its glycoprotein family members VEGF-A, -B, -C, and -D) is another important angiogenic factor that always upregulates in most cases with hepatocarcinoma [5]. The upregulation of VEGF in hepatocarcinoma is proved not only to increase tumor neovascularization but also to accelerate tumor growth via in vitro cell experiments and animal models. The role of VEGF is mediated mainly by two receptors: VEGF-R1 (also called Flt-1) and VEGF-R2 (also termed as KDR/Flk-1). Both VEGF-R1 and VEGF-R2 have tyrosine kinase activity and are normally expressed in hepatic parenchyma cells including endothelial cells of portal and sinusoidal tracts [5, 6]. In hepatocarcinoma, both mRNA and protein amount of them are increasing noticeably in the tumor tissues compared to peri-tumor tissues [25]. Some other factors, such as angiopoietin 1 and 2, involve in the regulation of angiogenesis in hepatocarcinoma (**Tables 1** and **2**) [5, 6, 13]. Together, increasing angiogenic potential but decreasing antiangiogenic potential facilitates hepatocarcinoma angiogenesis.

2.3 Angiogenesis biomarkers in hepatocarcinoma

In the past decades, several biomarkers, such as VEGF, angiogenin, and MVD, have been selected for elucidating angiogenic potential of hepatocarcinoma. **Table 3** summarized the potential of these biomarkers for hepatocarcinoma angiogenesis and angiogenesis-related tumor biological actions. Among these biomarkers, VEGF is concerned especially because of its clinic significance. For example, a hospital-based clinic samples analyses (including 7 cases with liver low-grade dysplastic nodule [DN], 8 cases with liver high-grade DN, 11 cases with early hepatocarcinoma, 17 cases with small hepatocarcinoma, and 21 cases with advanced hepatocarcinoma) by Park et al. [26] showed that the amount of VEGF increased gradually from low-grade DN to early hepatocarcinoma. Furthermore, this increasing expression of VEGF is significantly associated with neoangiogenesis (marked by MVD with CD34 staining) and cancer cell proliferation. Collectively, we can conclude that increasing VEGF expression and MVD are positively associated with tumor vascularization and the following tumor progression and poor survival of tumor cases. Furthermore, increasing evidence has exhibited that serum levels of VEGF are not only parallel with the amount in tumor tissues but also can predict therapy response of patients with hepatocarcinoma [29–32]. Thus, VEGF may be useful for improving therapeutic strategies of hepatocarcinoma based on the angiogenesis thesis.

No.	Study design	Samples	Results	Ref#
1	Hospital-based sample study	LGDs (n = 7), HGDs (n = 8), eHCCs (n = 11), shocks (n = 17), and aHCCs (n = 21)	(1) VEGF expression increases gradually from LGD to eHCC. (2) The sHCCs has an increasing neoangiogenesis and cell proliferation compared to aHCCs. (3) The levels of VEGF expression are positively associated with MVD (marked by CD34 staining).	[26]
2	Hospital-based sample study	HCCs (n = 60)	Amount of VEGF in the serum of patients positively correlates with that in the tumor tissues.	[27]
3	Hospital-based sample study	HCs (n = 20), CHs (n = 36), LCs (n = 77), and HCCs (n = 86)	Plasm VEGF levels are increasing in patients with HCC compared to in non-HCCs and this increase will more noticeable in cases with metastasis HCCs.	[28]
4	Hospital-based sample study	HCs (n = 30), LCs (n = 26), and HCCs (n = 52)	Plasm VEGF levels are increasing in patients with HCC compared to in non-HCCs and this increase will shorten the survival of HCCs.	[29]
5	Prospective study	HCCs (n = 100)	Plasm VEGF levels of HCC cases are related to tumor stage, postoperation recurrence, and blood invasion.	[30]

No.	Study design	Samples	Results	Ref#
6	Hospital-based sample study	HC (n = 15) and HCCs (n = 98)	Serum VEGF is a significant biomarker for HCC survival (including OS and RFS).	[31]
7	Prospective study	HCCs (n = 80)	Serum VEGF levels were correlated with clinical data, tumor response to TACE and survival results.	[32]
8	Hospital-based sample study	HCCs (n = 48)	TACE treatment can upregulate expression and bFGF in HCC tissues possibly due to hypoxia and ischemia.	[33]
9	Hospital-based sample study	HCCs (n = 38)	TACE treatment can upregulate expression and bFGF in HCC tissues possibly due to hypoxia and ischemia.	[34]
10	Hospital-based sample study	HCCs (n = 41)	Angiogenin mRNA in serum and tumor tissues positively associating with MVD and poor prognosis of cases	[35]
11	Hospital-based sample study	HCCs (n = 90)	MMP-2, MMP-9 and VEGF expression is positively correlated to the prognosis of HCC patients.	[36]
12	Hospital-based sample study	HCCs (n = 30)	The serum levels of Ang-2, HGF, IL-8, PDGF-BB, and VEGF were correlated with poor effects of sorafenib treatment in patients with HCC.	[37]
13	Hospital-based sample study	CHs (n = 79) and HCCs (n = 89)	(1) TEMs are involved in HCC angiogenesis. (2) The frequency of circulating TEMs was significantly higher in HCC than non-HCC patients. (3) The TEMs have higher diagnostic value for HCC than AFP, PIVKA-II and ANG-2.	[38]
14	Animal model	/	Mobilized EPCs participate in tumor angiogenesis of HCC	[39]

Abbreviations: *LGDs, patients with low-grade dysplasia; HGD, patients with high-grade dysplasia; eHCCs, patients with early hepatocellular carcinoma; HCC, hepatocellular carcinoma; sHCCs, patients with small HCC; aHCCs, patients with advanced HCC; HCCs, patients with HCC; HCs, healthy controls; LCs, patients with liver cirrhosis; VEGF, vascular endothelial growth factor; MVD, microvessel density; OS, overall survival; RFS, tumor reoccurrence-free survival; TACE, transarterial chemoembolization; bFGF, basic fibroblast growth factor; EPCs, bone marrow-derived endothelial progenitor cells; TEMs, TIE2-expressing monocytes/macrophages; Ang-2, angiopoietin-2; G-CSF, granulocyte colony-stimulating factor; HGF, hepatocyte growth factor; IL-8, interleukin-8.*

Table 3.
The potential of biomarkers for hepatocarcinoma angiogenesis and angiogenesis-related tumor biological actions.

3. DNA damage and DRR in hepatocarcinoma

3.1 DNA damage induced by risk factors for hepatocarcinoma

Multiple risk factors, including HBV and HCV infection, AFB1 exposure, ethanol consumption, and obesity, have been reported to correlate with hepatocarcinogenesis (**Figure 2**) [4]. These risk factors can induce multiple types of DNA damage, such as DNA single-stand break (SSB), double-strand break (DSB), base damage, DNA-adduct formation, oxidation damage, gene mutation, chromosomal aberration, and genomic instability [4]. Results from epidemiological and experimental studies show that viral-DNA damage relationship is characterized by:

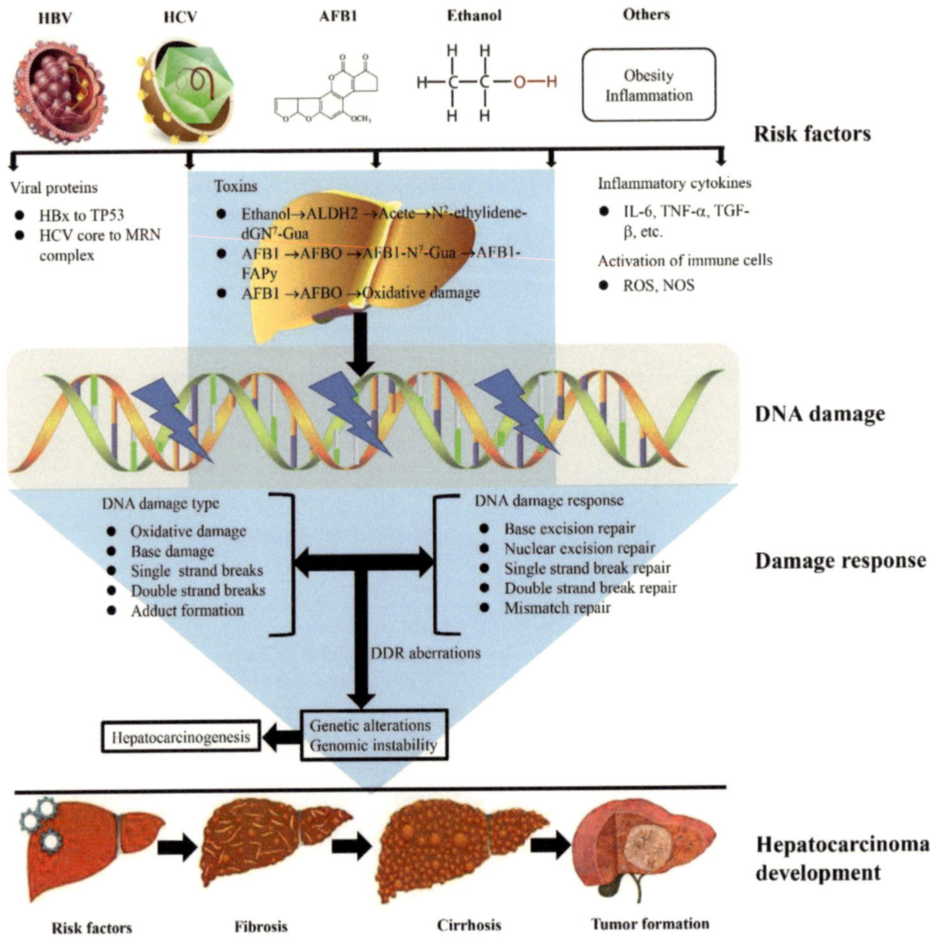

Figure 2.
Risk factors-induced DNA damage and damage repair response during hepatocarcinoma. **Abbreviations***: HBV, hepatitis B virus; HCV, hepatitis C virus; AFB1, aflatoxin B1; AFBO, AFB1-8,9-epoxide; IL, interleukin; TGF, transforming growth factor.*

(1) the integration of viral gene (such as HBx gene) into the genome of liver cells and resulting genomic instability of host cells [21, 24, 40, 41]; (2) TP53 mutation conducted by HBx integration resulting in abnormal cell response, including DNA repair, cell proliferation and cycle, and apoptosis potential [22]; (3) HCV core interfering the formation of Mre11/Rad50/Nbs1 (MRN) complex through the bind with Nbs1 [5]; (4) the inhibition of such DNA repair proteins as Ataxia telangiectasia mutated kinase (ATM) [42, 43]; and (5) inducing dysregulation of signal pathways, including Wnt/β-catenin pathway, sex steroid pathway, p38MAPK pathway, PI3K/Akt pathway, transforming growth factor β (TGFβ) pathway, NF-κB pathway, and so on [11].

For AFB1-induced DNA damage, adducts formation and gene mutations are concerned especially [44]. AFB1 is a known I-type chemical hepatocarcinogen produced mainly by *A. parasiticus* and *A. flavus* and a suspected risk factor for hepatocarcinoma in some dependent areas such as Sub-Saharan area, the southeast region of Asia, and the coast of southeast China. Results from prospective epidemiological and animal studies have exhibited that AFB1-induced DNA damage plays a vital role in the process of hepatocarcinoma caused by AFB1 exposure [40, 45]. Studies of AFB1 metabolism have further proved that cytochrome P450 (CYP) enzymes in hepatocytes can facilitate AFB1 into its epoxy compound, also termed as AFB1-8,9-epoxide (AFBe). AFBe can covalently bind to genomic DNA and ultimately induce multiple types of DNA damage [46, 47]. Increasing evidence exhibits that AFB1 can multiplicatively interact with HBV and/or HCV infection during hepatocarcinogenesis, and that, this multiplicative interaction may be associated with more noticeable DNA damage induced by both AFB1 exposure and HBV/HCV infection [23]. Epidemiological studies based on the case-control design with a large sample have proved that patients with chronic virus hepatitis (including B and C type) will feature increasing hepatocarcinoma risk under the conditions of high AFB1 exposure [46]. Furthermore, patients with high AFB1 often companies with chronic virus infection and faces higher frequency of gene mutation like TP53 and ras [47]. Interestingly, the mutation at the codon 249 of TP53 gene, namely G:C > T:A mutation resulting in the change of arginine to serine, has been identified as a relatively specifically change and named AFB1-induced hot-spot mutation [44]. This mutation may lead to the dysfunction of TP53 protein and abnormal cell actions like promoting cell growth, inhibiting cell apoptosis, and inhibiting transcription mediated by TP53 [40].

Other risk factors like alcohol intake also cause malignant transformation of hepatocytes. Chronic ethanol intake will significantly increase hepatocarcinoma risk (about five times) if more than 80 g/day × 10 years. Actually, less than this amount of uptake also increases cancer risk in spite of nonsignificance [48]. Although mechanisms are not still clear, increasing data have shown that chronic hepatic injury, abnormal regeneration, and cirrhosis may act some role in hepatocarcinogenesis [4]. Pathological and molecular biological studies display that acetaldehyde, an important metabolic product of ethanol, can bind to DNA and form DNA adducts. The DNA adduct formation caused could trigger replication errors and/or mutations in tumor suppressor genes and/or oncogene [4]. Additionally, oxidative DNA damage is more noticeable in tissues with hepatocarcinoma than peri-tumor tissues [40, 46]. However, it is unclear whether acetaldehyde-DNA adducts and oxidative damages are true carcinogens and how they trigger hepatocarcinogenesis [4, 49]. Therefore, future studies on DNA damage are needed to better validate these risk factors and detailed molecular mechanisms.

3.2 DRR in hepatocarcinoma

DNA damage will trigger DRR pathways, a kind of prompt signal event which can harmonize whether cells obtain cycle arrest for DNA repair or induce death for eliminating cells with severe DNA damage and genomic instability [4]. In human, cells develop several types of surveillance mechanisms consisting of SSB repair (SSBR), DSB repair (DSBR), base excision repair (BER), base mismatch repair (MMR), and nucleotide excision repair (NER) (**Figure 2**) [4, 40]. Among these DNA repair pathways, BER, MMR, and NER can repair base damage such as base mismatches, AFB1-DNA adducts, DNA pyrimidine dimers, and DNA damage induced by irradiation and anticancer drugs. SSBR can repair SSB that is a severe DNA damage, if not repaired quickly, will disrupt genic transcription and replication and ultimately results in lethal DNA damage [40]. DSBR pathway involves in homologous recombination (HR), single-strand annealing (SSA), and nonhomologous end joining (NHEJ). HR pathway can repair DSBs through an accurate repair method using the undamaged homologous chromosome or sister-chromatid as DNA repair temple; whereas NHEJ and SSA pathways are nonhomologous repair methods and usually lead to essential mutagenesis, so far

DRR pathway gene/ proteins	DRR pathway	Abnormal of DRR	Effects on hepatocarcinoma	Ref#
hOGG1	BER	Ser to Cys at codon 326	Increased hepatocarcinoma risk	[51]
XRCC1	BER and SSBR	Arg to His at codon 280 Arg to Gln at codon 399 Arg to Trp at codon 194	(1) Increasing individuals' susceptibility to HBV infection (2) Increasing individuals' susceptibility to hepatocarcinoma (3) Increasing amount of AFB1-DNA adducts in liver tissues (4) Increasing amount of adducts (including AFB1-DNA and AFB1-albumin adducts) in the peripheral WBCs (5) Increasing the frequency of TP53M (6) Increasing MVD	[52–56]
XRCC3	DSBR	Thr to Met at codon 241 rs1799796 A > G	(1) Increasing individuals' susceptibility to hepatocarcinoma (2) Increasing amount of AFB1-DNA adducts in liver tissues (3) Increasing amount of adducts (including AFB1-DNA and AFB1-albumin adducts) in the peripheral WBCs (4) Increasing the frequency of TP53M (5) Associating with hepatocarcinoma clinicopathological features (6) Increasing MVD	[57–59]
XRCC4	DSBR	rs28383151 G > A Ala to Ser at codon 247	(1) Increasing individuals' susceptibility to hepatocarcinoma (2) Increasing amount of AFB1-DNA adducts in liver tissues (3) Increasing amount of adducts (including AFB1-DNA and AFB1-albumin adducts) in the peripheral WBCs (4) Increasing the frequency of TP53M (5) Associating with hepatocarcinoma clinicopathological features (6) Increasing MVD	[20, 21, 60–63]
XRCC5	DSBR	rs16855458 C > A rs9288516 T > A XRCC5 expression	(1) Increasing individuals' susceptibility to HBV infection (2) Increasing individuals' susceptibility to hepatocarcinoma (3) Associating with biological actions of hepatocarcinoma cells, such as increasing XRCC5 expression inhibiting cancer cells proliferation (4) Functioning as a tumor suppressor by inducing S-phase arrest in a TP53-dependent pathway	[64–69]
XRCC6	DSBR	XRCC6 expression	(1) Increasing individuals' susceptibility to hepatocarcinoma (2) Decreasing Toll-like receptor 4 (TLR4) against hepatocarcinogenesis (3) Increasing DNA damage, and promoting programmed cell death in TLR4-deficient livers (4) Early diagnostic value for hepatocarcinoma	[70–73]

DRR pathway gene/ proteins	DRR pathway	Abnormal of DRR	Effects on hepatocarcinoma	Ref#
XRCC7	DSBR	rs7003908 T > G	(1) Increasing individuals' susceptibility to AFB1 exposure (2) Increasing individuals' susceptibility to hepatocarcinoma (3) Increasing amount of AFB1-DNA adducts in liver tissues (4) Increasing amount of adducts (including AFB1-DNA and AFB1-albumin adducts) in the peripheral WBCs (5) Increasing the frequency of TP53M (6) Interacting with AFB1 exposure during hepatocarcinogenesis (7) Increasing MVD	[21, 74, 75]
DNA-PKcs	DSBR	Amount in liver tissues	Implying hepatocarcinoma-specificity	[76]
TP53	DRR pathway	Genic mutations such as TP53M, Arg to His at codon 273, Arg to His at codon 175, Cys to Tyr at codon 135, and Arg to Trp at codon 248	1. Implying individuals' AFB1 exposure 2. Associating with hepatocarcinoma risk 3. Increasing individuals' susceptibility to hepatocarcinoma 4. Decreasing DRR potential and increasing DNA damage	[40, 45, 77, 78]
XPC	NER	XPC expression Lys to Gln at codon 939	(1) Increasing individuals' susceptibility to hepatocarcinoma (2) Increasing amount of AFB1-DNA adducts in liver tissues (3) Increasing amount of adducts (including AFB1-DNA and AFB1-albumin adducts) in the peripheral WBCs (4) Increasing the frequency of TP53M and decreasing DRR potential (5) Associating with hepatocarcinoma clinicopathological features (6) Increasing XPC expression (7) Increasing MVD	[21, 79–81]
XPD	NER	Lys to Gln at codon 751	(1) Increasing individuals' susceptibility to hepatocarcinoma (2) Increasing amount of AFB1-DNA adducts in liver tissues (3) Increasing amount of adducts (including AFB1-DNA and AFB1-albumin adducts) in the peripheral WBCs (4) Increasing the frequency of TP53M and decreasing DRR potential (5) Interacting with gender during hepatocarcinoma (6) Increasing MVD	[21, 82]
Rad50	NER	Rad50 hook domain	Strongly influencing Mre11 complex-dependent DRR signaling, tissue homeostasis, and tumorigenesis	[83]
Nbs1	NER	Rs1805794 C > G Mutations in Nbs1	(1) Increasing hepatocarcinoma risk (2) Associating with TP53 inactivation	[84–87]
PARP-1	BER	DRR potential	(1) Modifying biological actions of hepatocarcinoma cells (2) A novel promising diagnostic marker for hepatocarcinoma	[88–90]

DRR pathway gene/ proteins	DRR pathway	Abnormal of DRR	Effects on hepatocarcinoma	Ref#
Rad10	NER	rs11615 C > T ERCC1–4533 G > A ERCC1–8092 C > A	(1) Increasing hepatocarcinoma risk (2) The amount of ERCC1 expression in tissues with hepatocarcinoma decreases cancer cells' sensitivity on anti-cancer drugs (3) Predicting the outcome of hepatocarcinoma patients receiving TACE treatment	[91–93]
ATM	HR and ENEJ	Ser to Ala at codon 1981 Ser to Ala at codon 1893 Ser to Ala at codon 367 Ser to Ala at codon 2996 Autophosphorylation at codon 1981 Ser	(1) The functional deficiency in radioresistant DNA synthesis and substrate phosphorylation such as TP53, Chk2, Nbs1, and SMCI (2) Increasing cells' sensitivity to risk factors and risk factors-induced DNA damage such as adduct formation and chromosome aberrations (3)The functional dysregulation for G2/M checkpoint (4) Extending activations of DNA damage signaling pathways to reach S phase arrest in hepatocarcinoma cells (5) Leading to ATM unable to be released from other ATM molecules, and increasing gene mutation risk	[94–100]

Abbreviations: *hOGG1, human oxoguanine glycosylase 1; XRCC1, X-ray repair cross complementing 1; BER, base excision repair; SSBR, single-strand break repair; HBV, hepatitis B virus; XRCC3, X-ray repair cross complementing 3; AFB1, aflatoxin B1; DSBR, double-strand break repair; WBC, white blood cell; TP53M, hot-spot mutation at codon 249 of TP53 gene; DNA-PKcs, DNA-activated protein kinase catalytic subunit; XRCC4, X-ray repair cross complementing 4; XRCC5, X-ray repair cross complementing 5; XRCC6, X ray repair cross complementing 6; XRCC7, X-ray repair cross complementing 7; XPC, xeroderma pigmentosum, complementation group C; XPD, xeroderma pigmentosum, complementation group D; NER, nucleotide excision repair; PARP-1, poly(ADP-ribose) polymerase 1; ATM, Ataxia telangiectasia mutated kinase.*

Table 4.
The association between abnormal DRR potential and hepatocarcinogenesis.

as to induce chromosomal aberrations, abnormal cell cycle, and/or uncontrolled cell proliferation [50]. During DRR pathways, DNA repair genes play a central role [4]. Dysregulation of DRR caused by DNA repair genic mutations or low DNA repair capacity will increase hepatocarcinoma risk. **Table 4** summarized the effects of abnormal DRR in hepatocarcinogenesis. This evidence shows that dysregulation of DRR resulting from mutations in DNA repair genes and corresponding dysfunctions may promote hepatocarcinogenesis through the following pathways: (1) increasing individuals' susceptibility to risk factors such as hepatitis virus infection and AFB1 exposure [40, 60, 101]; (2) increasing individuals' susceptibility to cancer [45]; (3) increasing amount of carcinogens-DNA adducts in liver tissues [40]; (4) increasing amount of adducts (such as AFB1-DNA and AFB1-albumin adducts) in the peripheral WBCs and affecting immune reaction [61]; (5) increasing the frequency of tumor suppressor genes or oncogenes like Ras and TP53M [40, 47, 52, 61, 79]; and (6) interacting with risk factors during hepatocarcinogenesis [23]. Thus, the potential of DRR pathways should play an important function for hepatocarcinogenesis.

4. Hepatocarcinoma angiogenesis induced by DRR

Risk factors induced DNA damages and dysregulated DRRs are regarded as molecular events [4]. In human, risk factors for hepatocarcinoma can manifest acute and chronic DNA damage. Acute and noticeable DNA damages often lead to severe chromosome aberration and even cell death, whereas chronic DNA damages are the earliest molecular change in hepatocytes and ultimately result in hepatocarcinoma [40]. In the past decades, angiogenesis induced by dysregulation of DRR pathways may act as a vital role in the process of hepatocarcinoma. Evidence from epidemiological and clinicopathological studies has shown that higher potential of angiogenesis is in the liver of patients with chronic DNA damage and low DRR capacity [40, 102–105]. For example, Pastukh et al. [102] investigated the association between recruitment of DNA repair enzymes involving in BER pathway and VEGF expression via a chromatin immunoprecipitation technique. They found that hypoxia-induced reactive oxygen species (ROS) stress caused promoter base modifications targeted to hypoxic response elements (HREs) and increased VEGF expression. During this modification, 8-oxoguanine (8-oxodG, an oxidative DNA damage product) in VEGF promoter was temporally correlated with binding of human 8-oxodG glycosylase 1 (hOGG1, a BER repair enzyme), HIF-1α, redox effector factor-1, endonuclease one, and breaks in DNA strands. If 8-oxodG was decreased in the promoter region of VEGF, VEGF expression would downregulate [102]. Recent molecular epidemiological studies have further proved that genetic variants in hOGG1 genes increase hepatocarcinoma risk and modify the prognosis of this malignancy [103–105]. Collectively, these data suggest that increasing ROS like 8-oxodG resulting from low DRR capacity may promote angiogenesis.

Studies from high HBV and HCV infection and high AFB1 exposure area also display that the degrees of DNA damages are positively associated with MVD in tumor tissues from hepatocarcinoma [20, 55, 75, 79, 82]. For example, Lu et al. [20] investigated the effects of XRCC4 expression in tumor tissues on clinicopathological features and prognosis of hepatocarcinoma and found that decreasing XRCC4 expression was related to low DRR capacity, causing the formation of DNA adducts and TP53M. The dysregulation of XRCC4 may promote tumor proliferation and increase MVD. Several other studies further show that the low DRR capacity resulting from significant mutations in coding region of DNA repair genes (such as XRCC4, XRCC1, XPC, XPD, and XRCC7) increases MVD (**Table 4**) [21, 40, 52, 55, 59, 61, 62, 79, 80, 82]. Results from Lu et al. [20] and our studies [61, 62] showed that genetic alterations in the coding regions of XRCC4 gene (including Ala to Ser at codon 247 and Thr to Ala at codon 56) can decrease levels of XRCC4 protein expression and cause increasing amount of AFB1-DNA adducts and mutative frequency of TP53 gene in tissues with hepatocarcinoma. They also found that the amount of AFB1-induced DNA adducts, including 8,9-dihydro-8-(N^7-guanyl)-9-hydroxy-AFB1 (AFB1-N^7-Gua) and formamidopyridine AFB1 adduct (AFB1-FAPy), was positively associated with the number of microvessels (a biomarker for angiogenesis). Results from our studies [79, 106, 107] furthermore displayed that three low DNA repair markers related to AFB1, including tumor risk, TP53M frequency, and AFB1-FAPy adduct amount, were significantly correlated with the number of microvessels in liver tissues. These individuals with high AFB1-FAPy adduct level in liver tissues had an increasing risk of high MVD than those low adduct level (OR = 1.68, 95% CI = 1.45–2.87) [106]. Liu et al. [108] and Wang et al. [109] further proved that the upregulation of microRNA-429 and microRNA-24 expression in tissues with hepatocarcinoma not only increased the amount of AFB1-DNA adducts and the number of microvessels but also grew tumor metastasis risk via vessels and shorted patients' survival. Recent evidence has shown that microRNA-24/microRNA-429 can modify the capacity of DDR via controlling Nbs1 (a regulator of DRR) [110, 111] and angiogenesis via regulating the crosstalk between the pro-contractile transforming growth factor-β/bone morphogenetic protein (TGF-β/BMP) signal (inducing a quiescent 'contractile' phenotype) and the pro-synthetic platelet-derived growth factor (PDGF) signal (causing a proliferative 'synthetic' phenotype) [112, 113]. This suggests that microRNA-24/microRNA-429 may play an important regulative role between DRR capacity and angiogenesis. Taken together, this evidence proves that low DRR-induced MVD augmentation is regulated by the amount of DNA damage.

Evidence from in vitro and in vivo studies further shows that dysregulation of DRRs and signaling to cell cycle checkpoints (CCCs) may modify hepatocarcinoma angiogenesis. CCCs involving in DRRs mainly encompass G1/S and G2/M checkpoint [114]. During G1/S checkpoint, both ATR and ATM act as central activators for DRR via inducing the phosphorylation of p53 protein which can activate p21 (a Cdk inhibitor). ATM/TP53/P21 pathway also plays an important function controlling G2/M procession [114]. The dysregulation of these factors and signal pathways can change the status of angiogenesis [115–119]. For example, Qin et al. [115] found that E2F1, an important cell cycle regulator, can modify angiogenesis via controlling VEGF expression by p53-dependent way. In this control model, deficient phenotype of E2F1 will result in VEGF overexpression, while its positive phenotype decreases VEGF expression [115]. Factors controlling cell shape and cytosol can regulate the cycle of vessel endothelial cells and angiogenesis [116, 117]. In mice model with the deficiency of BCL-2 (an important regulatory factor in DDRs), cells featured increasing DNA damage [118]; the inhibition of BCL-2 will result in the arrest of cells in S phrase and suppression of tumor angiogenesis [119]. In an integrated genomic study (including 5 hepatocarcinoma patients with hepatitis D visus [HDV] and 7 HDV-positive cirrhosis cases), Diaz et al. [120] investigated the association between HDV-related hepatocarcinoma and potential signal pathways involved in DNA damage and repair and cell cycle and found significant interactions of DDR/cell cycle-related genes, such as BRCA1, BARD1, CDK1, CDKN2C, CCNA2, CCNB1, CCNE2, GSK3B, H2AFX, MSH2, NPM1, PRKDC, and TOP2A. Results from the t-SNP (*t*-distributed stochastic neighbor embedding analyses) further exhibited that HUS1, BRCA1, BARD1, GADD45, DNA-damage-induced 14-3-3σ, and MSH2 gene involving in DRRs valuably scored with regulatory genes (such as ATM, TP53, NO, and epidermal growth factor), which involve in G2/M checkpoint and angiogenesis [120]. The dysregulation of HUS1 and corresponding genotoxin-activated checkpoint complex (also termed as Rad9-Rad1-Hus1complex) will cause abnormal DRR capacity and cell cycle in response to DNA damage and promote the alteration of hematogenous metastatic phenotype for hepatocarcinoma [121, 122]. The genetic alterations and abnormal expression of BRCA1 and GADD45 (two important regulatory factors in DRR and apoptosis pathways) in hepatocytes can also change TP53-dependent CCCs and VEGF expression [123, 124]. Altogether, these studies have proved that the dysregulation of DDRs can cause the abnormal regulation of CCCs and change the status of hepatocarcinoma angiogenesis.

Detailed molecular mechanisms of DRR dysregulation promoting hepatocarcinoma angiogenesis have still not been fully understood. Several possible pathways may play some important roles. First, DNA damage agents induce NO synthase and increase the expression of VEGF and HGF [125, 126]. Second, DNA damage agents like AFB1 cause the mutations of such genes as TP53, ras, and DNA repair genes. Activation of oncogenes and inactivation of tumor suppression genes and

DNA repair genes lead to uncontrolled expression of genes involving in angiogenesis such as VEGF and Ang-1/2 [5, 6]. Third, genetic alterations in DRR pathways may alter the microenvironment of tumor and promote angiogenesis [127–129]. Fourth, the abnormal DRRs may accelerate the accumulation of DNA damages and trigger the dysregulation of angiogenesis-related genes and the progression of hepatocarcinoma. Finally, some metabolic products (such as AFBO) or nucleotide sequences (HBx) of DNA agents can bind to genomic DNA of hepatocytes and may increase the activation of VEGF HREs [22, 40, 41, 45]. Taken together, under the conditions of low DRR capacity and/or chronic risk factors, DNA damages will accumulate in hepatocytes and ultimately induce hepatocarcinogenesis and tumor angiogenesis.

5. Summary and further direction

Abnormal angiogenesis and DNA damages/DRRs are two important pathophysiological events in the process of hepatocarcinogenesis. Recently, it has become a growing evidence of DNA damage and repair and angiogenesis in hepatocarcinogenesis. Low DRR capacity resulting genetic or obtained alterations may lead to the accumulation of DNA damages and induce angiogenesis and ultimately promote hepatocarcinoma development. The main challenge for this field is the explanations of molecular basis and regulative signal pathways of DNA damages/DRRs interacting with angiogenesis during hepatocarcinogenesis. A better understanding of hypervascular feature and corresponding mechanisms of hepatocarcinoma on the basis of DNA damage/DRR pathway may be helpful for the medical researchers and clinic doctors exploring and validating hepatocarcinogenesis but also for them designing safe and efficient antiangiogenic drugs.

Acknowledgements

We thank Dr. Yuan-Feng Zhou for literature collection.

Conflicts of interest and source of funding

The authors declare no competing financial interests. This study was supported in part by the National Natural Science Foundation of China (Nos. 81860489, 81760502, 81572353, 81372639, 81472243, 81660495, and 81460423), the Innovation Program of Guangxi Municipal Education Department (Nos. 201204LX674 and 201204LX324), Innovation Program of Guangxi Health Department (No. Z2013781), the Natural Science Foundation of Guangxi (Nos. 2017GXNSFAA198002, 2017GXNSFGA198002, 2016GXNSFDA380003, 2015GXNSFAA139223, 2013GXNSFAA019251, 2014GXNSFDA118021, and 2014GXNSFAA118144), Research Program of Guangxi "Zhouyue Scholar" (No. 2017-38), Research Program of Guangxi Specially-invited Expert (No. 2017-6th), the "12th Five" Planning Program of Guangxi Education Science (No. 2015C397), the Innovative Program of Guangxi Graduate Education (No. JGY2015139), Research Program of Guangxi Clinic Research Center of Hepatobiliary Diseases (No.AD17129025), and Open Research Program from Molecular Immunity Study Room Involving in Acute & Severe Diseases in Guangxi Colleges and Universities (Nos. kfkt20160062 and kfkt20160063).

Abbreviations

AFB1	aflatoxin B1
Ang-2	angiopoietin-2
ATM	ataxia telangiectasia mutated kinase
BER	base excision repair
bFGF	basic fibroblast growth factor
DNA-PKcs	DNA-activated protein kinase catalytic subunit
DSBR	double-strand break repair
DRR	DNA damage repair response
G-CSF	granulocyte colony-stimulating factor
HBV	hepatitis B virus
HCV	hepatitis C virus
MVD	microvessel density
NER	nucleotide excision repair
HGF	hepatocyte growth factor
hOGG1	human oxoguanine glycosylase 1
IL-8	interleukin-8
PARP-1	poly(ADP-ribose) polymerase 1
SSBR	single-strand break repair
TEMs	TIE2-expressing monocytes/macrophages
TP53M	hot-spot mutation at codon 249 of TP53 gene
VEGF	vascular endothelial growth factor
XRCC1	X-ray repair cross complementing 1
XRCC3	X-ray repair cross complementing 3
XRCC4	X-ray repair cross complementing 4
XRCC5	X-ray repair cross complementing 5
XRCC6	X-ray repair cross complementing 6
XRCC7	X-ray repair cross complementing 7
XPC	xeroderma pigmentosum, complementation group C
XPD	xeroderma pigmentosum, complementation group D

Author details

Xi-Dai Long[1,2,3*†], Zhou-Ximao Long[4†], Xiao-Ying Huang[2], Jin-Guang Yao[2], Qiang Xia[1] and Yan Deng[5]

1 Department of Liver Surgery, Ren Ji Hospital, School of Medicine, Shanghai Jiao Tong University, Shanghai, China

2 Department of Pathology, The Affiliated Hospital of Youjiang Medical University for Nationalities, Baise, China

3 Guangxi Clinic Research Center of Hepatobiliary Diseases, Baise, China

4 Zhoupu Middle School, East China Normal University, Shanghai, China

5 Department of Epidemiology, Youjiang Medical University for Nationalities, Baise, China

*Address all correspondence to: sjtulongxd@263.net

† These authors contributed equally to this work

References

[1] Torre LA, Bray F, Siegel RL, Ferlay J, Lortet-Tieulent J, Jemal A. Global cancer statistics, 2012. CA: A Cancer Journal for Clinicians. 2015;**65**:87-108. DOI: 10.3322/caac.21262

[2] Blum HE, Spangenberg HC. Hepatocellular carcinoma: An update. Archives of Iranian Medicine. 2007;**10**:361-371. DOI: 07103/AIM.0015

[3] Aravalli RN, Cressman EN, Steer CJ. Cellular and molecular mechanisms of hepatocellular carcinoma: An update. Archives of Toxicology. 2013;**87**:227-247. DOI: 10.1007/s00204-012-0931-2

[4] Yang SF, Chang CW, Wei RJ, Shiue YL, Wang SN, Yeh YT. Involvement of DNA damage response pathways in hepatocellular carcinoma. BioMed Research International. 2014;**2014**:153867. DOI: 10.1155/2014/153867

[5] Semela D, Dufour JF. Angiogenesis and hepatocellular carcinoma. Journal of Hepatology. 2004;**41**:864-880. DOI: 10.1016/j.jhep.2004.09.006

[6] Sun HC, Tang ZY. Angiogenesis in hepatocellular carcinoma: The retrospectives and perspectives. Journal of Cancer Research and Clinical Oncology. 2004;**130**:307-319. DOI: 10.1007/s00432-003-0530-y

[7] Sugimachi K, Tanaka S, Terashi T, Taguchi K, Rikimaru T, Sugimachi K. The mechanisms of angiogenesis in hepatocellular carcinoma: Angiogenic switch during tumor progression. Surgery. 2002;**131**:S135-S141. DOI: 10.1067/msy.2002.119365

[8] Machado MV, Janeiro A, Miltenberger-Miltenyi G, Cortez-Pinto H. Genetic polymorphisms of proangiogenic factors seem to favor hepatocellular carcinoma development in alcoholic cirrhosis. European Journal of Gastroenterology & Hepatology. 2014;**26**:438-443. DOI: 10.1097/MEG.0000000000000044

[9] He Y, Ni J, Chen S, Jiang Y, Jia S, Gao Y. The vascular endothelial growth factor-2549 insertion/deletion polymorphism is not associated with susceptibility to hepatocellular carcinoma in Chinese. DNA and Cell Biology. 2010;**29**:393-396. DOI: 10.1089/dna.2009.1015

[10] Kong SY, Park JW, Lee JA, Park JE, Park KW, Hong EK, et al. Association between vascular endothelial growth factor gene polymorphisms and survival in hepatocellular carcinoma patients. Hepatology. 2007;**46**:446-455. DOI: 10.1002/hep.21720

[11] Chaparro M, Sanz-Cameno P, Trapero-Marugan M, Garcia-Buey L, Moreno-Otero R. Mechanisms of angiogenesis in chronic inflammatory liver disease. Annals of Hepatology. 2007;**6**:208-213. DOI: PMID18007549

[12] Wietecha MS, Cerny WL, DiPietro LA. Mechanisms of vessel regression: Toward an understanding of the resolution of angiogenesis. Current Topics in Microbiology and Immunology. 2013;**367**:3-32. DOI: 10.1007/82_2012_287

[13] Medina J, Arroyo AG, Sanchez-Madrid F, Moreno-Otero R. Angiogenesis in chronic inflammatory liver disease. Hepatology. 2004;**39**:1185-1195. DOI: 10.1002/hep.20193

[14] Kim KR, Moon HE, Kim KW. Hypoxia-induced angiogenesis in human hepatocellular carcinoma. Journal of Molecular Medicine (Berlin, Germany). 2002;**80**:703-714. DOI: 10.1007/s00109-002-0380-0

[15] Chiu DK, Tse AP, Xu IM, Di Cui J, Lai RK, Li LL, et al. Hypoxia inducible factor HIF-1 promotes myeloid-derived suppressor cells accumulation through ENTPD2/CD39L1 in hepatocellular carcinoma. Nature Communications. 2017;**8**:517. DOI: 10.1038/s41467-017-00530-7

[16] Mandl M, Depping R. ARNT is a potential direct HIF-1 target gene in human Hep3B hepatocellular carcinoma cells. Cancer Cell International. 2017;**17**:77. DOI: 10.1186/s12935-017-0446-2

[17] Shneor D, Folberg R, Pe'er J, Honigman A, Frenkel S. Stable knockdown of CREB, HIF-1 and HIF-2 by replication-competent retroviruses abrogates the responses to hypoxia in hepatocellular carcinoma. Cancer Gene Therapy. 2017;**24**:64-74. DOI: 10.1038/cgt.2016.68

[18] Jiao HK, Xu Y, Li J, Wang W, Mei Z, Long XD, et al. Prognostic significance of Cbx4 expression and its beneficial effect for transarterial chemoembolization in hepatocellular carcinoma. Cell Death & Disease. 2015;**6**:e1689. DOI: 10.1038/cddis.2015.57

[19] Li J, Xu Y, Long XD, Wang W, Jiao HK, Mei Z, et al. Cbx4 governs HIF-1alpha to potentiate angiogenesis of hepatocellular carcinoma by its SUMO E3 ligase activity. Cancer Cell. 2014;**25**:118-131. DOI: 10.1016/j.ccr.2013.12.008

[20] Lu J, Wang XZ, Zhang TQ, Huang XY, Yao JG, Wang C, et al. Prognostic significance of XRCC4 expression in hepatocellular carcinoma. Oncotarget. 2017;**8**:87955-87970. DOI: 10.18632/oncotarget.21360

[21] Yao JG, Huang XY, Long XD. Interaction of DNA repair gene polymorphisms and aflatoxin B1 in the risk of hepatocellular carcinoma. International Journal of Clinical and Experimental Pathology. 2014;**7**:6231-6244. DOI: PMC4203246

[22] Dewantoro O, Gani RA, Akbar N. Hepatocarcinogenesis in viral hepatitis B infection: The role of HBx and p53. Acta Medica Indonesiana. 2006;**38**:154-159. DOI: PMID16953033

[23] Moudgil V, Redhu D, Dhanda S, Singh J. A review of molecular mechanisms in the development of hepatocellular carcinoma by aflatoxin and hepatitis B and C viruses. Journal of Environmental Pathology, Toxicology and Oncology. 2013;**32**:165-175. DOI: 10.1615/JEnvironPatholToxicolOncol.2013007166

[24] Liu LP, Hu BG, Ye C, Ho RL, Chen GG, Lai PB. HBx mutants differentially affect the activation of hypoxia-inducible factor-1alpha in hepatocellular carcinoma. British Journal of Cancer. 2014;**110**:1066-1073. DOI: 10.1038/bjc.2013.787

[25] O'Connor JP, Jayson GC. Do imaging biomarkers relate to outcome in patients treated with VEGF inhibitors? Clinical Cancer Research. 2012;**18**:6588-6598. DOI: 10.1158/1078-0432.CCR-12-1501

[26] Park YN, Kim YB, Yang KM, Park C. Increased expression of vascular endothelial growth factor and angiogenesis in the early stage of multistep hepatocarcinogenesis. Archives of Pathology & Laboratory Medicine. 2000;**124**:1061-1065. DOI: 10.1043/0003-9985(2000)124<1061:IEOVEG>2.0.CO;2

[27] Poon RT, Lau CP, Cheung ST, Yu WC, Fan ST. Quantitative correlation of serum levels and tumor expression of vascular endothelial growth factor in patients with hepatocellular carcinoma. Cancer Research. 2003;**63**:3121-3126. DOI: PMID12810638

[28] Jinno K, Tanimizu M, Hyodo I, Nishikawa Y, Hosokawa Y, Doi T,

et al. Circulating vascular endothelial growth factor (VEGF) is a possible tumor marker for metastasis in human hepatocellular carcinoma. Journal of Gastroenterology. 1998;**33**:376-382. DOI: PMID9658317

[29] Kim SJ, Choi IK, Park KH, Yoon SY, Oh SC, Seo JH, et al. Serum vascular endothelial growth factor per platelet count in hepatocellular carcinoma: Correlations with clinical parameters and survival. Japanese Journal of Clinical Oncology. 2004;**34**:184-190. DOI: PMID15121753

[30] Poon RT, Ng IO, Lau C, Zhu LX, Yu WC, Lo CM, et al. Serum vascular endothelial growth factor predicts venous invasion in hepatocellular carcinoma: A prospective study. Annals of Surgery. 2001;**233**:227-235. DOI: PMC1421205

[31] Chao Y, Li CP, Chau GY, Chen CP, King KL, Lui WY, et al. Prognostic significance of vascular endothelial growth factor, basic fibroblast growth factor, and angiogenin in patients with resectable hepatocellular carcinoma after surgery. Annals of Surgical Oncology. 2003;**10**:355-362. DOI: 10.1245/ASO.2003.10.002

[32] Poon RT, Lau C, Yu WC, Fan ST, Wong J. High serum levels of vascular endothelial growth factor predict poor response to transarterial chemoembolization in hepatocellular carcinoma: A prospective study. Oncology Reports. 2004;**11**:1077-1084. DOI: 10.3892/or.11.5.1077

[33] Liao X, Yi J, Li X, Yang Z, Deng W, Tian G. Expression of angiogenic factors in hepatocellular carcinoma after transcatheter arterial chemoembolization. Journal of Huazhong University of Science and Technology. Medical Sciences. 2003;**23**:280-282. DOI: PMID14526434

[34] Suzuki H, Mori M, Kawaguchi C, Adachi M, Miura S, Ishii H. Serum vascular endothelial growth factor in the course of transcatheter arterial embolization of hepatocellular carcinoma. International Journal of Oncology. 1999;**14**:1087-1090. DOI: 10.3892/ijo.14.6.1087

[35] Hisai H, Kato J, Kobune M, Murakami T, Miyanishi K, Takahashi M, et al. Increased expression of angiogenin in hepatocellular carcinoma in correlation with tumor vascularity. Clinical Cancer Research. 2003;**9**: 4852-4859. DOI: PMID14581357

[36] Guo RP, Zhong C, Shi M, Zhang CQ, Wei W, Zhang YQ, et al. Clinical value of apoptosis and angiogenesis factors in estimating the prognosis of hepatocellular carcinoma. Journal of Cancer Research and Clinical Oncology. 2006;**132**:547-555. DOI: 10.1007/s00432-006-0097-5

[37] Miyahara K, Nouso K, Tomoda T, Kobayashi S, Hagihara H, Kuwaki K, et al. Predicting the treatment effect of sorafenib using serum angiogenesis markers in patients with hepatocellular carcinoma. Journal of Gastroenterology and Hepatology. 2011;**26**:1604-1611. DOI: 10.1111/j.1440-1746.2011.06887.x

[38] Matsubara T, Kanto T, Kuroda S, Yoshio S, Higashitani K, Kakita N, et al. TIE2-expressing monocytes as a diagnostic marker for hepatocellular carcinoma correlates with angiogenesis. Hepatology. 2013;**57**:1416-1425. DOI: 10.1002/hep.25965

[39] Sun XT, Yuan XW, Zhu HT, Deng ZM, Yu DC, Zhou X, et al. Endothelial precursor cells promote angiogenesis in hepatocellular carcinoma. World Journal of Gastroenterology. 2012;**18**:4925-4933. DOI: 10.3748/wjg.v18.i35.4925

[40] Long XD, Yao JD, Yang Q, Huang CH, Liao P, Nong LG, et al. Polymorphisms of DNA repair genes and toxicological effects of aflatoxin B1 exposure. In: Faulkner AG, editor.

Aflatoxins: Food Sources, Occurrence and Toxicological Effects. 1. New York: Nova Science Publishers; 2014. pp. 125-156. DOI: 978-1-63117-298-4

[41] Niller HH, Ay E, Banati F, Demcsak A, Takacs M, Minarovits J. Wild type HBx and truncated HBx: Pleiotropic regulators driving sequential genetic and epigenetic steps of hepatocarcinogenesis and progression of HBV-associated neoplasms. Reviews in Medical Virology. 2016;**26**:57-73. DOI: 10.1002/rmv.1864

[42] Huang CY, Hsieh FS, Wang CY, Chen LJ, Chang SS, Tsai MH, et al. Palbociclib enhances radiosensitivity of hepatocellular carcinoma and cholangiocarcinoma via inhibiting ataxia telangiectasia-mutated kinase-mediated DNA damage response. European Journal of Cancer. 2018;**102**:10-22. DOI: 10.1016/j.ejca.2018.07.010

[43] Min J, Guo K, Suryadevara PK, Zhu F, Holbrook G, Chen Y, et al. Optimization of a novel series of ataxia-telangiectasia mutated kinase inhibitors as potential radiosensitizing agents. Journal of Medicinal Chemistry. 2016;**59**:559-577. DOI: 10.1021/acs.jmedchem.5b01092

[44] Kew MC. Aflatoxins as a cause of hepatocellular carcinoma. Journal of Gastrointestinal and Liver Diseases. 2013;**22**:305-310. DOI: PMID24078988

[45] Wu XM, Xi ZF, Lu J, Wang XZ, Zhang TQ, Huang XY, et al. Genetic single nucleotide polymorphisms (GSNPs) in the DNA repair genes and hepatocellular carcinoma related to aflatoxin B1 among Guangxiese population. In: Parine NR, editor. Genetic Polymorphisms. Vol. 1. Rijeka, Croatia: InTech; 2017. pp. 97-119. DOI: 10.5772/intechopen.69530

[46] Kensler TW, Roebuck BD, Wogan GN, Groopman JD. Aflatoxin: A 50-year odyssey of mechanistic and translational toxicology. Toxicological Sciences. 2011;**120**(Suppl 1):S28-S48. DOI: 10.1093/toxsci/kfq283

[47] Wang JS, Groopman JD. DNA damage by mycotoxins. Mutation Research. 1999;**424**:167-181. DOI: 10.1016/S0027-5107(99)00017-2

[48] Kubo S, Kinoshita H, Hirohashi K, Tanaka H, Tsukamoto T, Shuto T, et al. High malignancy of hepatocellular carcinoma in alcoholic patients with hepatitis C virus. Surgery. 1997;**121**:425-429. DOI: 10.1016/S0039-6060(97)90313-5

[49] Leshets M, Silas YBH, Lehming N, Pines O. Fumarase: From the TCA cycle to DNA damage response and tumor suppression. Frontiers in Molecular Biosciences. 2018;**5**:68. DOI: 10.3389/fmolb.2018.00068

[50] Davis AJ, Chen DJ. DNA double strand break repair via non-homologous end-joining. Translational Cancer Research. 2013;**2**:130-143. DOI: 10.3978/j.issn.2218-676X.2013.04.02

[51] Piciocchi M, Cardin R, Cillo U, Vitale A, Cappon A, Mescoli C, et al. Differential timing of oxidative DNA damage and telomere shortening in hepatitis C and B virus-related liver carcinogenesis. Translational Research. 2016;**168**:122-133. DOI: 10.1016/j.trsl.2015.08.012

[52] Long XD, Ma Y, Huang HD, Yao JG, Qu DY, Lu YL. Polymorphism of XRCC1 and the frequency of mutation in codon 249 of the p53 gene in hepatocellular carcinoma among Guangxi population, China. Molecular Carcinogenesis. 2008;**47**:295-300. DOI: 10.1002/mc.20384

[53] Li LP, Wu W, Li XH, Song SS. The XRCC1 Arg280His gene polymorphism and hepatocellular carcinoma risk: A meta-analysis. Asian Pacific Journal of

Cancer Prevention. 2013;**14**:2033-2036. DOI: PMID23679314

[54] Li W, Yang F, Gui Y, Bian J. DNA repair gene XRCC1 Arg194Trp polymorphism and susceptibility to hepatocellular carcinoma: A meta-analysis. Oncology Letters. 2014;**8**:1725-1730. DOI: 10.3892/ol.2014.2351

[55] Long XD, Ma Y, Wei YP, Deng ZL. The polymorphisms of GSTM1, GSTT1, HYL1*2, and XRCC1, and aflatoxin B1-related hepatocellular carcinoma in Guangxi population, China. Hepatology Research. 2006;**36**:48-55. DOI: 10.1016/j.hepres.2006.06.004

[56] Zeng XY, Huang JM, Xu JW, Xu Y, Yu HP, Ji L, et al. Meta-analysis demonstrates lack of a relationship between XRCC1-399 gene polymorphisms and susceptibility to hepatocellular carcinoma. Genetics and Molecular Research. 2013;**12**:1916-1923. DOI: 10.4238/2013.March.15.5

[57] Avadanei ER, Giusca SE, Negura L, Caruntu ID. Single nucleotide polymorphisms of XRCC3 gene in hepatocellular carcinoma–relationship with clinicopathological features. Polish Journal of Pathology. 2018;**69**:73-81. DOI: 10.5114/pjp.2018.75340

[58] Ji RB, Qian YS, Hu AR, Hu YR. DNA repair gene XRCC3 T241M polymorphism and susceptibility to hepatocellular carcinoma in a Chinese population: A meta-analysis. Genetics and Molecular Research. 2015;**14**:15988-15996. DOI: 10.4238/2015.December.7.11

[59] Long XD, Ma Y, Qu DY, Liu YG, Huang ZQ, Huang YZ, et al. The polymorphism of XRCC3 codon 241 and AFB1-related hepatocellular carcinoma in Guangxi population, China. Annals of Epidemiology. 2008;**18**:572-578. DOI: 10.1016/j.annepidem.2008.03.003

[60] Makkoch J, Praianantathavorn K, Sopipong W, Chuaypen N, Tangkijvanich P, Payungporn S. Genetic Variations in XRCC4 (rs1805377) and ATF6 (rs2070150) are not associated with hepatocellular carcinoma in Thai patients with hepatitis B virus infection. Asian Pacific Journal of Cancer Prevention. 2016;**17**:591-595. DOI: PMID26925648

[61] Long XD, Zhao D, Wang C, Huang XY, Yao JG, Ma Y, et al. Genetic polymorphisms in DNA repair genes XRCC4 and XRCC5 and aflatoxin B1-related hepatocellular carcinoma. Epidemiology. 2013;**24**:671-681. DOI: 10.1097/EDE.0b013e31829d2744

[62] Long XD, Yao JG, Zeng Z, Ma Y, Huang XY, Wei ZH, et al. Polymorphisms in the coding region of X-ray repair complementing group 4 and aflatoxin B1-related hepatocellular carcinoma. Hepatology. 2013;**58**:171-181. DOI: 10.1002/hep.26311

[63] Jung SW, Park NH, Shin JW, Park BR, Kim CJ, Lee JE, et al. Polymorphisms of DNA repair genes in Korean hepatocellular carcinoma patients with chronic hepatitis B: Possible implications on survival. Journal of Hepatology. 2012;**57**:621-627. DOI: 10.1016/j.jhep.2012.04.039

[64] Xu Y, Liu AJ, Gao YX, Hu MG, Zhao GD, Zhao ZM, et al. Expression of Ku86 and presence of Ku86 antibody as biomarkers of hepatitis B virus related hepatocellular carcinoma. Digestive Diseases and Sciences. 2014;**59**:614-622. DOI: 10.1007/s10620-013-2941-1

[65] Wang Z, Lin H, Hua F, Hu ZW. Repairing DNA damage by XRCC6/KU70 reverses TLR4-deficiency-worsened HCC development via restoring senescence and autophagic flux. Autophagy. 2013;**9**:925-927. DOI: 10.4161/auto.24229

[66] Li R, Yang Y, An Y, Zhou Y, Liu Y, Yu Q, et al. Genetic polymorphisms in DNA double-strand break repair genes

XRCC5, XRCC6 and susceptibility to hepatocellular carcinoma. Carcinogenesis. 2011;**32**:530-536. DOI: 10.1093/carcin/bgr018

[67] Kim E, Li K, Lieu C, Tong S, Kawai S, Fukutomi T, et al. Expression of apolipoprotein C-IV is regulated by Ku antigen/peroxisome proliferator-activated receptor gamma complex and correlates with liver steatosis. Journal of Hepatology. 2008;**49**:787-798. DOI: 10.1016/j.jhep.2008.06.029

[68] Reliene R, Goad ME, Schiestl RH. Developmental cell death in the liver and newborn lethality of Ku86 deficient mice suppressed by antioxidant N-acetyl-cysteine. DNA Repair (Amst). 2006;**5**:1392-1397. DOI: 10.1016/j.dnarep.2006.06.007

[69] Muguruma M, Nishimura J, Jin M, Kashida Y, Moto M, Takahashi M, et al. Molecular pathological analysis for determining the possible mechanism of piperonyl butoxide-induced hepatocarcinogenesis in mice. Toxicology. 2006;**228**:178-187. DOI: 10.1016/j.tox.2006.08.029

[70] Chu L, Zhang X, Wang G, Zhou W, Du Z, Liu A, et al. Serum anti-Ku86: A potential biomarker for early detection of hepatocellular carcinoma. Zhonghua Zhong Liu Za Zhi. 2014;**36**:123-127. DOI: PMID24796461

[71] Wang Z, Yan J, Lin H, Hua F, Wang X, Liu H, et al. Toll-like receptor 4 activity protects against hepatocellular tumorigenesis and progression by regulating expression of DNA repair protein Ku70 in mice. Hepatology. 2013;**57**:1869-1881. DOI: 10.1002/hep.26234

[72] Hsu CM, Yang MD, Chang WS, Jeng LB, Lee MH, Lu MC, et al. The contribution of XRCC6/Ku70 to hepatocellular carcinoma in Taiwan. Anticancer Research. 2013;**33**:529-535. DOI: PMID23393345

[73] Nomura F, Sogawa K, Noda K, Seimiya M, Matsushita K, Miura T, et al. Serum anti-Ku86 is a potential biomarker for early detection of hepatitis C virus-related hepatocellular carcinoma. Biochemical and Biophysical Research Communications. 2012;**421**:837-843. DOI: 10.1016/j.bbrc.2012.04.099

[74] Hsieh YH, Chang WS, Tsai CW, Tsai JP, Hsu CM, Jeng LB, et al. DNA double-strand break repair gene XRCC7 genotypes were associated with hepatocellular carcinoma risk in Taiwanese males and alcohol drinkers. Tumour Biology. 2015;**36**:4101-4106. DOI: 10.1007/s13277-014-2934-5

[75] Long XD, Yao JG, Huang YZ, Huang XY, Ban FZ, Yao LM, et al. DNA repair gene XRCC7 polymorphisms (rs#7003908 and rs#10109984) and hepatocellular carcinoma related to AFB1 exposure among Guangxi population, China. Hepatology Research. 2011;**41**:1085-1093. DOI: 10.1111/j.1872-034X.2011.00866.x

[76] Pascale RM, Joseph C, Latte G, Evert M, Feo F, Calvisi DF. DNA-PKcs: A promising therapeutic target in human hepatocellular carcinoma? DNA Repair (Amst). 2016;**47**:12-20. DOI: 10.1016/j.dnarep.2016.10.004

[77] Song H, Hollstein M, Xu Y. p53 gain-of-function cancer mutants induce genetic instability by inactivating ATM. Nature Cell Biology. 2007;**9**:573-580. DOI: 10.1038/ncb1571

[78] Dong P, Karaayvaz M, Jia N, Kaneuchi M, Hamada J, Watari H, et al. Mutant p53 gain-of-function induces epithelial-mesenchymal transition through modulation of the miR-130b-ZEB1 axis. Oncogene. 2013;**32**:3286-3295. DOI: 10.1038/onc.2012.334

[79] Long XD, Huang HD, Huang XY, Yao JG, Xia Q. XPC codon 939 polymorphism is associated with

susceptibility to DNA damage induced by aflatoxin B1 exposure. International Journal of Clinical and Experimental Medicine. 2015;**8**:1197-1204. DOI: PMC4358568

[80] Long XD, Ma Y, Zhou YF, Ma AM, Fu GH. Polymorphism in xeroderma pigmentosum complementation group C codon 939 and aflatoxin B1-related hepatocellular carcinoma in the Guangxi population. Hepatology. 2010;**52**:1301-1309. DOI: 10.1002/hep.23807

[81] Long XD, Ma Y, Huang YZ, Yi Y, Liang QX, Ma AM, et al. Genetic polymorphisms in DNA repair genes XPC, XPD, and XRCC4, and susceptibility to *Helicobacter pylori* infection-related gastric antrum adenocarcinoma in Guangxi population, China. Molecular Carcinogenesis. 2010;**49**:611-618. DOI: 10.1002/mc.20630

[82] Long XD, Ma Y, Zhou YF, Yao JG, Ban FZ, Huang YZ, et al. XPD Codon 312 and 751 polymorphisms, and AFB1 exposure, and hepatocellular carcinoma risk. BMC Cancer. 2009;**9**:400. DOI: 10.1186/1471-2407-9-400

[83] Roset R, Inagaki A, Hohl M, Brenet F, Lafrance-Vanasse J, Lange J, et al. The Rad50 hook domain regulates DNA damage signaling and tumorigenesis. Genes & Development. 2014;**28**:451-462. DOI: 10.1101/gad.236745.113

[84] Kim JH, Grosbart M, Anand R, Wyman C, Cejka P, Petrini JHJ. The Mre11-Nbs1 interface is essential for viability and tumor suppression. Cell Reports. 2017;**18**:496-507. DOI: 10.1016/j.celrep.2016.12.035

[85] Wang Y, Li M, Long J, Shi XY, Li Q, Chen J, et al. Clinical significance of increased expression of Nijmegen breakage syndrome gene (NBS1) in human primary liver cancer. Hepatology International. 2014;**8**:250-259. DOI: 10.1007/s12072-013-9500-x

[86] Wang Y, Hong Y, Li M, Long J, Zhao YP, Zhang JX, et al. Mutation inactivation of Nijmegen breakage syndrome gene (NBS1) in hepatocellular carcinoma and intrahepatic cholangiocarcinoma. PLoS One. 2013;**8**:e82426. DOI: 10.1371/journal.pone.0082426

[87] Huang MD, Chen XF, Xu G, Wu QQ, Zhang JH, Chen GF, et al. Genetic variation in the NBS1 gene is associated with hepatic cancer risk in a Chinese population. DNA and Cell Biology. 2012;**31**:678-682. DOI: 10.1089/dna.2011.1421

[88] Li J, Dou D, Li P, Luo W, Lv W, Zhang C, et al. PARP-1 serves as a novel molecular marker for hepatocellular carcinoma in a Southern Chinese Zhuang population. Tumour Biology. 2017;**39**:1010428317706914. DOI: 10.1177/1010428317706914

[89] Mao X, Du S, Yang Z, Zhang L, Peng X, Jiang N, et al. Inhibitors of PARP-1 exert inhibitory effects on the biological characteristics of hepatocellular carcinoma cells in vitro. Molecular Medicine Reports. 2017;**16**:208-214. DOI: 10.3892/mmr.2017.6568

[90] Luo Q, Li Y, Deng J, Zhang Z. PARP-1 inhibitor sensitizes arsenic trioxide in hepatocellular carcinoma cells via abrogation of G2/M checkpoint and suppression of DNA damage repair. Chemico-Biological Interactions. 2015;**226**:12-22. DOI: 10.1016/j.cbi.2014.12.007

[91] Chen L, Liu MM, Liu H, Lu D, Zhao XD, Yang XJ. ERCC1 and XRCC1 but not XPA single nucleotide polymorphisms correlate with response to chemotherapy in endometrial carcinoma. OncoTargets and Therapy. 2016;**9**:7019-7028. DOI: 10.2147/OTT.S110976

[92] Hu ZJ, Xue JF, Zhang XY, Shi XS, Zhou H. Relationship between genetic polymorphism of ERCC1

and susceptibility to liver cancer. Zhonghua Liu Xing Bing Xue Za Zhi. 2010;**31**:1288-1291. DOI: 10.3760/cma.j.issn.0254-6450.2010.11.020

[93] Li Y, Ou C, Shu H, Zhao H, Zhu B. The ERCC1-4533/8092, TNF-alpha 238/308 polymorphisms and the risk of hepatocellular carcinoma in Guangxi Zhuang populations of China: Case-control study. Medicine (Baltimore). 2016;**95**:e5217. DOI: 10.1097/MD.0000000000005217

[94] Liu J, Liu Y, Meng L, Ji B, Yang D. Synergistic antitumor effect of sorafenib in combination with ATM inhibitor in hepatocellular carcinoma cells. International Journal of Medical Sciences. 2017;**14**:523-529. DOI: 10.7150/ijms.19033

[95] Ma CQ, Yang Y, Wang JM, Du GS, Shen Q, Liu Y, et al. The aPKCiota blocking agent ATM negatively regulates EMT and invasion of hepatocellular carcinoma. Cell Death & Disease. 2014;**5**:e1129. DOI: 10.1038/cddis.2014.91

[96] Mansoori AA, Jain SK. Molecular links between alcohol and tobacco induced DNA damage, gene polymorphisms and patho-physiological consequences: A systematic review of hepatic carcinogenesis. Asian Pacific Journal of Cancer Prevention. 2015;**16**:4803-4812. DOI: PMID26163595

[97] Gu DL, Chen YH, Shih JH, Lin CH, Jou YS, Chen CF. Target genes discovery through copy number alteration analysis in human hepatocellular carcinoma. World Journal of Gastroenterology. 2013;**19**:8873-8879. DOI: 10.3748/wjg.v19.i47.8873

[98] Huang S, Zhang Y, Zeng T. Effect of ATM-111 (G>A) polymorphism on cancer risk: A meta-analysis. Genetic Testing and Molecular Biomarkers. 2016;**20**:359-366. DOI: 10.1089/gtmb.2015.0320

[99] Vorechovsky I. Mutation analysis of large genomic regions in tumor DNA using single-strand conformation polymorphism. Lessons from the ATM gene. Methods in Molecular Medicine. 2002;**68**:115-124. DOI: PMID11901497

[100] Thorstenson YR, Shen P, Tusher VG, Wayne TL, Davis RW, Chu G, et al. Global analysis of ATM polymorphism reveals significant functional constraint. American Journal of Human Genetics. 2001;**69**:396-412. DOI: 10.1086/321296

[101] Yu L, Liu X, Han C, Lu S, Zhu G, Su H, et al. XRCC1 rs25487 genetic variant and TP53 mutation at codon 249 predict clinical outcomes of hepatitis B virus-related hepatocellular carcinoma after hepatectomy: A cohort study for 10 years' follow up. Hepatology Research. 2016;**46**:765-774. DOI: 10.1111/hepr.12611

[102] Pastukh V, Roberts JT, Clark DW, Bardwell GC, Patel M, Al-Mehdi AB, et al. An oxidative DNA "damage" and repair mechanism localized in the VEGF promoter is important for hypoxia-induced VEGF mRNA expression. American Journal of Physiology. Lung Cellular and Molecular Physiology. 2015;**309**:L1367-L1375. DOI: 10.1152/ajplung.00236.2015

[103] Guo J, Yang J, Li Y. Association of hOGG1 Ser326Cys polymorphism with susceptibility to hepatocellular carcinoma. International Journal of Clinical and Experimental Medicine. 2015;**8**:8977-8985. DOI: PMC4537974

[104] Sakamoto T, Higaki Y, Hara M, Ichiba M, Horita M, Mizuta T, et al. hOGG1 Ser326Cys polymorphism and risk of hepatocellular carcinoma among Japanese. Journal of Epidemiology. 2006;**16**:233-239. DOI: 10.2188/jea.16.233

[105] Wang W, Dang S, Li Y, Sun M, Jia X, Wang R, et al. hOGG1 Ser326Cys polymorphism and risk of

hepatocellular carcinoma among East Asians: A meta-analysis. PLoS One. 2013;**8**:e60178. DOI: 10.1371/journal.pone.0060178

[106] Long XD, Yao JD, Yang Q, Huang CH, Liao P, Nong LG, et al. Polymorphisms of DNA repair genes and toxicological effects of aflatoxin B1 exposure. In: Faulkner AG, editor. Aflatoxins: Food Sources, Occurrence and Toxicological Effects. 1st ed. New York: Nova Science Publishers; 2014. pp. 107-124

[107] Long XD, Huang HD, Xia Q. The polymorphism of XRCC3 codon 241 and the hotspot mutation in the TP53 gene in hepatocellular carcinoma induced by aflatoxin B1. Journal of Tumor. 2014;**2**:272-277. DOI: 10.6051/j.issn.1819-6187.2014.02.57

[108] Liu YX, Long XD, Xi ZF, Ma Y, Huang XY, Yao JG, et al. MicroRNA-24 modulates aflatoxin B1-related hepatocellular carcinoma prognosis and tumorigenesis. BioMed Research International. 2014;**2014**:482926. DOI: 10.1155/2014/482926

[109] Huang XY, Yao JG, Huang HD, Wang C, Ma Y, Xia Q, et al. MicroRNA-429 modulates hepatocellular carcinoma prognosis and tumorigenesis. Gastroenterology Research and Practice. 2013;**2013**:804128. DOI: 10.1155/2013/804128

[110] Lovric J, Mano M, Zentilin L, Eulalio A, Zacchigna S, Giacca M. Terminal differentiation of cardiac and skeletal myocytes induces permissivity to AAV transduction by relieving inhibition imposed by DNA damage response proteins. Molecular Therapy. 2012;**20**:2087-2097. DOI: 10.1038/mt.2012.144

[111] Kasza Z, Fredlund Fuchs P, Tamm C, Eriksson AS, O'Callaghan P, Heindryckx F, et al. MicroRNA-24 suppression of N-deacetylase/N-sulfotransferase-1 (NDST1) reduces endothelial cell responsiveness to vascular endothelial growth factor A (VEGFA). The Journal of Biological Chemistry. 2013;**288**:25956-25963. DOI: 10.1074/jbc.M113.484360

[112] Chan MC, Hilyard AC, Wu C, Davis BN, Hill NS, Lal A, et al. Molecular basis for antagonism between PDGF and the TGFbeta family of signalling pathways by control of miR-24 expression. The EMBO Journal. 2010;**29**:559-573. DOI: 10.1038/emboj.2009.370

[113] Zhou Q, Anderson C, Zhang H, Li X, Inglis F, Jayagopal A, et al. Repression of choroidal neovascularization through actin cytoskeleton pathways by microRNA-24. Molecular Therapy. 2014;**22**:378-389. DOI: 10.1038/mt.2013.243

[114] Jeggo PA, Lobrich M. Contribution of DNA repair and cell cycle checkpoint arrest to the maintenance of genomic stability. DNA Repair (Amst). 2006;**5**:1192-1198. DOI: 10.1016/j.dnarep.2006.05.011

[115] Qin G, Kishore R, Dolan CM, Silver M, Wecker A, Luedemann CN, et al. Cell cycle regulator E2F1 modulates angiogenesis via p53-dependent transcriptional control of VEGF. Proceedings of the National Academy of Sciences of the United States of America. 2006;**103**:11015-11020. DOI: 10.1073/pnas.0509533103

[116] Herbert SP, Odell AF, Ponnambalam S, Walker JH. Activation of cytosolic phospholipase A2-{alpha} as a novel mechanism regulating endothelial cell cycle progression and angiogenesis. The Journal of Biological Chemistry. 2009;**284**:5784-5796. DOI: 10.1074/jbc.M807282200

[117] Ingber DE, Prusty D, Sun Z, Betensky H, Wang N. Cell shape, cytoskeletal mechanics, and cell cycle

control in angiogenesis. Journal of Biomechanics. 1995;**28**:1471-1484. DOI: 10.1016/0021-9290(95)00095-X

[118] Gillardon F, Moll I, Meyer M, Michaelidis TM. Alterations in cell death and cell cycle progression in the UV-irradiated epidermis of bcl-2-deficient mice. Cell Death and Differentiation. 1999;**6**:55-60. DOI: 10.1038/sj.cdd.4400455

[119] Ashimori N, Zeitlin BD, Zhang Z, Warner K, Turkienicz IM, Spalding AC, et al. TW-37, a small-molecule inhibitor of Bcl-2, mediates S-phase cell cycle arrest and suppresses head and neck tumor angiogenesis. Molecular Cancer Therapeutics. 2009;**8**:893-903. DOI: 10.1158/1535-7163.MCT-08-1078

[120] Diaz G, Engle RE, Tice A, Melis M, Montenegro S, Rodriguez-Canales J, et al. Molecular signature and mechanisms of hepatitis D virus-associated hepatocellular carcinoma. Molecular Cancer Research. 2018;**16**:1406-1419. DOI: 10.1158/1541-7786.MCR-18-0012

[121] Zhou ZQ, Zhao JJ, Chen CL, Liu Y, Zeng JX, Wu ZR, et al. HUS1 checkpoint clamp component (HUS1) is a potential tumor suppressor in primary hepatocellular carcinoma. Molecular Carcinogenesis. 2018. DOI: 10.1002/mc.22908 [Ahead of print]

[122] Broustas CG, Hopkins KM, Panigrahi SK, Wang L, Virk RK, Lieberman HB. RAD9A promotes metastatic phenotypes through transcriptional regulation of anterior gradient 2 (AGR2). Carcinogenesis. 2018. DOI: 10.1093/carcin/bgy131 [Ahead of print]

[123] Chen Q, Wang L, Jiang M, Huang J, Jiang Z, Feng H, et al. E2F1 interactive with BRCA1 pathway induces HCC two different small molecule metabolism or cell cycle regulation via mitochondrion or CD4+T to cytosol. Journal of Cellular Physiology. 2018;**233**:1213-1221. DOI: 10.1002/jcp.25988

[124] Gramantieri L, Chieco P, Giovannini C, Lacchini M, Trere D, Grazi GL, et al. GADD45-alpha expression in cirrhosis and hepatocellular carcinoma: Relationship with DNA repair and proliferation. Human Pathology. 2005;**36**:1154-1162. DOI: 10.1016/j.humpath.2005.07.017

[125] Majano PL, Garcia-Monzon C, Lopez-Cabrera M, Lara-Pezzi E, Fernandez-Ruiz E, Garcia-Iglesias C, et al. Inducible nitric oxide synthase expression in chronic viral hepatitis. Evidence for a virus-induced gene upregulation. The Journal of Clinical Investigation. 1998;**101**:1343-1352. DOI: 10.1172/JCI774

[126] Shimoda K, Mori M, Shibuta K, Banner BF, Barnard GF. Vascular endothelial growth factor/vascular permeability factor mRNA expression in patients with chronic hepatitis C and hepatocellular carcinoma. International Journal of Oncology. 1999;**14**:353-359. DOI: 10.3892/ijo.14.2.353

[127] Si M, Lang J. The roles of metallothioneins in carcinogenesis. Journal of Hematology & Oncology. 2018;**11**:107. DOI: 10.1186/s13045-018-0645-x

[128] Lezina L, Spriggs RV, Beck D, Jones C, Dudek KM, Bzura A, et al. CD40L/IL-4-stimulated CLL demonstrates variation in translational regulation of DNA damage response genes including ATM. Blood Advances. 2018;**2**:1869-1881. DOI: 10.1182/bloodadvances.2017015560

[129] Tehrani SS, Karimian A, Parsian H, Majidinia M, Yousefi B. Multiple functions of long non-coding RNAs in oxidative stress, DNA damage response and cancer progression. Journal of Cellular Biochemistry. 2018;**119**:223-236. DOI: 10.1002/jcb.26217

Chapter 10

Natural Drugs in DNA Repair

Thulasi G. Pillai, Cherupally K. Krishnan Nair and P. Uma Devi

Abstract

Natural products have been used in medicine right from the ancient civilisation. Natural products are used in many types of diseases, together with chemotherapy and radiotherapy. Many products are used against cancer. Many diseases are genetically derived. The drugs which have the capacity to act at genome level gains significant importance in any disease scenario. The genetic information essential for the identity and function of eukaryotic cells exist in DNA and during the lifetime of the cell DNA can be repeatedly damaged due to different factors. The stability and the fidelity of the replication process are meant to be the most remarkable features of the genetic material. The stability can be affected at any time. Compound which can enhance the DNA repair are applicable in many disease condition. Our study was focussed on the DNA repair enhancing property of a glucan from the macro fungi *Ganoderma lucidum*. Comet assay and chromosomal aberrations in mouse bone marrow were used as end points of study. Glucan was found to have DNA repair enhancing property in human lymphocytes.

Keywords: natural products, *Ganoderma lucidum*, glucan, mushroom, DNA repair

1. Introduction

The word 'Natural' has gained tremendous importance in the twenty-first century. Products obtained from nature are known to be natural. The Father of Medicine, Hippocrates has quoted that 'Let your food be our medicine and medicine be our food'. The incorporation of medicinal herbs and extract as food has been practiced long ago. In the present scenario, herbals are seen as potential medicine for a variety of diseases often viewed to super cede the pharmacological efficacy of allopathic drugs [1]. Natural products has become an extremely valuable commodity for the world today. The developing countries miss the modern medicine as they cannot afford it. Natural drugs were already there is use in Chinese medicine, Indian Ayurveda, Arabic Unani medicine and various other indigenous medicine. The two most important classics describing about more than 700 botanicals along with their classification, pharmacological and therapeutic properties are Charak Samhita and Sushrut Samhita (100–500 BC) [2, 3]. Recent reports have substantiated the general belief that traditional medicine is affordable as compared to modern medicine [4]. Natural products play a major role as 'drugs' and as 'lead structures' for the development of synthetic molecules [5]. Ancient people were fully aware of rich potential of herbs for curing different types of ailments. The twentieth century made invaluable contributions to the domain of medical sciences. The discovery of the fascinating molecule, DNA double helix and completion of human genome project were marvellous achievements that had no parallel.

IntechOpen

Different modalities of DNA repair mechanisms are offered by natural drugs in mammalian system like base excision repair (BER), nucleotide excision repair (NER), mismatch repair (MMR), SSB repair, which includes BER and DNA-PK-mediated ligation; DSB repair, which includes NHEJ and HR; inter-strand cross-link repair and DPCs (DNA-protein cross links) repair. The drugs act even as a biological catalyst where the rate of the repair process is enhanced [6]. An important cell pathology determinant is the rate of DNA repair. Shortened lifespan and increased cancer incidence has been observed in experimental animals with genetic deficiencies in DNA repair. Mice deficient in the dominant NHEJ pathway and in telomere maintenance mechanisms get lymphoma and infections more often, and consequently have shorter lifespans than wild-type mice [7]. Mice with deficient key repair mechanisms and DNA helices unwinding transcription protein have premature onset of aging-related diseases and shortening of lifespan [8]. Few natural products with DNA protective activity are phenolic compounds, essential oils, alkaloids, caratenoids, glutathione and glucans. Polyphenols and phenolic compounds have the capacity to donate electrons and scavenge free radicals [9, 10].

Phenolic compounds have the capacity to donate electrons and directly scavenge free radicals [9, 10]. The extracts of *Geranium sanguineum* are rich with polyphenol compounds are found to exhibit anti-mutagenic and free radical scavenging capacities [11, 12]. Essential oils, are antioxidants. The essential oil from ginger is a natural antioxidant [13]. Alkaloids, are antioxidants. Carotenoids are lipophilic compounds. Lycopene present in tomatoes and other red fruits like red carrots, red bell peppers, watermelons, and papayas has good antioxidant capacity [14]. Glutathione is a free radical scavenger by either reacting directly with free radical molecules or by acting as proton donor for protection of active molecules as DNA [15]. Glucan is an important carbohydrate from plants, bacteria and fungi. It is discussed in detail here due to their diverse activity. Somehow the antioxidant activity is related to DNA repair mechanism as most of the compound which can repair DNA damage are found possess antioxidant capacity.

Macro fungi are distinguished as important natural resources with therapeutic potential. Studies were conducted on the glucan isolated from the medicinal mushroom and the macrofungi, *Ganoderma lucidum*. *Ganoderma* is popularly known as 'The mushroom of longevity and immortality'1. *Ganoderma lucidum*, commonly known as reishi, a mushroom like fungus which grows on logs or tree stumps is one of the most popular medicinal mushrooms in China, Japan and the United States (**Figure 1**). It has a shiny, hard, asymmetrical cap that ranges in colour from yellow to black. Species of the genus *Ganoderma* P. Karst (Ganodermatales) are important wood decaying mushrooms occurring throughout the world, mainly on tropical trees. Over 250 species of this mushrooms are known. The fruiting

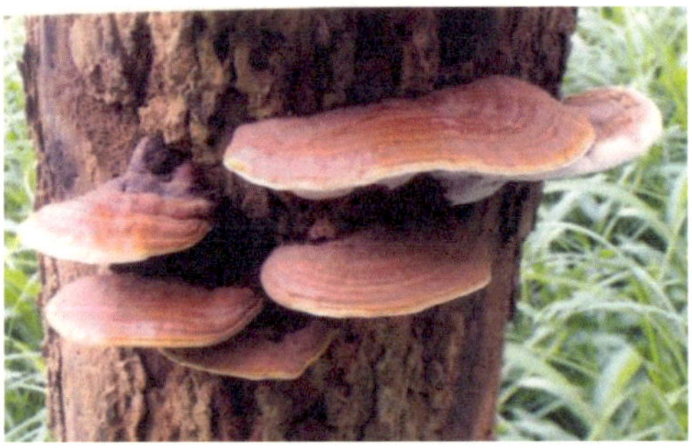

Figure 1.
Ganoderma lucidum growing in wild.

bodies of *Ganoderma lucidum* contain a variety of chemical substances. The polysaccharides of *G. lucidum* are the other major source of its biological activity and therapeutic use. This mushroom has attracted great attention owing to its antitumor and hypoglycemic activities [16]. Many fungal polysaccharides have been reported to be active in humans. More than 180 chemical substances have been isolated from *Ganoderma*, which include polysaccharides, triterpenes, nucleosides, ergosterols, fatty acids, proteins, peptides and trace elements. *Ganoderma* has been extensively used as mushroom of immortality in China and other Asian countries. *Ganoderma* has been reported to have numerous pharmacological effects including immunomodulating, anti-inflammatory, analgesic, anticancer, anti-lipidemic and hepatoprotective antihypertensive effects [8, 17]. It is widely accepted that pharmacological effects of *Ganoderma* depends on its colour, on the stage of development and the environment in which it grows. The fruiting bodies of *Ganoderma lucidum*, commonly known as reishi have long been prescribed in Chinese medicine as a tonic and sedative [18]. In Chinese folklore reishi has been regarded as a panacea for all types of diseases, perhaps owing to its demonstrated efficacy as a popular medicine. *Ganoderma* is also used in treating conditions of the nervous system. The ability of bioactive polysaccharides and polysaccharide-bound proteins to modulate immune cells can be due to the structural diversity and variability of these macromolecules. The bioactive glucanes and proteoglucans isolated from medicinal mushrooms are the most promising class of immunoceutics. Unlike proteins and nucleic acids, polysaccharides contain repetitive structural features which are polymers of monosaccharide residues joined to each other by glycosidic linkages. Glucan appear to be beneficial to humans with impaired immune systems, and those suffering from infectious diseases and cancer, as well as in helping patient recovery from chemotherapy and radiotherapy.

The basic mechanism of DNA replication, recombination and DNA repair are conserved throughout evolution. The complementarity of strands of DNA and the double stranded nature of DNA plays the major role in all the process. Damage to DNA by physical, chemical and biological factors influences the extraordinary accuracy of the entire process. At each cell division a handful of error is introduced per billion bp. Treatment modalities for cancer like chemo and radiotherapy affect DNA in many ways. Drugs of natural origin are capable of increasing the rate of DNA repair. The chapter will focus on the natural drugs and their influence on DNA repair mechanism. In the hierarchy of targets of reproductive death, DNA must be surely placed at the top, though membrane damage should be considered as the second important target with eukaryotic cells which contain their DNA in the nucleus, little lethal damage is observed as long as the radiation is absorbed only by the outer membrane and cytoplasm. There is a drastic increase as soon as the ionizing radiation reaches the nucleus and hence DNA. The DNA damages produced by ionizing radiation can be intra- or inter-strand cross linking and single and double strand breaks (**Figures 2** and **3**). The cellular reactions include halt in cell cycle, advancement at cell cycle checkpoints and the stimulation of DNA repair. An unrepaired or misrepaired DNA damage can result in genetic or genomic variability, changes in cellular individuality and role, cell death, and in multi-cellular organisms, neoplastic transformation.

Humanities use of mushrooms extends as early to 5000 B.C. About 2000 species of edible mushrooms are known all over the world. The total production of the edible mushroom is about 3.75 million tonnes. However they are rich source of high quality protein, vitamins and minerals. The average protein content is 10–40% on dry weight basis and low in fat content. Extracts and powders of mushrooms (mycelia and sporocarps) in the form of sugar coated tablets are being marketed on commercial scale for treatment of diseases such as diabetes, cancer, etc. Medicinal macro fungi modulate immune system and possess antitumor, antimicrobial,

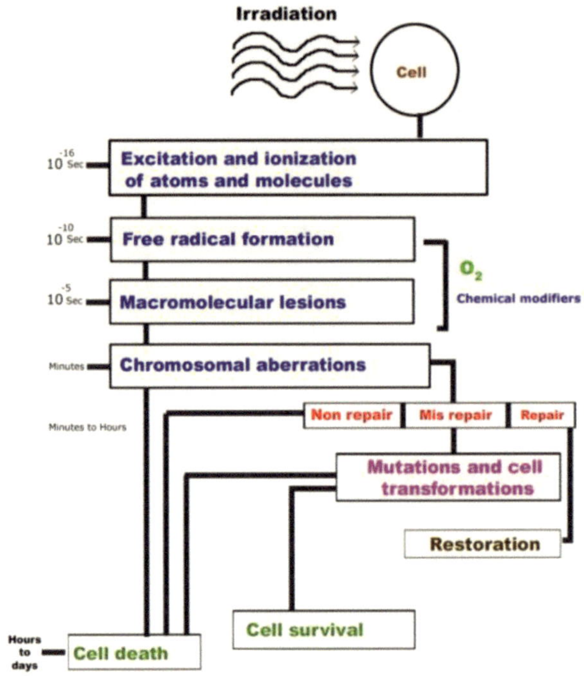

Figure 2.
Effect of radiation on cell.

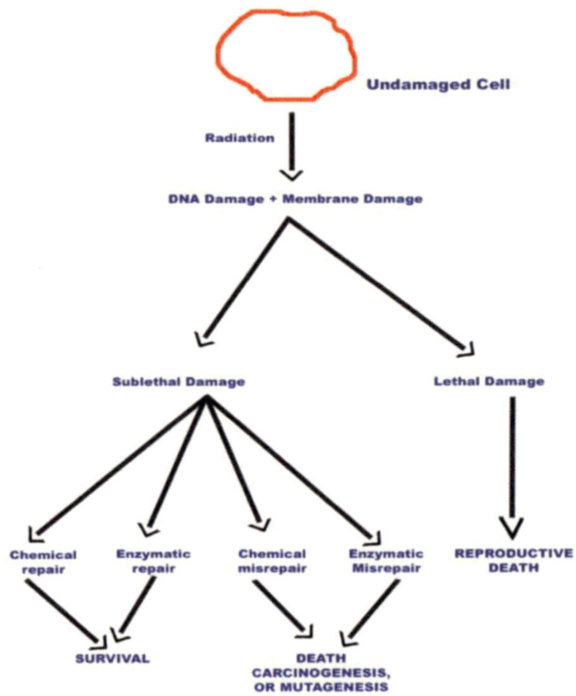

Figure 3.
Different types of damages in cell after radiation exposure.

anti-inflammatory activities. Attempts are done to explore the use of mushrooms and their metabolites for the treatment of a variety of human ailments [19]. More than 100 medicinal mushrooms have been identified.

Ganoderma lucidum, commonly known as reishi, the mushroom of immortality is one of the most popular medicinal mushrooms. The fruiting bodies of *Ganoderma lucidum* contain a variety of chemical substances including polysaccharides, triterpenes, nucleosides, ergosterols, fatty acids, proteins, peptides and trace elements. The polysaccharides of *G. lucidum* are the other major source of its biological activity and therapeutic use. This mushroom has attracted great attention owing to its antitumor and hypoglycemic activities [6]. Many fungal glucan have been reported to be active in humans.

2. Materials and methods

2.1 Animals

Swiss albino mice, were kept for a week under environmentally controlled conditions with access to standard food and water. Recommendations of the ethical Committee for the Purpose of Control and Supervision of Experiments on Animals (CPCSEA) instituted by the Animal Welfare Division of the Government of India were followed.

2.2 Irradiation

Gamma cell facility of Bhabha Atomic Research Centre, Trombay was used for irradiation. Whole body irradiation to mice was given to unanesthetized animals, which were kept in well-ventilated Perspex boxes and was exposed at a dose rate of 1 Gy/min. *Ex vivo* irradiation of human peripheral leukocytes was done in Junior Theratron unit with a dose rate of approximately 0.4 Gy/min. Chemicals were obtained from Sigma Chemicals (St. Louis, Missouri) and purchased from Merck India Ltd., Mumbai.

3. Methods

3.1 Isolation of glucan

Ganoderma lucidum were collected from Southern parts of India. The polysaccharides were isolated from the fruiting bodies by the method of Mizuno [20]. Purification of the compound was done by ion-exchange chromatography. Qualitative confirmation was done by anthrone [21] and phenol sulphuric acid reagent [22]. Further characterization of the compound was done by IR and NMR, mass spectra, gel filtration and acid hydrolysis.

3.2 Comet assay

Comet assay was performed by the method of Singh with modifications [23]. DNA damage in blood leukocytes was estimated. Ten microliters of heparinised whole blood, is mixed with 200 μl of low melting point agarose at 37°C and layered on frosted slides pre-coated with 200 μl high melting point agarose. The slides were pre-chilled in lysing solution and the standard protocol was followed [24].

CASP software was used for the quantitation of the DNA strand breaks of the stored images by which the percentage DNA in tail, tail length, tail moment, and olive tail moment [25]. The tail length of comet specifies the extent of damage as the smaller molecules move faster on the agarose gel. The longer tails of the comets indicate that the strand breaks are more frequent. The tail moment normalizes the difference in the size of the nucleus studied, which is product of the percent DNA in the tail of the comet and tail length. Calculation of olive tail moment distance of centre of gravity of DNA is considered rather than usual tail length.

3.3 Metaphase preparation

Six groups of six animals each were used. At 22 h after irradiation all the animals were injected i.p. with 0.025 colchicine and sacrificed 2 h later by cervical dislocation. Bone marrow from the femur was aspirated, washed in saline, treated hypotonically (0.565% KCl), at 37°C for 30 min, fixed in 3:1::methanol:acetic acid, spread on clean slides and stained with 4% Giemsa [26].

The aberrations were scored with the help of a light microscope. Per animal 500 metaphases were scored. Chromatid breaks, chromosome breaks, fragments, rings and dicentrics as well as cells showing polyploidy and severely damaged cells (SDC), cells with 10 or more aberrations of any type, the different types of aberrations were scored. In 'chromosome type' aberration, breaks involved both the chromatids and in 'chromatid type' aberration involved only one chromatid. Fragments are those deleted portion having no apparent relation to any particular chromosome [27]. Data are mean ± (S.E).

3.4 Treatment of animals

Group I—double distilled water (DDW).
Group II—300 mg/kg body wt. of amifostine i.p. (30 min prior to irradiation).
Group III—20 mg/kg body wt. of glucan orally (5 min after irradiation).
Group IV—DDW + 4 Gy radiation (RT).
Group V—300 mg/kg body wt. of amifostine (30 min before irradiation) + RT 4 Gy.
Group VI—RT 4 Gy + 20 mg/kg body wt. glucan orally (5 min after irradiation).

4. Results and discussion

The compound isolated from *G. lucidum* answered anthrone and phenol sulphuric tests giving typical colour reactions indicating the presence of carbohydrates. From the IR spectrum, pyranoid form was suggested to be present due to the presence of three absorption bands at 1153.4, 1091.6 and 1029.9 cm^{-1}. In the HNMR spectrum H^{-1} signals were observed at less than 4.8 ppm (4.762, 4.683, 4.667, 4.658, 4.402 ppm), which suggest that component sugars have beta configuration. From gel filtration chromatography, the molecular weight of the compound was found to be 1.5×10^6 Daltons. From the acid hydrolysis treatment for the detection of monosaccharides, the sugars present in the compound were found to be glucose, mannose and rhamnose. The compound was identified to be beta-glucan.

4.1 DNA repair enhancement

The repair process in lymphocytes was found to be enhanced by the glucan at 50 μg/ml concentration. The percent DNA, tail length, tail moment and olive tail moment was reduced significantly. At 2 Gy 0 min, the comet parameters increased. Fifteen minutes after irradiation the comet parameters were reduced. The presence of glucan reduced the comet parameters further. After 2 h of irradiation the comet parameters were reduced by the glucan to the control level (**Figure 4** and **Table 1**).

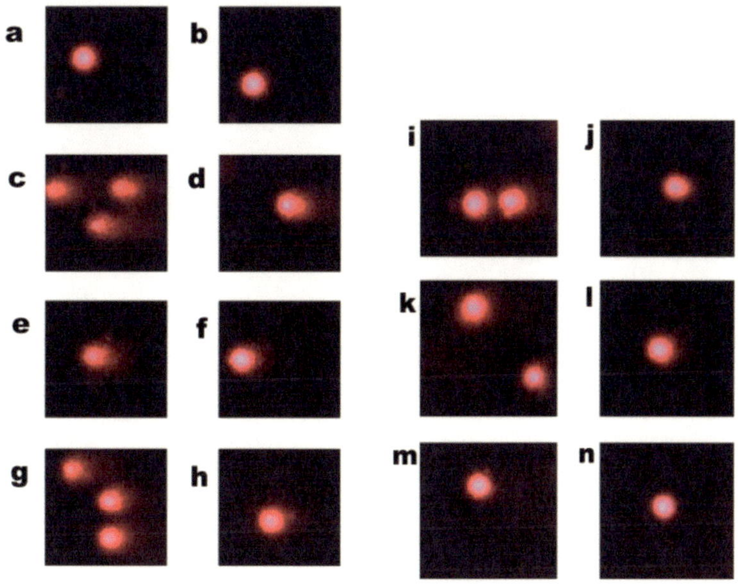

Figure 4.
DNA repair enhancement by glucan in human lymphocytes (comet assay). Untreated: (a) control; (c) 2 Gy 0 min; (e) 2 Gy 15 min; (g) 2 Gy 30 min; (i) 2 Gy 45 min; (k) 2 Gy 60 min; (m) 2 Gy 120 min. Treated with glucan: (b) control; (d) 2 Gy 0 min; (f) 2 Gy 15 min; (h) 2 Gy 30 min; (j)2 Gy 45 min; (l) 2 Gy 60 min; (n) 2 Gy 120 min.

Treatment (per 500 cells)	Fragments	Chromatid break	Chromosome break	Rings	Dicentrics
DDW (control)	6.3 ± 2.5	0.16 ± 2.5	0	0	0
Amifostine (alone)	8.0 ± 1.7	2.3 ± 0.3	0	0	0
Glucan (alone)	7.3 ± 0.8	1.0 ± 0.5	0	0	0
RT 4 Gy (alone)	384.1 ± 16.4[g]	13 ± 2.3[g]	8.5 ± 1.5[g]	3.8 ± 0.6[g]	11.3 ± 1.6[g]
RT 4 Gy + amifostine	31.5 ± 4.0[a,i]	9.5 ± 1.8[e]	2.3 ± 0.4[b,i]	0.8 ± 0.4[b]	2.1 ± 0.4[a,i]
RT 4 Gy + glucan	38.6 ± 4.6[a]	8.1 ± 0.7[e,k]	2.8 ± 0.4[a]	0.8 ± 0.3[b]	1.3 ± 0.4[a]

Datas are mean ± S.E. n = 6.
[a]*P < 0.0001.*
[b]*P < 0.001.*
[c]*P < 0.01.*
[d]*P < 0.05.*
[e]*Marginally significant, compared to RT alone.*
[f]*P < 0.05 compared to RT + amifostine.*
[g]*P < 0.0001 compared to DDW.*
[h]*P < 0.001 compared to amifostine alone.*
[i]*P < 0.01 compared to amifostine alone.*
[j]*P < 0.05 compared to amifostine alone.*
[k]*P < 0.0001 compared to glucan alone.*
[l]*P < 0.001 compared to glucan alone.*

Table 1.
*Effect of **G. lucidum** glucan and amifostine on the induction of different chromosomal aberrations in mouse bone marrow after whole body γ-irradiation (4 Gy).*

4.2 Chromosomal aberrations

Sham treated control showed 1% aberrant cells. Compared to control glucan or amifostine alone did not induce any significant changes. There was significant increase in the percentage of aberrant cells treated with radiation. Treatment with glucan after irradiation and amifostine before irradiation resulted in significant

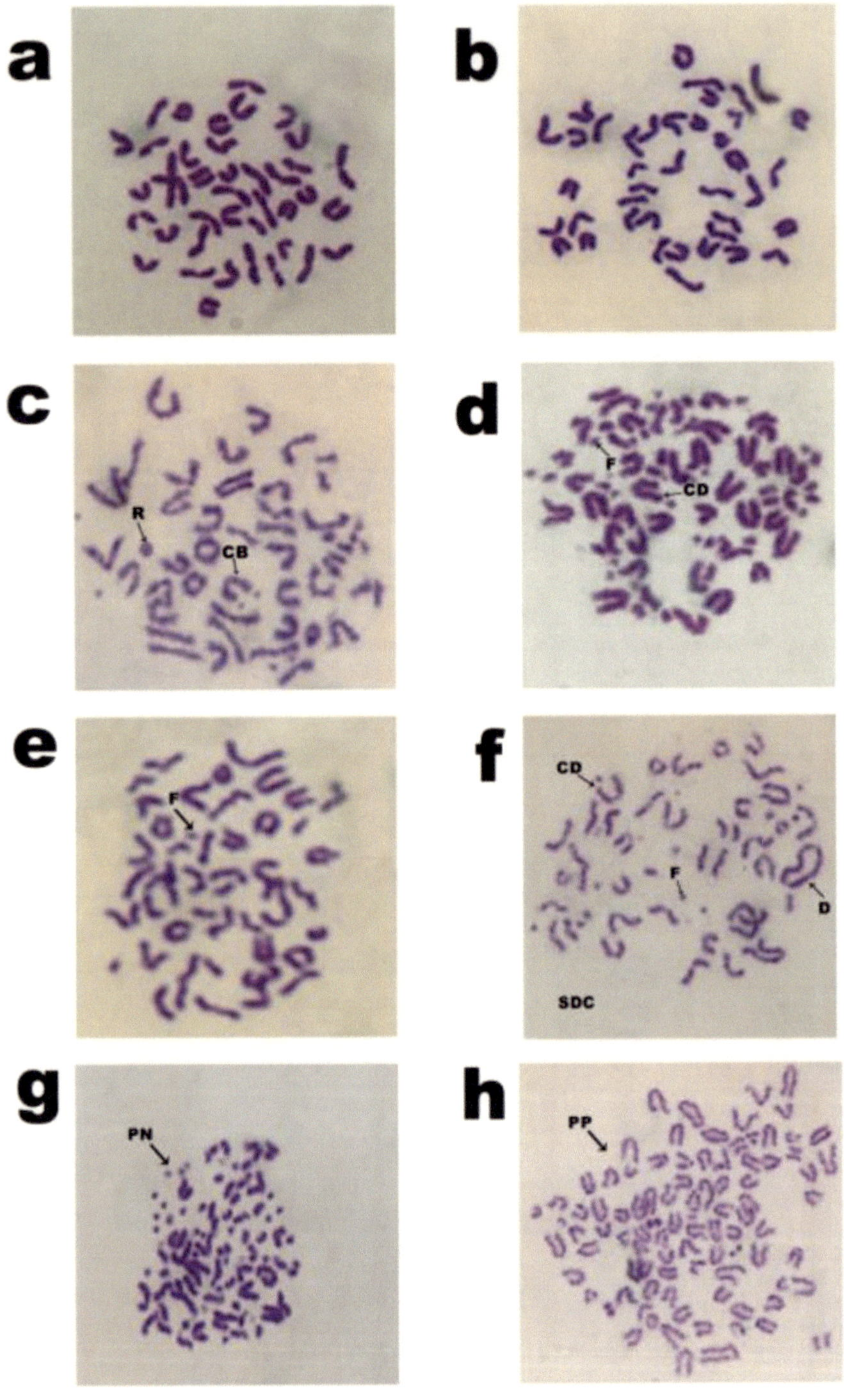

Figure 5.
Different types of chromosomal aberrations in mouse bone marrow. F, fragments; CD, chromatid break; CB, chromosome break; PN, pulverisation; SDC, severe damaged cell; PP, polyploidy; D, dicentrics; R, rings.

decrease in the percentage of aberrant cells and number of aberrations per cell compared to the group which received radiation alone. A decrease in all types of aberrations, as well as polyploidy and cells with pulverisation was observed. The number of severe damaged cells (SDC) significantly reduced to about 1.5 times after glucan treatment. The number of cells with multiple and complex damage was

Treatment	Polyploidy	SDC	Pulverised cells
DDW (control)	0	0	0
Amifostine (alone) (300 mg/kg body wt.)	0.6 ± 0.66	0	0
Glucan (alone) (20 mg/kg body wt.)	0	0	0
RT 4 Gy (alone)	4.8 ± 0.60^{g}	14 ± 1.3^{g}	10.6 ± 1.3^{g}
RT 4 Gy + amifostine (300 mg/kg body wt.)	0.83 ± 0.40^{a}	$3.6 \pm 0.71^{a,i}$	$1.6 \pm 0.33^{a,j}$
RT 4 Gy + glucan 20 mg/kg body wt.)	0.5 ± 0.22^{a}	$2.0 \pm 0^{a,f}$	$1.5 \pm 0.22^{a,l}$

Datas are mean ± S.E. n = 6.
[a]*P < 0.0001.*
[b]*P < 0.001.*
[c]*P < 0.01.*
[d]*P < 0.05.*
[e]*Marginally significant, compared to RT alone.*
[f]*P < 0.05 compared to RT + amifostine.*
[g]*P < 0.0001 compared to DDW.*
[h]*P < 0.001 compared to amifostine alone.*
[i]*P < 0.01 compared to amifostine alone.*
[j]*P < 0.05 compared to amifostine alone.*
[k]*P < 0.0001 compared to glucan alone.*
[l]*P < 0.001 compared to glucan alone.*

Table 2.
Effect of G. lucidum polysaccharides and amifostine on the induction of polyploidy, SDC and pulverization in mouse bone marrow after whole body γ-irradiation (4 Gy).

Time	Olive tail moment without glucan	Olive tail moment with glucan
0 Gy 0 min	3.9444 ± 0.2582	3.677 ± 0.2362
2 Gy 0 min	26.1602 ± 0.5566	26.001 ± 0.3345
2 Gy 15 min	15.6947 ± 0.5193	15.0996 ± 0.7832
2 Gy 30 min	10.0415 ± 0.5287	7.9954 ± 0.57714
2 Gy 45 min	7.2821 ± 0.5541	6.1824 ± 0.5673
2 Gy 60 min	7.5109 ± 0.5966	4.4504 ± 0.3189
2 Gy 120 min	6.2424 ± 0.3847	3.6330 ± 0.3214

Table 3.
Effect of glucan on enhancement of DNA repair in human lymphocytes after 2 Gy gamma irradiation (comet assay).

significantly decreased by glucan post-treatment indicating that the former may help in the repair of the DNA breaks (**Figure 5**, **Tables 2** and **3**).

The lifespan of cells to radiation leading to a loss of cell viability can be greatly influenced by the ability of cells to repair injured DNA. The hazard in mammals exposed to ionizing radiation is to the haemopoetic system. Radiation induced damage to DNA can temporarily affect DNA replication allowing repair to happen involving a well-coordinated event of DNA repair enzymes such as DNA repair polymerase, DNA ligase and PARP [28]. The factors that influence the response of living cells to radiation are the DNA repair status, the physiological state of cells, the presence of oxygen and chemicals as well as pre and post-irradiation treatments [29].

By examining the comet parameters of human peripheral blood leucocytes the effect of polysaccharides on DNA repair was ascertained. Through the initial 30 min, most of the DNA repair processes were completed. The presence of polysaccharide boosted the process of DNA repair. The comet parameters were more at 30 min post-irradiation, in irradiated control and polysaccharide treated group which can be attributed to the commencement of excision repair process [30]. After 45 min there was not much difference in the comet parameters, in control group. The comet parameters kept on reducing in the presence of polysaccharides and at 120 min the comet parameters were almost similar to the unirradiated control. Re-joining of DNA strand breaks by most cell types is known to be a rapid process within few seconds-minutes [31] and this kinetics are seen in comet assay too. In freshly isolated lymphocytes repair by Hydrogen peroxide induced breaks takes place very slowly which can be due to the additional DNA breakage as a result of quick exposure to atmospheric oxygen in the repair incubation period [32]. At the same time repair of endonuclease III- or FPG-sensitive sites (i.e., oxidized purine and pyrimidines) by base excision repair, is much slower process, taking few hours [33].

Background levels of DNA damage in normal cells, the variation in DNA repair capacity within human populations, and the regulation of DNA repair at the molecular level within the nucleus can be monitored by comet assay [34].

5. Conclusion

The integrity of DNA molecule at structural level has to be protected and preserved for the effectual transmission of the genetic information contained to progeny. Distinctions in the arrangement of nucleotides or changes in the configuration of bases or sugars, in the double helix of DNA can impede the replication or transcription of genome.

Multilation to DNA molecule is the crucial factor for cell death. Mechanisms of repair of damaged DNA molecules play a vital role in cell survival. No medicine has been invented that could successively be applied in DNA damage. Our study indicates that the polysaccharides from *G. lucidum* enhance the repair process.

5.1 Advances in area of DNA repair

Prevention is better than cure and cancer induction is greatly influenced by nutrition. The unaffordable discovery cost and failures at the completion of discovery pipeline makes medicines arbitrary to the developing countries. Newer technologies like reverse pharmacology, systems biology which are charming give innovation opportunities based on investigational wisdom and universal viewpoint of translation medicine. Chemotherapy and SSRI revolutionised longevity and quality of life in therapeutics. The Human Genome Project opened understanding towards personalised medicine. Glucan from *G. lucidum* possess immunomodulating activities and regulate a number of undiscovered cellular genes. New studies are needed to unravel these molecular targets giving insights into the interactions of the fungi like *G. lucidum* with our body system and provide strategies for the discovery of effective and safe approaches for drugs from natural sources.

Glucan was isolated from the mushroom *Ganoderma lucidum*, a basidiomycete white rot macro fungus that has been used extensively for therapeutic use in China and Japan for years. The compound was characterised by different chromatographic techniques, done by IR, NMR, and paper chromatography, gel filtration chromatography and spectroscopic techniques like infra-red spectrum and nuclear magnetic resonance spectrum.

The molecular weight of the isolated glucan was 1.6×10^6 Daltons. The rate of DNA repair in the presence and absence of the compound was determined. Comet assay was performed using the method of Singh in human lymphocytes. Chromosomal aberration was studied in mouse bone marrow. After radiation exposure, the comet parameters, percent DNA, tail length, tail moment and olive tail moment were changed in the presence of glucan. Chromosomal aberrations and individual aberrations were also reduced by glucan. The result of present investigation reveals the potential application of glucan from *G. lucidum* in increasing the rate of DNA repair which makes it useful in medical scenario.

The path of science is always fascinating giving deep intuitions with new technologies. The term 'DNA repair' gained more significance in last decade. The beautiful discoveries in essential mechanisms of DNA repair extended Nobel prize in Chemistry in 2015 to T. Lindahl, P. Modrich and A. Sancar. Their discovery defined three pathways that essentially correct DNA damage, protecting the integrity of genetic code assuring perfect replication through generations allowing correct cell division. The mechanisms behind base excision repair, mismatch repair and nucleotide excision repair was explained. Since then the number of drugs and targeted pathways has increased remarkably. The DNA repair enzyme was declared as the molecule of the year in 1994. Though the studies from model organisms serve as a basis to elucidate of repair mechanism, the utilisation of cutting edge technology has channelled in a new era of DNA repair research. The DNA repair pathways have also become better understood. The accessibility of a wide-ranging spectrum of drugs with known molecular targets will provide the rationale to use those drugs in relation to various disease conditions and to combine DNA damaging agents with the appropriate DNA repairing agent. The journey of DNA repair continues. Our current research is carried out in this direction.

Author details

Thulasi G. Pillai[1]*, Cherupally K. Krishnan Nair[2] and P. Uma Devi[3]

1 Department of Life sciences, Model College, Dombivli, Mumbai, India

2 St. Gregorios Dental College and Research Centre, India

3 Independent Scientist

*Address all correspondence to: thulasigpillai@gmail.com

References

[1] Sharma RK and Arora R. Herbal Drugs, A 21st Century Perspective. New Delhi: Jaypee Brothers Medical Publishers (P) Ltd.; 2006

[2] Samhita C. Translation, Chaukhambha Orientalia. New Delhi: Munshorama manoharlal Publishers; 1995

[3] Gogate VM. Ayurvedic Pharmacology and Therapeutics of Medicinal Plants. Mumbai: Bharatiya Vidhya Bhavan's SPARC; 2000

[4] Wonderling D et al. Cost effectiveness analysis of a randomised trial of acupuncture for chronic headache in primary care. British Medical Journal. 2004;**328**:747-752

[5] Harvey A. Strategies for discovering drugs from previously known unexplored natural products. Drug Discovery Today. 2000;**5**:294-300

[6] Pillai TG, Nair CKK, Janardhanan KK. Enhancement of repair of radiation induced DNA strand breaks in human cells by *Ganoderma* mushroom polysaccharides. Food Chemistry. 2010;**119**(3):1040-1043

[7] Dolle ME, Busuttil RA, Garcia AM, Wijnhoven S, van Drunen E, Niedernhofer LJ, et al. Increased genomic instability is not a prerequisite for shortened lifespan in DNA repair deficient mice. Mutation Research. 2006;**596**:22-35

[8] Espejel S, Martin M, Klatt P, Martin-Caballero J, Flores JM, Blasco MA. Shorter telomeres, accelerated ageing and increased lymphoma in DNA-PKcs-deficient mice. EMBO Reports. 2004;**5**:503-509

[9] Sharma P, Jha AB, Dubey RS, Pessarakli M. Reactive oxygen species, oxidative damage, and antioxidative defense mechanism in plants under stressful conditions. Journal of Botany. 2012:1-26

[10] Arora A, Byrem TM, Nair MG, Strasburg GM. Modulation of liposomal membrane fluidity by flavonoids and isoflavonoids. Archives of Biochemistry and Biophysics. 2000;**373**:102-109

[11] Grace SG, Logan BA. Energy dissipation and radical scavenging by the plant phenyl propanoid pathway. Philosophical Transactions of the Royal Society of London. Series B, Biological Sciences. 2000;**355**:1499-1510

[12] Kaur R, Arora S. Alkaloids-important therapeutic secondary metabolites of plant origin. Journal of Critical Reviews. 2015;**2**:1-8

[13] Sokmen M, Angelova M, Krumova E, Pashova S, Ivancheva S, et al. In vitro antioxidant acitivity of polyphenol extracts with antiviral properties from *Geranium sanguineum* L. Life Sciences. 2005;**2005**(76):2981-2993

[14] Kumari AJ, Venkateshwarlu G, Choukse MK, Anandan R. Effect of essential oil and aqueous extract of ginger (*Zingiber officinale*) on oxidative stability of fish oil-in-water emulsion. Journal of Food Processing & Technology. 2014;**6**:412

[15] Islamian JP, Mehrali H. Lycopene as a carotenoid provides radioprotectant and antioxidant effects by quenching radiation-induced free radical singlet oxygen: An overview. Cell Journal. 2015;**16**:386-391

[16] Gao YH, Zhou SH, Jiang WQ, Huang M, Dai XH. Effect of ganopoly, a *G. lucidum* polysaccharide extract on the immunological function in advanced stage cancer patents. Immunological Investigations. 2003;**5**:201-215

[17] Gao Y, Dai X, Chen G, Ye J, Zhou S. A randomized, placebo-controlled, multicenter study of *Ganoderma lucidum* (W. Curt.:Fr.) Lloyd (Aphylloromycetidae) polysaccharides (Ganopoly R) in patients with advanced lung cancer. International Journal of Medicinal Mushrooms. 2003;**4**:369-381

[18] Shiao MS, Lee KR, Lin LJ, Wang CT. Natural products and biological activities of the Chinese medical fungus, Ganoderma lucidum. In: Ho CT, Osawa T, Huang MT, Rosen RT, editor. Food phytochemicals for cancer prevention II: Teas, spices and herbs. Washington, DC: American Chemical Society. 1994;**4**:342-354

[19] Jong SC, Birmingham JM. Edible mushrooms in biotechnology. In: Proceeding of Asian Mycology Symposium, Seoul; 1992. pp. 18-35

[20] Mizuno T, Usui T, Tomoda M. Studies on the host-mediated antitumour polysaccharides. VI. Isolation and characterisation of antitumour active beta-D-glucan from mycelial cells of *Ganoderma applanatum*. Shizuoka Daigaku Nogakuba Kenkyu Hokoku. 1982;**32**:41-58

[21] Yemn EW, Wills AJ. The estimation of carbohydrate in plant extract by anthrone. The Biochemical Journal. 1954;**57**:508-514

[22] Dubois SM, Gilles GA, Hamilton JK. Colourimetric estimation of carbohydrates by phenol sulphuric acid method. Analytical Chemistry. 1956;**28**:350-356

[23] Chaubey RC, Bhilwade HN, Rajagopalan R, Bannur SV. Gamma ray induced DNA damage in human and mouse leukocytes measured by SCGE—Pro: Software developed for automated image analysis and data processing for comet assay. Mutation Research. 2000;**490**:187-197

[24] Umadevi P, Bisht KS, Vinita M. A comparitive study of radioprotection by Ocimum flavanoids and synthetic aminothiol protectors in the mouse. The British Journal of Radiology. 1998;**71**:782-784

[25] Bender MA, Awa AA, Brooks AL, Evans HJ, Groer PG, Littlefield LG, et al. Current status of cytogenetic procedures to detect and quantify previous exposures to radiation. Mutation Research. 1998;**196**:103-159

[26] Hanawalt PC, Cooper PC, Ganesan AK, Smith KC. DNA repair in bacteria and mammalian cells. Annual Review of Biochemistry. 1979;**48**:783-836

[27] Pasupathy K, Nair CKK, Kagiya TV. Effect of a hypoxic radiosensitizer AK 2123 on yeast *Saccharomyces cerevisiae*. Journal of Radiation Research. 2001;**42**:217-227

[28] Mendiola-Cruz MT, Morales-Ramirez P. Repair kinetics of γ-ray induced DNA damage determined by single cell gel electrophoresis. Mutation Research. 1999;**433**:45-52

[29] Frankenberg-Schwage VM. Review of repair kinetics for DNA damage induced in eukaryotic cells in vitro by ionizing radiation. Radiotherapy and Oncology. 1989;**14**:307-320

[30] Torbergsen AC, Collins AR. Recovery of human lymphocytes from oxidative DNA damage: The apparent enhancement of DNA repair by carotenoids is probably simply an antioxidant effect. European Journal of Nutrition. 2000;**39**:80-85

[31] Collins AR, Horvathova E. Oxidative DNA damage, antioxidant and DNA repair: Applications of comet assay. Biochemical Society Transactions. 2001;**29**:337-341

[32] Gantt R. A cell cycle associated pathway for repair of DNA—Protein crosslinks in mammalian cells. Mutation Research. 1987;**183**:75-87

[33] Pillai TG, Nair CKK, Janardhanan KK. Polysaccharides isolated from *Ganoderma lucidum* occurring in Southern parts of India, protects radiation induced damages both in vitro and in vivo. Environmental Toxicology and Pharmacology. 2008;**26**:80-85

[34] Saini N. The journey of DNA repair. Trends in Cancer. 2008;**1**:215-216